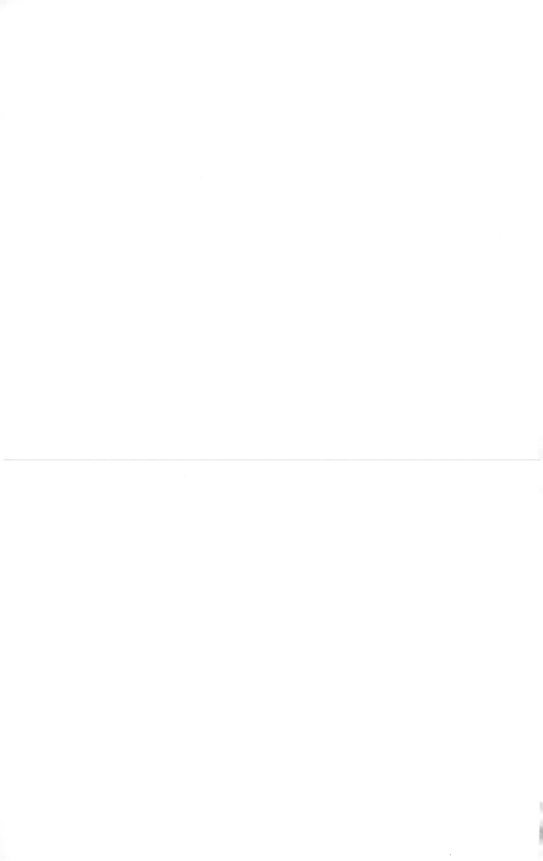

# Adolescent Undiagnosed and Rare Diseases

*Editors*

HEATHER TOTH
ROBERT KLIEGMAN
BRETT J. BORDINI

# MEDICAL CLINICS
# OF NORTH AMERICA

www.medical.theclinics.com

*Consulting Editor*
JACK ENDE

January 2024 • Volume 108 • Number 1

**ELSEVIER**

1600 John F. Kennedy Boulevard • Suite 1800 • Philadelphia, Pennsylvania, 19103-2899

http://www.theclinics.com

**MEDICAL CLINICS OF NORTH AMERICA Volume 108, Number 1**
**January 2024 ISSN 0025-7125, ISBN-13: 978-0-443-13079-3**

Editor: Taylor Hayes
Developmental Editor: Malvika Shah

Medical Clinics of North America (ISSN 0025-7125) is published bimonthly by Elsevier Inc., 360 Park Avenue South, New York, NY 10010-1710. Months of publication are January, March, May, July, September, and November. Business and editorial offices: 1600 John F. Kennedy Boulevard, Suite 1800, Philadelphia, PA 19103-2899. Periodicals postage paid at New York, NY, and additional mailing offices. Subscription prices are USD $336.00 per year (US individuals), $100.00 per year (US Students), $433.00 per year (Canadian individuals), $200.00 per year for (foreign students), $100.00 per year for (Canadian students), $479.00 per year (foreign individuals). For institutional access pricing please contact Customer Service via the contact information below. To receive student/resident rate, orders must be accompanied by name of affiliated institution, date of term, and the signature of program/residency coordinator on institution letterhead. Orders will be billed at individual rate until proof of status is received. Foreign air speed delivery is included in all Clinics' subscription prices. All prices are subject to change without notice. **POSTMASTER:** Send address changes to *Medical Clinics of North America*, Elsevier Health Sciences Division, Subscription Customer Service, 3251 Riverport Lane, Maryland Heights, MO 63043. **Customer Service: Telephone: 1-800-654-2452** (U.S. and Canada); **1-314-447-8871** (outside U.S. and Canada). **Fax: 314-447-8029. E-mail: journalscustomerserviceusa@elsevier.com** (for print support); **journalsonlinesupport-usa@elsevier.com** (for online support).

*Reprints.* For copies of 100 or more of articles in this publication, please contact the Commercial Reprints Department, Elsevier Inc., 360 Park Avenue South, New York, NY 10010-1710. Tel.: 212-633-3874; Fax: 212-633-3820; E-mail: reprints@elsevier.com.

*Medical Clinics of North America* is also published in Spanish by McGraw-Hill Interamericana Editores S. A., P.O. Box 5-237, 06500 Mexico, D.F., Mexico.

*Medical Clinics of North America* is covered in *MEDLINE/PubMed (Index Medicus), Current Contents, ASCA, Excerpta Medica, Science Citation Index,* and *ISI/BIOMED.*

## PROGRAM OBJECTIVE

The goal of the *Medical Clinics of North America* is to keep practicing physicians up to date with current clinical practice by providing timely articles reviewing the state of the art in patient care.

## TARGET AUDIENCE

All practicing physicians and other healthcare professionals.

## LEARNING OBJECTIVES

Upon completion of this activity, participants will be able to:
1. Review the origin of various disorders of adolescents and young adults.
2. Explain the importance of primary care providers' and subspecialists understanding of the pathophysiology and multidisciplinary nature of multisystem diseases.
3. Discuss factors that improve diagnostics yields.

## ACCREDITATION

The Elsevier Office of Continuing Medical Education (EOCME) is accredited by the Accreditation Council for Continuing Medical Education (ACCME) to provide continuing medical education for physicians.

The EOCME designates this journal-based CME activity for a maximum of 15 *AMA PRA Category 1 Credit*(s)™. Physicians should claim only the credit commensurate with the extent of their participation in the activity.

All other healthcare professionals requesting continuing education credit for this enduring material will be issued a certificate of participation.

## DISCLOSURE OF CONFLICTS OF INTEREST

The EOCME assesses conflict of interest with its instructors, faculty, planners, and other individuals who are in a position to control the content of CME activities. All relevant conflicts of interest that are identified are thoroughly vetted by EOCME for fair balance, scientific objectivity, and patient care recommendations. EOCME is committed to providing its learners with CME activities that promote improvements or quality in healthcare and not a specific proprietary business or a commercial interest.

**The planning committee, staff, authors, and editors listed below have identified no financial relationships or relationships to products or devices they or their spouse/life partner have with commercial interest related to the content of this CME activity:**

Louella Amos, MD; Bethany Auble, MD, MEd; Donald Basel, MD; Kristina Bolling, APNP; Brett J. Bordini, MD; Larisa Broglie, MD, MS; Ross Carson, MD; Dominic O. Co, MD, PhD; Jeanne Conner, APNP; Tejaswini Deshmukh, MD; Justin Dey, MD; Alejandra Escobar Vasco, MD; Kaitlin V. Kirkpatrick, MD; Robert M. Kliegman, MD; Meghan K. Konda, MD; Leah Lalor, MD; Michelle Littlejohn; James J. Nocton, MD; Merlin Packiam; Bridget A. Rafferty, MD, MPH, MFA; Alexander Raskin, MD; Allison Remiker, MD; Katie Ryan, MD, MPH; Vaishali Singh, MD; Joshua A. Steinberg, MD; Coral M. Stredny, MD; Pooja Thakrar, MD; Heather Toth, MD; Scott K. Van Why, MD; James Verbsky, MD, PhD; Ryan D. Walsh, MD; Hsi (Kevin) Yen, MD, MPH

**The planning committee, staff, authors, and editors listed below have identified financial relationships or relationships to products or devices they or their spouse/life partner have with commercial interest related to the content of this CME activity:**

Matthew Harmelink, MD: Consultant: Sarepta Therapeutics, Encoded Therapetics; Advisor: Biogen, Sarepta Therapeutics, Novartis AG, PTC Therapeutics; Speaker: Sarepta Therapeutics; Researcher: Sarepta Therapeutics, Biogen, Novartis AG, Genentech, Capricor Therapeutics

## UNAPPROVED/OFF-LABEL USE DISCLOSURE

The EOCME requires CME faculty to disclose to the participants;
1. When products or procedures being discussed are off-label, unlabelled, experimental, and/or investigational (not US Food and Drug Administration [FDA] approved); and
2. Any limitations on the information presented, such as data that are preliminary or that represent ongoing research, interim analyses, and/or unsupported opinions. Faculty may discuss information about pharmaceutical agents that is outside of FDA-approved labelling. This information is intended solely for CME and is not intended to promote off-label use of these medications. If you have any questions, contact the medical affairs department of the manufacturer for the most recent prescribing information.

**TO ENROLL**

To enroll in the *Medical Clinics of North America* Continuing Medical Education program, call customer service at 1-800-654-2452 or sign up online at http://www.theclinics.com/home/cme. The CME program is available to subscribers for an additional annual fee of USD 319.00.

**METHOD OF PARTICIPATION**

In order to claim credit, participants must complete the following;
1. Complete enrolment as indicated above.
2. Read the activity.
3. Complete the CME Test and Evaluation. Participants must achieve a score of 70% on the test. All CME Tests and Evaluations must be completed online.

**CME INQUIRIES/SPECIAL NEEDS**

For all CME inquiries or special needs, please contact elsevierCME@elsevier.com.

# MEDICAL CLINICS OF NORTH AMERICA

**FORTHCOMING ISSUES**

*March 2024*
**Sexually Transmitted Infections**
Susan Tuddenham, *Editor*

*May 2024*
**Patient Management with Stable
Ischemic Heart Disease**
Alexander Fanaroff and John Hirschfeld,
*Editors*

*July 2024*
**Allergy and Immunology**
Andrew Lutzkanin and Kristen M.
Lutzkanin, *Editors*

**RECENT ISSUES**

*November 2023*
**Current Challenges and New Directions in
Preventive Medicine**
Marie Krousel-Wood, *Editor*

*September 2023*
**Vascular Medicine**
Geno Merli and Raghu Kolluri, *Editors*

*July 2023*
**An Update in Nephrology**
Jeffrey Turner and Ursula Brewster, *Editors*

# Contributors

## CONSULTING EDITOR

**JACK ENDE, MD, MACP**
The Schaeffer Professor of Medicine, Perelman School of Medicine, University of Pennsylvania, Philadelphia, Pennsylvania

## EDITORS

**HEATHER TOTH, MD**
Professor and Hospitalist, Departments of Medicine and Pediatrics, Medical College of Wisconsin, Milwaukee, Wisconsin

**ROBERT KLIEGMAN, MD**
Professor and Chair Emeritus, Department of Pediatrics, Medical College of Wisconsin, Milwaukee, Wisconsin

**BRETT J. BORDINI, MD**
Associate Professor, Division of Hospital Medicine, Department of Pediatrics, Nelson Service for Undiagnosed and Rare Diseases, Medical College of Wisconsin, Milwaukee, Wisconsin

## AUTHORS

**LOUELLA AMOS, MD**
Associate Professor of Pediatrics, Division of Pulmonary and Sleep Medicine, Medical College of Wisconsin, Children's Wisconsin, Milwaukee, Wisconsin

**BETHANY AUBLE, MD, MEd**
Associate Professor of Pediatrics, Division of Endocrinology, Fellowship Director, Associate Program Director, Pediatrics Residency Program, Medical College of Wisconsin, Milwaukee, Wisconsin

**DONALD BASEL, MD**
Professor, Department of Pediatrics, Section Chief, Division of Medical Genetics, Medical College of Wisconsin, Milwaukee, Wisconsin

**KRISTINA BOLLING, APNP**
Advanced Practice Nurse Practitioner, Division of Allergy and Clinical Immunology, Department of Pediatrics, Medical College of Wisconsin, Children's Wisconsin, Milwaukee, Wisconsin

**BRETT J. BORDINI, MD**
Associate Professor, Division of Hospital Medicine, Department of Pediatrics, Nelson Service for Undiagnosed and Rare Diseases, Medical College of Wisconsin, Milwaukee, Wisconsin

**LARISA BROGLIE, MD, MS**
Assistant Professor, Division of Hematology/Oncology/Blood and Marrow Transplantation, Department of Pediatrics, Medical College of Wisconsin, Milwaukee, Wisconsin

**ROSS CARSON, MD**
Resident Physician, Department of Neurology, Boston Children's Hospital, Harvard Medical School, Boston, Massachusetts

**DOMINIC O. CO, MD, PhD**
Associate Professor, Division of Allergy, Immunology, Rheumatology, Department of Pediatrics, University of Wisconsin School of Medicine and Public Health, Clinical Science Center (CSC), Madison, Wisconsin

**JEANNE E. CONNER, MSN, RN, APNP**
Advanced Practice Nurse Practitioner, Division of Allergy and Clinical Immunology, Department of Pediatrics, Medical College of Wisconsin, Milwaukee, Wisconsin

**TEJASWINI DESHMUKH, MD**
Associate Professor, Department of Radiology, Division of Pediatric Radiology, Medical College of Wisconsin, Department of Pediatric Imaging, Milwaukee, Wisconsin

**JUSTIN DEY, MD**
Fellow, Pediatric Endocrinology, Medical College of Wisconsin Affiliated Hospitals, Milwaukee, Wisconsin

**MATTHEW HARMELINK, MD**
Associate Professor, Department of Neurology, Section of Child Neurology, Medical College of Wisconsin, Milwaukee, Wisconsin

**KAITLIN V. KIRKPATRICK, MD**
Fellow, Department of Pediatric Rheumatology, Medical College of Wisconsin, Children's Corporate Center, Milwaukee, Wisconsin

**MEGHAN K. KONDA, MD**
Instructor, Department of Neurology, Section of Child Neurology, Medical College of Wisconsin, Milwaukee, Wisconsin

**LEAH LALOR, MD**
Associate Professor of Dermatology and Pediatrics, Department of Dermatology, Division of Pediatric Dermatology, Medical College of Wisconsin, Milwaukee, Wisconsin

**JAMES J. NOCTON, MD**
Professor, Department of Pediatrics, Medical College of Wisconsin, Milwaukee, Wisconsin

**ASHLEY PHIMISTER, MD**
Division of Cardiology, Department of Pediatrics, Advanced Heart Failure and Transplantation, Medical College of Wisconsin, Milwaukee, Wisconsin

**BRIDGET A. RAFFERTY, MD, MPH, MFA**
Resident Physician, Department of Diagnostic Radiology, Medical College of Wisconsin, Milwaukee, Wisconsin

**ALEXANDER RASKIN, MD**
Assistant Professor, Department of Pediatrics, Division of Cardiology, Advanced Heart Failure and Transplantation, Medical College of Wisconsin, Milwaukee, Wisconsin

**ALLISON REMIKER, MD**
Assistant Professor of Pediatrics, Division of Hematology/Oncology/Blood and Marrow Transplantation, Department of Pediatrics, Medical College of Wisconsin, Children's Wisconsin, Milwaukee, Wisconsin

**KATHLEEN RYAN, MD, MPH**
Assistant Professor, Infectious Disease, Department of Pediatrics, Medical College of Wisconsin, Children's Hospital of Wisconsin, Wauwatosa, Wisconsin

**VAISHALI SINGH, MD**
Assistant Professor, Department of Pediatrics, Medical College of Wisconsin, Milwaukee, Wisconsin

**JOSHUA A. STEINBERG, MD**
Associate Professor, Division of Allergy and Clinical Immunology, Department of Pediatrics, Medical College of Wisconsin, Section of Allergy, Department of Medicine, Clement J. Zablocki Veterans' Affairs Medical Center, Milwaukee, Wisconsin

**CORAL M. STREDNY, MD**
Division of Epilepsy and Clinical Neurophysiology, Program in Neuroimmunology, Department of Neurology, Boston Children's Hospital, Harvard Medical School, Boston, Massachusetts

**JULIE-ANN TALANO, MD**
Associate Professor, Division of Hematology/Oncology/Blood and Marrow Transplantation, Department of Pediatrics, Medical College of Wisconsin, Milwaukee, Wisconsin

**POOJA THAKRAR, MD**
Associate Professor, Pediatric Imaging, Medical College of Wisconsin, Children's Wisconsin, Milwaukee, Wisconsin

**TRACEY THOMPSON, MD**
Pediatric Cardiology Fellow, Department of Pediatrics, Division of Cardiology, Advanced Heart Failure and Transplantation, Medical College of Wisconsin, Milwaukee, Wisconsin

**SCOTT K. VAN WHY, MD**
Professor, Department of Pediatrics, Medical College of Wisconsin, Milwaukee, Wisconsin

**ALEJANDRA ESCOBAR VASCO, MD**
Division of Hematology/Oncology/Blood and Marrow Transplantation, Department of Pediatrics, Medical College of Wisconsin, Milwaukee, Wisconsin

**JAMES VERBSKY, MD, PhD**
Professor of Pediatrics and Microbiology and Immunology, Division of Allergy and Clinical Immunology, Division of Rheumatology, Department of Pediatrics, Medical College of Wisconsin, Children's Wisconsin, Milwaukee, Wisconsin

**RYAN D. WALSH, MD**
Associate Professor of Ophthalmology and Neurology, Department of Neurology, Medical College of Wisconsin, Eye Institute–Froedtert Hospital, Milwaukee, Wisconsin

**HSI YEN, MD, MPH**
Pediatric Dermatology Fellow, Department of Dermatology, Division of Pediatric Dermatology, Medical College of Wisconsin, Milwaukee, Wisconsin

# Contents

**Foreword: Of Horses, Zebras, and the Diagnostic Process**      xv

Jack Ende

**Preface: Discovering Undiagnosed and Rare Diseases and their Mimics**      xvii

Heather Toth, Robert Kliegman, and Brett J. Bordini

**Attaining Diagnostic Excellence: How the Structure and Function of a Rare Disease Service Contribute to Ending the Diagnostic Odyssey**      1

Brett J. Bordini, Ryan D. Walsh, Donald Basel, and Tejaswini Deshmukh

Patients with rare or otherwise undiagnosed disorders frequently find themselves on a diagnostic odyssey, the often-prolonged journey toward diagnosis that can be characterized by significant physical, emotional, and financial hardship, as well as by diagnostic errors and delays. The wider availability of clinical exome sequencing has helped end many diagnostic odysseys, though diagnostic success rates of around 35% for exome sequencing leave many patients undiagnosed. Diagnostic yields can be improved via the implementation of advanced genetic testing modalities, though both these modalities and exome sequencing perform significantly better when paired with high-quality phenotypic data. Diagnostic centers of excellence can improve outcomes for patients on a diagnostic odyssey by providing a process and environment that address shortfalls in diagnostic access while providing high-quality phenotyping. Features of successful undiagnosed and rare disease evaluation teams are discussed and an illustrative case is provided.

**Monogenetic Etiologies of Diabetes**      15

Bethany Auble and Justin Dey

Maturity onset diabetes of the young (MODY) describes a group of non-autoimmune forms of diabetes that are characterized by mostly autosomal dominant, monogenic mutations resulting in decreased beta cell function in the pancreas. MODY accounts for roughly 1% to 5% of diabetes cases, and the optimal treatment for each MODY depends on the causative mutation. This article provides a review of MODY to aid providers with knowing what aspects of the history and physical exam should prompt further investigation for this group of conditions.

**Non-syndromic and Syndromic Severe Acne in Adolescent Patients**      27

Hsi Yen and Leah Lalor

Acne is a common skin disorder in adolescents. However, severe acne that is persistent and refractory to conventional treatment or has other associated symptoms should raise suspicion for non-syndromic or syndromic acne.

**Unusual Presentations of Systemic Lupus Erythematosus**    43

Kaitlin V. Kirkpatrick and James J. Nocton

Systemic lupus erythematosus (SLE) often develops during adolescence, may affect any organ system, and may present with a wide variety of signs and symptoms. It is critical to recognize the unusual manifestations of SLE in order to make a prompt diagnosis. Earlier diagnosis allows for appropriate treatment and ultimately decreases morbidity and mortality.

**Adolescent Onset of Acute Heart Failure**    59

Tracey Thompson, Ashley Phimister, and Alexander Raskin

Heart failure in adolescents can manifest due to a multitude of causes. Presentation is often quite variable ranging from asymptomatic to decompensated heart failure or sudden cardiac death. Because of the diverse nature of this disease, a thoughtful and extensive evaluation is critical to establishing the diagnosis and treatment plan. Identifying and addressing reversible pathologies often leads to functional cardiac recovery. Some disease states are irreversible and progressive, requiring chronic heart failure management and potentially advanced therapies such as transplantation.

**Fever of Unknown Origin**    79

Kathleen Ryan

Fever of unknown origin in adolescents is a challenging disease state for which potential underlying etiology can include infectious, non-infectious inflammatory, and malignancy processes. Careful and thorough history (including exposure history), serial examination, and targeted laboratory and imaging testing is critical for these patients. In adolescents in which an etiology is discovered, infectious etiology remains the most prevalent, followed by non-infectious inflammatory diseases. In patients with non-diagnostic overall reassuring work up, the prognosis is typically self-limiting and favorable.

**Acquired Demyelinating Syndromes**    93

Dominic O. Co

Acquired demyelinating syndromes (ADS) are a heterogenous group of inflammatory demyelinating conditions that include presentations of optic neuritis, transverse myelitis, and acute demyelinating encephalomyelitis. They can be monophasic or can develop into relapsing episodes of the initial demyelinating event or evolve to include other types of demyelination. Significant progress has been made in differentiating subtypes of ADS that differ in their tendency to relapse and in which anti-inflammatory therapies are effective. Differentiating between these subtypes is important for the optimal management of these patients. Clinical features, labs (especially autoantibodies), and MRI findings can help to differentiate between the different ADS.

**Common Variable Immunodeficiency**    107

Allison Remiker, Kristina Bolling, and James Verbsky

Common variable immunodeficiency (CVID) is the most common primary immune deficiency characterized by impaired production of specific immunoglobulin. The clinical manifestations are heterogeneous including acquisition of recurrent bacterial infections after a period of wellness, lymphoproliferation, autoimmunity, pulmonary disease, liver disease, enteropathy, granulomas, and an increased risk of malignancy. The etiology of CVID is largely unknown, with a considerable number of patients having an underlying genetic defect causing immune dysregulation. The antibody deficiency found in CVID is treated with lifelong immunoglobulin therapy, which is preventative of the majority of infections when given regularly.

## Approach to Idiopathic Anaphylaxis in Adolescents    123

Jeanne E. Conner and Joshua A. Steinberg

Anaphylaxis is a potentially-life threatening condition. Adolescents are particularly vulnerable due to increased risk-taking behaviors, poor disease management, and minimized perception of risk. Although most anaphylaxis can be attributed to food, drug, or venom allergy via a detailed history and confirmatory studies, in nearly 1 in 5 cases, the cause may not be obvious. Clinical differentials including rare allergens, cofactors, mast-cell disorders, and mimic disorders can increase the likelihood of discovering of the cause of anaphylaxis.

## Monogenic Etiology of Hypertension    157

Vaishali Singh and Scott K. Van Why

Monogenic hypertension encompasses a group of conditions wherein single gene mutations result in increased renal sodium reabsorption manifesting as low renin hypertension. As these diseases are rare, their contribution to hypertension in children and adolescents is often overlooked. Precise diagnosis is essential in those who have not been found to have more common identifiable causes of hypertension in adolescents, since treatment strategies for these rare conditions are specific and different from antihypertensive regimens for the other more common causes of hypertension in this age group. The objective of this review is to provide insight to the rare, monogenic forms of hypertension.

## Adolescent Onset of Muscle Weakness    173

Meghan K. Konda and Matthew Harmelink

Pediatric adolescent muscle weakness can be from a variety of causes. Methodical diagnostic evaluation can lead to the category of diseases whereby phenotypic overlap requires either specialized care or broad testing patterns. However, having the ultimate diagnosis is important for prognostication.

## Hemophagocytic Lymphohistiocytosis in Adolescents and Young Adults: Genetic Predisposition and Secondary Disease    189

Alejandra Escobar Vasco, Julie-Ann Talano, and Larisa Broglie

Hemophagocytic lymphohistiocytosis (HLH) is a disorder of impaired immune regulation resulting in hyperinflammation that is ultimately fatal if not treated. HLH is categorized into familial disease, caused by genetic mutations affecting the function of cytotoxic T lymphocytes and natural killer cells, and secondary disease, triggered by infections, malignancies, rheumatologic disorders, or immune deficiency. Adolescent and young adults with HLH represent a unique population with specific diagnostic challenges. Here we review the diagnostic criteria, possible etiologies, pathophysiology, and management of HLH with focus on the adolescent population.

**Severe, Refractory Seizures: New-Onset Refractory Status Epilepticus and Febrile Infection-Related Epilepsy Syndrome**                                                 201

Ross Carson and Coral M. Stredny

NORSE (new-onset refractory status epilepticus) and FIRES (febrile infection-related epilepsy syndrome) represent presentations of new-onset status epilepticus without apparent underlying structural, metabolic, or toxic etiology. The cause of NORSE/FIRES remains cryptogenic in up to half of cases, and an abnormal response of the innate immune system has been implicated. Consensus guidelines recommend broad diagnostic investigation and empiric treatment with immunotherapy. NORSE/FIRES is associated with poor outcomes including cognitive impairment and epilepsy, but early recognition and treatment may be important for improving outcomes.

**Later Onset Congenital Central Hypoventilation Syndrome**                                 215

Louella Amos

Congenital central hypoventilation syndrome (CCHS) is a rare disorder of the autonomic nervous system involving multiple organ systems, with the hallmark symptom of respiratory failure due to aberrant central control of breathing resulting in hypoxemia and hypercapnia. Later onset CCHS (LOCCHS) is defined as the diagnosis of CCHS in children older than 1 month. Molecular genetic testing for *PHOX2B* variants has led not only to increased diagnosis of neonates with CCHS but also the increased identification of older children, adolescents, and adults with LOCCHS who may have a milder clinical presentation of this multisystem disease.

**Chronic Recurrent Multifocal Osteomyelitis**                                                 227

Bridget A. Rafferty and Pooja Thakrar

Chronic recurrent multifocal osteomyelitis (CRMO) is an underrecognized autoinflammatory disease affecting the skeletal system. Its vague symptoms are often first attributed to growing pains, infection, or malignancy, which can lead to a delay in diagnosis for days to years. Untreated CRMO has the potential to cause debilitating skeletal deformities, arthritis, and chronic pain; hence early recognition and treatment are paramount. MRI is the gold standard for diagnosis. Treatment consists of various anti-inflammatory medications and may also include bisphosphonates if vulnerable skeletal sites are involved. Even when treated, the disease may have a relapsing course lasting years.

# Foreword

# Of Horses, Zebras, and the Diagnostic Process

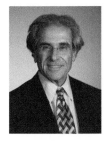

Jack Ende, MD, MACP
*Consulting Editor*

For this special issue of *Medical Clinics of North America*, our guest editors, Drs Toth, Kliegman, and Bordini, provide a fascinating collection of curated cases and diagnostic dilemmas that remind us that, yes, zebras are less common than horses, but they're out there. And part of the challenge all clinicians face is to identify then, or at least appreciate, when something is not typical. Quite a challenge for the busy clinician, eh? But as our guest editors state, "none of us is as smart as all of us," suggesting that we should have a low threshold to discuss unusual cases with colleagues, or to refer them to specialists and even to units dedicated to diagnosing rare diseases, such as the ones described in this issue.

But when? At what stage in the diagnostic process should clinicians realize that this case is not like others they have seen? The answer, of course, will be different for different cases, but considering this question provides us with an opportunity to think about the diagnostic process.

We know from research on clinical reasoning that the diagnosticians utilize one of two pathways, although clinicians can—and indeed, should—move from one pathway to the other. The first pathway is intuitive, in which clinical data are gathered and formulated into an illness script, familiar to the clinician, that is, something already in his or her repertoire of past cases, enabling early hypothesis generation, and then, confirmation. This method is fast, often requiring sparse use of resources and, understandably, is more available to the expert compared with the novice. It is also subject to biases. The second pathway is more deliberative and analytic, and relies on evidence-based algorithms, and typically takes more time and consumes more resources.

These processes are not mutually exclusive. Indeed, one of the distinguishing characteristics of the most expert diagnosticians is that they appreciate when to move to a

Med Clin N Am 108 (2024) xv–xvi
https://doi.org/10.1016/j.mcna.2023.09.001
0025-7125/24/© 2023 Published by Elsevier Inc.

more analytical approach, typically when they recognize that things are "not working out" either diagnostically or therapeutically.

That may help us understand just when to consider that a patient has a rare or even previously undiagnosed condition. This issue presents an array of such cases from which we can learn not just about the described clinical entities but also about the diagnostic process itself.

Jack Ende, MD, MACP
Perelman School of Medicine
of the University of Pennsylvania
Philadelphia, PA, USA

*E-mail address:*
jack.ende@pennmedicine.upenn.edu

# Preface

# Discovering Undiagnosed and Rare Diseases and their Mimics

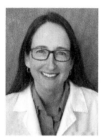 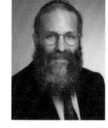 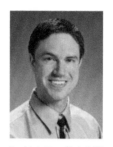

Heather Toth, MD        Robert Kliegman, MD        Brett J. Bordini, MD

*Editors*

"None of us is as smart as all of us" is the motto or aphorism we remind ourselves when discussing undiagnosed and challenging cases that are referred to our Undiagnosed and Rare Disease Program. Undiagnosed and rare diseases often create diagnostic delay and dilemmas for the practitioner, although more important is the physical, emotional, and financial hardships for the patients and their families. This issue of *Medical Clinics of North America* highlights the importance of diagnostic dilemmas, disease mimics, and unusual manifestations of common diseases and rare disorders that may present as a more common disease in adolescents. In addition, we address diagnostic

https://doi.org/10.1016/j.mcna.2023.06.019
0025-7125/24/© 2023 Published by Elsevier Inc.
medical.theclinics.com

and cognitive errors and emphasize the importance of emerging technology and utilizing the greater availability of molecular genetic testing.

Heather Toth, MD
Departments of Medicine and Pediatrics
Medical College of Wisconsin
9200 West Wisconsin Avenue
Milwaukee, WI 53226, USA

Robert Kliegman, MD
Department of Pediatrics
Medical College of Wisconsin
9200 West Wisconsin Avenue
Milwaukee, WI 53226, USA

Brett J. Bordini, MD
Department of Pediatrics
Medical College of Wisconsin
9200 West Wisconsin Avenue
Milwaukee, WI 53226, USA

*E-mail addresses:*
htoth@mcw.edu (H. Toth)
rkliegma@mcw.edu (R. Kliegman)
bbordini@mcw.edu (B.J. Bordini)

# Attaining Diagnostic Excellence
## How the Structure and Function of a Rare Disease Service Contribute to Ending the Diagnostic Odyssey

Brett J. Bordini, MD[a],*, Ryan D. Walsh, MD[b,c], Donald Basel, MD[d],
Tejaswini Deshmukh, MD[e,f]

KEYWORDS

- Undiagnosed diseases • Rare diseases • Diagnostic odyssey • Diagnostic access
- Phenotyping

KEY POINTS

- Patients with rare and otherwise undiagnosed disorders frequently face significant diagnostic delays and physical, emotional, and financial burdens.
- Undiagnosed and rare disease diagnostic centers of excellence can shorten the diagnostic odyssey by providing high-quality phenotyping and addressing shortfalls in diagnostic access.
- The diagnostic yield of advanced molecular genetic studies is enhanced via an environment and processes that mitigate diagnostic error and produce high-quality phenotyping.

Over 350 million individuals globally live with one of the more than 7000 identified rare diseases, a total that surpasses the number affected by many common disorders.[1] In the United States, nearly 30 million people are affected by a rare disease and its attendant physical, emotional, and financial hardships.[2] The economic burden of rare diseases is significant: an analysis of the annual financial impact of 379 rare disorders in

[a] Department of Pediatrics, Division of Hospital Medicine, Nelson Service for Undiagnosed and Rare Diseases, Medical College of Wisconsin; [b] Department of Neurology, Medical College of Wisconsin; [c] Eye Institute – Froedtert Hospital, 925 North 87th Street, Milwaukee, WI 53226, USA; [d] Department of Pediatrics, Section Chief, Division of Medical Genetics, Medical College of Wisconsin, 9000 West Wisconsin Avenue MC716, Milwaukee, WI 53226, USA; [e] Department of Radiology, Division of Pediatric Radiology, Medical College of Wisconsin; [f] Department of Pediatric Imaging, 9000 West Wisconsin Avenue, Milwaukee, WI 53226, USA
* Corresponding author. Children's Corporate Center, 999 North 92nd Street Suite C560, Milwaukee, WI 53226.
*E-mail address:* bbordini@mcw.edu

Med Clin N Am 108 (2024) 1–14
https://doi.org/10.1016/j.mcna.2023.06.013
0025-7125/24/© 2023 Elsevier Inc. All rights reserved.

the United States, representing just over half of American individuals with a rare disease, estimated nearly a trillion dollars in direct medical and indirect associated expenses.[3] The costs of rare disease diagnosis and care significantly exceed those for more common disorders,[4,5] though attaining diagnosis and implementing specific treatment plans lower these costs.[6] However, over 95% of rare disorders lack specific disease-directed therapies,[7] and with over 200 additional rare disorders identified annually,[2] diagnosis is crucial to improving individual, family, and systems outcomes by allowing for further understanding of pathophysiologic mechanisms, clarification of genotype–phenotype correlations, provision of focused genetic counseling, creation of patient and family support networks, and exploration of novel therapies.[8,9]

Despite this diagnostic imperative, most individuals with a rare disease find themselves on a *diagnostic odyssey*, the journey of experiencing unexplained symptoms, seeking evaluation, experiencing symptom evolution, and seeking further evaluation, all in an attempt to obtain an accurate diagnosis.[10] While over half of rare diseases affect the pediatric population and while nearly 80% of all rare diseases are believed to have a genetic etiology,[11] the diagnostic odyssey is often prolonged, on the order of years even in children and adolescents,[9,12] in spite of advances in and the greater availability of molecular genetic testing. Compounding most diagnostic odysseys is *diagnostic error*, if in no other form than a delayed or missed diagnosis.[13,14]

Recognizing the critical role of diagnosis in improving outcomes for individuals with rare disorders, the National Institutes of Health (NIH) Office of Rare Diseases Research, the NIH Clinical Center, and the National Human Genome Research Institute established the NIH Undiagnosed Diseases Program in 2008 to aid in the diagnosis and treatment of patients with rare or otherwise undiagnosed disorders. In 2012, the program was extended to a network of 7 clinical sites, a coordinating center, and a series of core laboratories to comprise the Undiagnosed Diseases Network (UDN).[15] In the decade since then, the network has added additional clinical sites and further clinical and research laboratory cores. This process mirrored similar independent as well as coordinated efforts both within the United States and internationally, creating an infrastructure of diagnostic centers of excellence for collaborative diagnostic and therapeutic efforts for patients with rare diseases.

Since its inception, the UDN has evaluated hundreds of patients, with initial reviews of these evaluations revealing an overall diagnostic success rate of around 30%.[16] As these UDN experiences often involved patients with previous nondiagnostic exome sequencing, these reviews highlighted the potential limitations of exome sequencing in the evaluation of patients with undiagnosed disorders, with exome sequencing at the time offering diagnostic yields typically no greater than 35%.[17] Subsequent efforts both within the UDN and among the greater rare disease evaluation community highlighted the essential role of moving "beyond the exome" and incorporating additional methods and diagnostic modalities to increase diagnostic yield.[18] Periodic sequencing reanalysis, short-read genome sequencing, long-read sequencing, transcriptomics, metabolomics, methylation studies, pan-genome referencing, matchmaking, and functional studies have all emerged as a handful of additional advanced modalities that have increased diagnostic yield in patients with previous nondiagnostic clinical sequencing.[17–19]

While many of these advanced diagnostic modalities are still not widely clinically available, there is increasing parity with respect to their incorporation into the evaluation of patients with undiagnosed disorders.[17,20] As this technological gap closes, improved diagnostic yields will become increasingly dependent on *high-quality phenotyping*, wherein a detailed list of objective physical and laboratory findings, semi-objective symptoms and findings, and subjective symptoms is generated and verified and paired with data analysis tools that generate probability-matched descriptive terms. High-quality phenotyping has been instrumental in ending the diagnostic odyssey in up to 40% of cases that have had previous nondiagnostic clinical exome sequencing[18,21,22] and should be one of the primary goals of a rare disease evaluation. Patients on a diagnostic odyssey are frequently subject to numerous cognitive biases that introduce error into their diagnostic formulation and management plans. Frequent among them is *diagnostic momentum*, in which diagnostic labels are copied forward and perpetuated over time without being adequately questioned, despite those labels oftentimes being outdated, incomplete, or even inaccurate.[10] These labels can take on a life of their own, obscuring the true phenotype and prolonging the diagnostic odyssey if they are not regularly and actively clarified in an objective manner that replaces presumed diagnoses with descriptions of the essential phenomena at hand. This process should incorporate the use of Human Phenotype Ontology (HPO) terms when possible such as "atrial septal defect" as using more HPO terms in generating the clinical phenotype and then in filtering and interpreting sequencing data improves the diagnostic success rate, though the yield of this approach appears to plateau beyond the use of approximately 5 HPO terms.[21,23]

Furthermore, shortening the length of the diagnostic odyssey will require improving *diagnostic access*, the ability to be evaluated in a health care environment with the requisite knowledge, experience, and resources capable of producing a timely, accurate, and satisfactory explanation for patient signs and symptoms.[10,24,25] Impaired diagnostic access may be a function of limited availability of specialist consultation or specialized testing, inability to access a rare disease center secondary to travel, financial, or illness-related constraints, or an acute or critical illness necessitating a rapid evaluation during a hospitalization. Local diagnostic centers of excellence programs can address the diagnostic needs of acutely and critically ill patients, serve as a complimentary referral pipeline for patients unable to travel to national evaluation centers, and meet the diagnostic needs of patients who may not have readily available specialists or specialized testing.

## A FRAMEWORK FOR SUCCESSFUL RARE DISEASE EVALUATION TEAMS

As diagnostic technology parity increases, attaining excellence in diagnosis will depend on creating a process and an environment that address shortfalls in diagnostic access and provide high-quality phenotype clarification to inform the diagnostic process and the interpretation of advanced diagnostic modalities. In the decade since the creation of our undiagnosed and rare disease (URD) evaluation site, we have created a system that has led to a diagnostic success rate among the highest in the nation and have developed collaborative relationships with other specialists and centers of excellence to best meet the needs of patients with rare or otherwise undiagnosed disorders. We propose a model process and environment for a successful URD team.

1. *A patient referral is received.* Patients present to our institution for URD evaluation via either external referral or inpatient consultation. Located on the grounds of the Milwaukee Regional Medical Center that includes the main campus of the Medical College of Wisconsin, Children's Wisconsin is a large freestanding academic children's hospital with regional, national, and international patient populations. Since its inception in 2013, our service has evaluated approximately 300 patients and families from 22 states and 2 foreign nations with an aggregated clinical and molecular diagnostic rate of 40%. Our team includes representatives from 31 clinical specialties, mostly pediatric, with a handful of adult generalists and specialists. We additionally have a research genetic counselor, a research coordinator, and

a research nurse within the Division of Pediatric Genetics. Furthermore, we have established research collaborations with basic sciences researchers and our genomic sciences and precision medicine center, which serves as a core for multi-OMIC investigations, including next-generation exome and genome sequencing, RNA sequencing, reduced-representation bisulfite sequencing, assay for transposase-accessible chromatin (ATAC)-sequencing, and chromatin immunoprecipitation (ChIP)-sequencing. The core additionally offers full tissue services; single-cell technologies are available although are mostly reserved for rare oncology investigations.

2. *A member of our core clinical team reviews the consultation request, along with the entirety of the patient's medical record, inclusive of records from institutions where the patient has received care previously.* This process is deliberate and meant to engage a more analytical approach to diagnosis that minimizes cognitive biases that could or have contributed to diagnostic delays and errors.[10,26,27] When possible, actual copies of any studies performed previously at other institutions are obtained—including biopsy tissue—and are re-reviewed by our staff. Doing so provides not only phenotypic refinement; in some cases, this review process has uncovered findings that were diagnostic and previously not appreciated, such as a subtle intracranial mass on computed tomography of the head. The core clinician then summarizes the aggregated data and conducts a telephone or virtual visit with the patient and family to obtain and clarify any additional history.

3. *Based on this initial case review, an ad hoc evaluation team is assembled, involving members not only from disciplines pertinent to the patient's presenting concerns and medical history, but also from disciplines that may not be directly related.* The aphorism that drives every one of our diagnostic evaluations is that "none of us is as smart as all of us." This team-based approach enhances diagnostic accuracy beyond that achieved by individual senior expert clinicians, as collective intelligence-based medical decision-making has consistently and significantly outperformed even the most accurate individual diagnosticians in many clinical contexts.[28–30] While these meetings have oftentimes been at their most robustly productive when conducted in person, based on the urgency of the patient's illness, or more recently, given the constraints of conducting large in-person meetings during the coronavirus pandemic, these meetings have been conducted virtually as well. In advance of this meeting, evaluation team members are expected to familiarize themselves with as much of the patient's medical record as possible.

4. *The assembled evaluation team reviews the data as a group to produce the group phenotype, which consists of a descriptive list of essential phenomena, be they objective findings, semi-objective, or subjective.* Previously-applied diagnostic labels are removed in favor of these phenomenological descriptors so as to interrupt diagnostic momentum and better illustrate potential unifying pathophysiologic mechanisms in what is referred to as a *differential pathophysiology*. The phenomenological descriptors are then categorized based on which are likely to represent primary pathology, which represent morbidity secondary to that pathology, which findings may be true though unrelated to the underlying disease, and which may be consequences of therapy or otherwise iatrogenic.[10] The use of HPO terms is encouraged.

5. *Based on the group phenotype and differential pathophysiology, a differential diagnosis and evaluation plan are generated.* The plan often involves the patient being seen by subspecialists to expand the history, clarify physical examination findings, and focus further testing. This process may involve the uncovering of

pathognomonic or otherwise rare findings, such as our geneticist noticing hyper-trichosis cubiti in a patient, directing a focused evaluation for Weidemann–Steiner syndrome and the identification of a pathogenic variant in *KMT2A*, or our neuro-muscular neurologist noting spinal rigidity in a patient with skeletal muscle weak-ness and cardiomyopathy, ultimately suggesting a *BAG3*-related myofibrillar myopathy.[31] An additional benefit of these subspecialty evaluations is to focus the use of specialized testing and minimize unnecessary testing. Concurrent with these evaluations is obtaining any more generalized testing as agreed upon by group consensus, such as routine chemistries or plain radiography; how-ever, specialized or invasive testing such as biopsies or molecular genetic studies is usually performed only after these initial subspecialty visits have refined the phenotype further and focused the differential diagnosis.

6. *Constant communication is maintained throughout the evaluation.* Siloed commu-nication often leads to siloed thinking, wherein the entire scope of a patient's phenotype may be missed by specialists subconsciously restricting their medical decision-making to disease processes and pathophysiologic mechanisms rele-vant only to their specialty. All members of the evaluation team communicate throughout the evaluation, whether that consists of seeing the patient in tandem during combined multidisciplinary visits or communicating immediately via tele-phone or e-mail at the conclusion of each visit to share diagnostic impressions. A daily summary is also generated by the core clinician at the end of each day's evaluation, so that all team members can suggest and make any necessary adjustments to the evaluation plan.

7. *An access center coordinator is critical to the success of any evaluation.* Our ac-cess center coordinator is actively involved throughout the entirety of a patient's evaluation, from the time a referral is placed to the moment a patient receives a diagnosis and is transitioned into the realm of diagnosis-specific care. The access center coordinator maintains our patient care database, monitoring the progress of every patient through our evaluation process, and coordinates all outpatient ap-pointments and studies or scheduled elective inpatient diagnostic evaluations. Furthermore, the access center coordinator is responsible for obtaining and collating all outside medical records for review. Without these key data and this essential logistical organization, our evaluations would be subject to fragmenta-tion and unnecessary delays.

8. *A medical librarian is an essential member of any rare disease evaluation team.* As the pace of advancement in the biomedical sciences continues to quicken, it is increasingly challenging for any individual clinician to remain abreast of the latest developments in every discipline that may be pertinent to a patient with an undi-agnosed condition. A medical librarian plays a crucial role in clarifying medical literature queries and identifying the highest quality evidence to drive evaluation and management. Our medical librarian actively participates in all large-group case reviews and is included in all communications during active patient evalua-tions, oftentimes assisting in finding literature to help with test selection and inter-pretation in real time.

9. *Recurring case review sessions and sequencing data reanalysis increase diag-nostic yield.* The core clinicians and any available members of the larger team meet quarterly for a "case review." Successful diagnostic evaluations are dis-cussed to share lessons learned and identify potential pointers and pitfalls for similar future patient presentations. Evaluations-in-progress are summarized to ensure agreement on and comprehensiveness of the evaluation plan, and recent referrals are previewed to ensure adequate representation in the composition of

the evaluation team. Patients with nondiagnostic sequencing results have their sequencing data re-analyzed on a scheduled, recurring basis, and this process has resulted in variants of uncertain significance being reclassified as pathogenic, as well as in the identification of new potentially pathogenic variants.

10. *The application of advanced diagnostic modalities is regularly considered for patients who remain undiagnosed.* For patients with nondiagnostic exome sequencing, our team regularly considers the role of next-generation genome sequencing, long-read sequencing, RNA sequencing and proteomics, metabolomics, variant classification, and candidate gene analysis. Recurring case discussion meetings are held between our clinicians and our genomic sciences and precision medicine personnel to determine when and how such approaches can best be applied.

11. *Nongenetic disease as well as heritable disorders for which a genetic mechanism has not yet been identified should always be part of the discussion.* While approximately 80% of rare diseases have a genetic etiology,[11] the possibility of nongenetic disease is always considered in the differential diagnosis and testing strategy. Here, defining pathophysiologic mechanisms is of the utmost importance, particularly for autoimmune and autoinflammatory conditions, many of which lack identified associated genes. Careful selection of biopsy specimens and thoughtful application of assays designed to demonstrate function and capture dysfunction, such as mitochondrial enzyme analysis or immunophenotyping, can clarify the phenotype and even suggest the possibility of novel genetic disorders.

This approach requires extensive clinical and research infrastructure and the recognition that not all services rendered will generate commensurate clinical revenue. Grant and philanthropic support are often required, especially when insurance coverage is incomplete[32] and faculty time investment in rare disease evaluations becomes significant.[22] However, when this process functions optimally, it can greatly increase the chances of ending a diagnostic odyssey well beyond that offered by clinical sequencing alone.[13,22] A previous patient evaluation case from our service is illustrative:

An 11-year-old previously healthy and typically developing child presented with right eye monocular vision loss. The past medical history was unremarkable: recommended childhood immunizations had been administered on schedule and the only prior surgical procedure was an orolabial frenectomy at 1 week of age. Routine childhood illnesses consisted of several episodes of infectious gastroenteritis and the occasional uncomplicated upper respiratory tract infection. No illnesses were recalled in the months preceding the onset of vision loss, though mother recalled a transient dysconjugate gaze on several occasions in the previous 2 months, suggesting vision loss had already developed at least a couple of months prior to the child alerting the parents of a visual concern.

Family history was notable for the father and a paternal uncle both having previous cutaneous eruptions that were diagnosed as tinea versicolor. They both also had a history of patellar subluxation. A maternal uncle had immunoglobulin (Ig)A vasculitis, and a maternal cousin had hypermobility. Regarding eye disease, the paternal grandfather had cataracts and the maternal grandfather had cataracts and an epiretinal membrane. In terms of social history, the patient lives with mother, father, and an older healthy sibling in a larger city with access to municipal water and sewer service in their home. There are no nearby large-scale industrial or agricultural facilities and the patient has not been around domesticated or agricultural animals. Parental occupations involve no significant exposure risks and there is no smoke exposure.

Review of travel and any additional exposures reveals that the patient and family have been to south Asia twice, most recently several years prior to symptom onset. They stayed mostly within a city while there, though did some travel into more rural locations. The patient and family experienced no illnesses during those travels or within the months after returning. The family took several camping trips in the summer and fall preceding the onset of vision loss. They deny any known tick exposure or the use of fresh water sources for drinking water or cooking.

The patient was seen within 24 hours of symptom onset by an ophthalmologist in the local emergency department and was diagnosed with right eye vision loss that was likely chronic in nature given that some degree of optic nerve thinning was appreciated. A dedicated follow-up evaluation in ophthalmology clinic revealed right eye monocular blindness (no light perception) with visual acuity of 20/20 in the left eye. Protective eyeglasses were prescribed. MRI of the brain and orbits revealed T2 enhancement of the intraorbital, intracanalicular, and prechiasmatic portions of the right optic nerve suggestive of a presumptive diagnosis of right optic neuritis (**Fig. 1**). The patient was hospitalized for a 5-day course of parenteral corticosteroids.

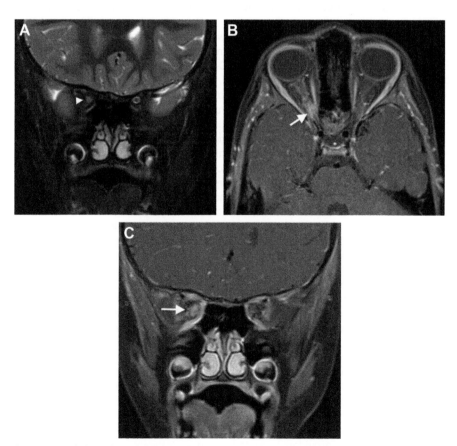

**Fig. 1.** MRI of the orbits. (*A*) Coronal T2WI shows right optic nerve atrophy (*white arrowhead*). (*B*) Axial and (*C*) coronal contrast-enhanced fat-suppressed T1WI reveal thickening and enhancement of the right optic sheath and subtle enhancement of the optic nerve (posterior intraorbital and intracanalicular segments) (*white arrows*).

Diagnostic evaluation was notable for negative serum assays for anti-myelin oligodendrocyte glycoprotein (MOG) antibodies, anti-aquaporin-4 antibodies, systemic lupus erythematosus, and Lyme disease. Cerebrospinal fluid was negative for distinct oligoclonal bands. The patient was discharged home on an oral steroid taper and was seen in neuro-ophthalmology clinic after a several week interval, where examination revealed possible though minimal light and motion perception in the right eye and continued 20/20 visual acuity in the left eye. A later follow-up examination revealed similar findings with light perception and possible motion perception in the right eye. The steroid taper was quickened given a lack of vision recovery in the right eye.

A second opinion was obtained after several months, where the diagnostic formulation was suggestive of atypical optic neuritis. Repeat MRI showed no change in the enhancement of the right optic nerve. Ophthalmology consultation was then obtained at a third institution, where the diagnostic formulation was suggestive of neuromyelitis optica spectrum disorder (NMOSD). When an MRI of the brain and orbits was unchanged from previous, the patient was hospitalized and received 7 courses of therapeutic plasma exchange (PLEX) over a 2-week period, with intravenous immunoglobulin or rituximab discussed as additional potential therapeutic options. Repeat testing, obtained prior to the PLEX, was negative for anti-aquaporin-4 antibodies, anti-MOG antibodies, and Lyme disease. Serum and cerebrospinal fluid tests for sarcoidosis were negative, cerebrospinal fluid cytology was negative for malignancy or other abnormalities, and a gene panel for Leber hereditary optic neuropathy was negative. Erythrocyte sedimentation rate (ESR) and C-reactive protein (CRP) levels, checked on multiple occasions, were uniformly bland.

Several months later, the patient developed a small, discolored eruption on the forehead with seborrhea-like changes on the scalp and was diagnosed with tinea versicolor; this lesion resolved readily with topical antifungals. MRI of the brain, orbits, and entire spine revealed no changes in the right optic nerve enhancement and otherwise revealed no other lesions. Serial optical coherence tomography (OCT) demonstrated progressive thinning of the right optic nerve.

One year after initial presentation, the patient was referred to our URD program for further evaluation. Our access center coordinator obtained the entirety of the patient's medical record across all institutions that had previously conducted evaluations, and this record was reviewed by one of our core clinicians. Digital copies of all relevant imaging studies were obtained and reinterpreted by our neuroradiology staff. Following this initial review, a multidisciplinary care team was assembled, consisting of representatives of pediatric hospital medicine, genetics, ophthalmology and neuro-ophthalmology, hematology, oncology, bone marrow transplant, rheumatology, complex immunodeficiency, neurology, neuro-immunology, neuroradiology, and pathology. The history and the results of all previous diagnostic evaluations and therapeutic interventions were reviewed in detail to generate a comprehensive phenotype, which was then used to formulate hypotheses regarding potential unifying pathophysiologic mechanisms. Given the persistent optic nerve enhancement on serial imaging despite multiple immunosuppressive and immunomodulatory treatments, additional differential diagnostic considerations included infiltrative processes such as optic pathway tumors, lymphoma, Langerhans cell histiocytosis, central nervous system hemophagocytic lymphohistiocytosis, and additional mimics of optic neuritis.

To investigate these possibilities, the patient was seen in clinic by one of our core clinicians as well as by providers in neurology, ophthalmology, and genetics. Physical examination was notable for visual acuities of only light and motion perception in the right eye and 20/20 in the left eye. The previously noted lesion that had been labeled as tinea versicolor was not present. A shotty lymph node was noted in the left postauricular region, with no overlying skin changes. The remainder of the physical evaluation revealed no abnormalities. Based on the initial pre-visit case conference and these first specialist evaluations, the diagnostic evaluation consisted of fluoro-deoxyglucose (FDG)-PET-MRI, which revealed a tiny focus of mildly increased FDG avidity along the left postauricular scalp without a definite correlate on MR images, which was felt to be nonspecific and likely corresponding to the lymph node noted on examination. Mildly increased radiotracer uptake was noted symmetrically in the bilateral extraocular muscles (**Fig. 2**).

Lumbar puncture opening pressure was normal at 18 cm of water. Cerebrospinal fluid examination demonstrated 1 total nucleated cell and 0 red blood cells with a differential showing 59% lymphocytes and 41% monocytes. Cerebrospinal fluid protein was 12, and glucose was 43 with a corresponding serum glucose of 88. The cerebrospinal fluid cytology was negative for malignancy and hemophagocytosis. Angiotensin-converting enzyme level in the cerebrospinal fluid was 7, which was normal.

A complete blood count was normal. Hematopathology slide review was negative for malignancy. Coagulation studies revealed a partial thromboplastin time of 35.2 (upper limit of normal 35.0), though the remainder was normal, including fibrinogen. Procalcitonin and CRP were below threshold of detection; ESR was 5 and ferritin 16.3. A comprehensive metabolic profile was notable only for sodium of 146. Lactate dehydrogenase level was 644 and uric acid was 1.9, both within the reference range of normal.

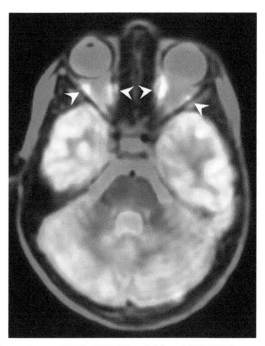

**Fig. 2.** [18]F-fluorodeoxyglucose (FDG)-PET-MRI: axial fused PET-MRI image reveals physiologic avid radiotracer uptake in the bilateral extraocular muscles (*white arrowheads*). No abnormal uptake corresponding with the right optic nerve or sheath abnormality seen on MRI.

Given the consideration of infiltrative processes and that hemophagocytic lympho-histiocytosis was a diagnostic possibility, a soluble interleukin-2 (IL-2) receptor level was checked and was normal at 478.6; Chemokine (C-X-C motif) ligand 9 (CXCL9) level was 217, also normal. Perforin/granzyme assay had natural killer cells demonstrating normal expression levels of perforin and granzyme B; mild B cell lymphopenia was noted. A familial hemophagocytic lymphohistiocytosis gene panel was sent and ultimately returned normal, as did *CTLA4* testing.

Throughout and following these initial evaluations, the multidisciplinary team communicated continuously, discussing and refining diagnostic impressions and formulating best next steps in the evaluation. With respect to findings on the PET-MRI, the posterior auricular scalp had no overlying skin changes to suggest Langerhans cell histiocytosis or other superficial dermatologic lesion. On examination, a very normal texture and sized lymph node was noted in that area (<0.5 cm) and no other adenopathy was noted elsewhere. Given the low degree of enhancement on imaging, the lack of overlying skin changes, and the normal appearance and texture on examination, impressions favored a physiologic to slightly reactive posterior auricular node that warranted serial observation though did not appear associated with an underlying disease process. Recommendations included the notion that should additional similar lesions develop or should this specific lesion evolve in a fashion more suggestive of a systemic process, then biopsy of this lesion or another typical lesion should be considered.

With respect to the extraocular muscle enhancement on the PET scan, these muscles were uniformly normal appearing on all the previous conventional MRIs, and the patient had no symptoms or other findings to suggest a bilateral inflammatory process in the extraocular muscles. This finding was ultimately felt to be physiologic in nature.

At this point in the evaluation, the persistent MRI enhancement along the right optic nerve remained the major concerning data point. If that enhancement had resolved, the most appropriate diagnostic label would likely have been seronegative neuromyelitis optica spectrum disorder. However, the persistent gadolinium enhancement, particularly after a course of parenteral steroids and multiple rounds of PLEX, was felt to be rather atypical for any variety of inflammatory or demyelinating optic neuropathy (including NMOSD) and suggested alternate hypotheses, particularly an infiltrative process.

To further the diagnostic evaluation, several approaches were considered:

1. *Continue to follow serial exams and imaging.* This approach could risk misdiagnosis of an alternate process, such as infiltrative lesions. This approach also does not proactively address the possibility that if this is an inflammatory process, the next episode of inflammation could occur in the seeing eye, could be just as resistant to treatment as the right eye was, and leave the patient completely blind.
2. *Treat empirically with an alternate immunomodulatory approach, using an agent like rituximab.* This approach assumes that the diagnosis of optic neuritis is correct, which it may not be. This approach would also put the patient at risk for complications related to such treatment modalities, such as infection or malignancy.
3. *Biopsy the area of enhancement in the optic nerve/optic nerve sheath.* Given the persistent enhancement on MRI, the potential yield of biopsy was considered high. The risk of this approach is related to the inherent risk associated with optic nerve sheath biopsy: infection or worsening of vision. At this point, the patient was already blind in that eye, and, based on serial OCT exams, there was severe optic atrophy indicating that there was very little prospect of regaining any functional sight in that eye. This approach was considered the best chance to capture an

alternate pathophysiology, though an additional risk would be a nondiagnostic biopsy.

4. *Biopsy a more-accessible alternate site that may be related to the process in the optic nerve, such as the lymph node behind the left ear.* Were there more evidence of systemic inflammation, or had the imaging characteristics or physical findings been more concerning, one could argue this approach, but given the lack of physical findings and the low degree of enhancement on the PET-MRI, it was felt that this approach would be low yield, and that it may be better to follow that lymph node clinically over time and surveil for new external spots that might be more amenable to biopsy.

Of these approaches, referral to neuro-ophthalmology and oculoplastics for discussion of biopsy was recommended. From these evaluations, it was felt that the location of optic nerve enhancement would be challenging to biopsy. Ongoing discussions regarding the imaging findings and differential diagnosis among the team revealed that the primary locus of enhancement on MRI was felt to be within the optic sheath itself, eliciting concern for optic nerve sheath meningioma. As this tumor type would not typically take up fluorodeoxyglucose (FDG) tracer, a gallium-68 DOTATATE PET-MRI scan was recommended and revealed abnormal DOTATATE uptake along the right optic nerve, in the region of abnormal enhancement on MRI, highly suggestive of *optic nerve sheath meningioma* (**Fig. 3**). Germline testing for neurofibromatosis was negative. The patient was subsequently referred to neuro-oncology for further management.

This case illustrates the role and the value of collaborative phenotyping and diagnosis. The label of optic neuritis had developed its own diagnostic momentum, persisting as the prevailing working diagnosis despite the lack of response to

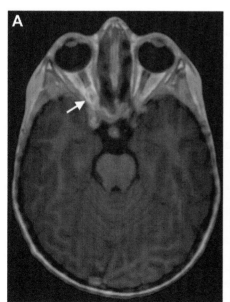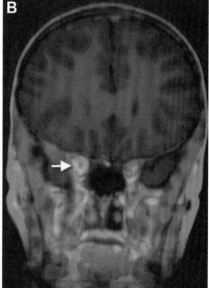

**Fig. 3.** Gallium-68 DOTATATE PET-MRI. (*A*) Axial and (*B*) coronal fused PET-MRI images reveal abnormal radiotracer uptake within the right posterior optic nerve and sheath (*white arrows*), corresponding with the MRI abnormality.

conventional therapeutic approaches to optic neuritis. This label was instead worked backwards to descriptors of essential phenomena—right-sided monocular vision loss, progressive thinning of the right optic nerve, absent signs of systemic inflammation, and persistent gadolinium enhancement on serial imaging despite multiple broad anti-inflammatory treatments. Using these essential phenomena descriptors, a differential pathophysiology was generated that included infiltrative lesions, and during the evaluation process, constant communication among the team members and frequent reinterpretation of clinical data resulted in the proposal of a DOTATATE scan to investigate for optic nerve sheath meningioma, ultimately ending the diagnostic odyssey. Of note, the sporadic nature of this diagnosis highlights the importance of considering nongenetic diagnoses in patients with rare or otherwise undiagnosed disorders.

Although individually rare, in aggregate rare diseases affect a great number of individuals and result in significant physical, emotional, and financial burden. Over the last decade, major advancements in the global approach to rare diseases, paired with breakthroughs in diagnostic modalities, have eased that burden, though as the number of recognized rare diseases continues to increase, there is a growing need for enhanced access to optimized diagnosis and increased diagnostic yields for existing diagnostic modalities. These goals will be best achieved by an approach that centers the patient in a collaborative team-based evaluation at institutions that utilize a structured approach to wed enhanced, high-quality phenotypic data to sophisticated molecular diagnostics and address shortfalls in diagnostic access by providing timely and comprehensive evaluations when and where patient needs arise.

## CLINICS CARE POINTS

- Undiagnosed and rare disease diagnostic centers of excellence focus on high-quality phenotyping and improving diagnostic access.
- A structured team-based approach with constant collaborative communication improves diagnostic yield in patients with undiagnosed and rare disorders.
- Both advanced genetic testing and the possibility of non-genetic disease should be considered in patients who remain undiagnosed.

## DISCLOSURE

The authors have no relevant financial relationships to disclose.

## REFERENCES

1. Nguengang Wakap S, Lambert DM, Olry A, et al. Estimating cumulative point prevalence of rare diseases: analysis of the Orphanet database. Eur J Hum Genet 2020;28(2):165–73.
2. Haendel M, Vasilevsky N, Unni D, et al. How many rare diseases are there? Nat Rev Drug Discov 2020;19(2):77–8.
3. Yang G, Cintina I, Pariser A, et al. The national economic burden of rare disease in the United States in 2019. Orphanet J Rare Dis 2022;17(1):163.
4. Richards J, Korgenski EK, Srivastava R, et al. Costs of the diagnostic odyssey in children with inherited leukodystrophies. Neurology 2015;85(13):1167–70.
5. Report: Economic Burden of Rare Diseases Is 10 Times Higher Than Mass Market Diseases. AJMC. Published March 2, 2022. Available at: https://www.ajmc.

com/view/report-economic-burden-of-rare-diseases-is-10-times-higher-than-mass-market-diseases. Accessed May 22, 2023.

6. Andreu P, Karam J, Child C, et al. The Burden of Rare Diseases: An Economic Evaluation. Available at: https://chiesirarediseases.com/assets/pdf/chiesiglobalrare diseases.whitepaper.feb.-2022_production-proof.pdf. Accessed May 25, 2023.

7. Kaufmann P, Pariser AR, Austin C. From scientific discovery to treatments for rare diseases – the view from the National Center for Advancing Translational Sciences – Office of Rare Diseases Research. Orphanet J Rare Dis 2018;13(1):196.

8. Splinter K, Adams DR, Bacino CA, et al. Effect of Genetic Diagnosis on Patients with Previously Undiagnosed Disease. N Engl J Med 2018;379(22):2131-9.

9. Wu AC, McMahon P, Lu C. Ending the Diagnostic Odyssey: Is whole genome sequencing the answer? JAMA Pediatr 2020;174(9):821-2.

10. Bordini BJ. Undiagnosed and Rare Diseases in Critical Care: The Role of Diagnostic Access. Crit Care Clin 2022;38(2):159-71.

11. Batshaw ML, Groft SC, Krischer JP. Research Into Rare Diseases of Childhood. JAMA 2014;311(17):1729-30.

12. Sawyer SL, Hartley T, Dyment DA, et al. Utility of whole-exome sequencing for those near the end of the diagnostic odyssey: time to address gaps in care. Clin Genet 2016;89(3):275-84.

13. Gainotti S, Mascalzoni D, Bros-Facer V, et al. Meeting Patients' Right to the Correct Diagnosis: Ongoing International Initiatives on Undiagnosed Rare Diseases and Ethical and Social Issues. Int J Environ Res Public Health 2018;15(10). https://doi.org/10.3390/ijerph15102072.

14. Eurordis. European Organisation for Rare Diseases. What is a rare disease? Available at: www.eurordis.org/article.php3?id_article=252. Accessed November 27, 2021.

15. Undiagnosed Diseases Network (UDN). Genome.gov. Published September 14, 2022. Available at: https://www.genome.gov/Funded-Programs-Projects/Undiagnosed-Diseases-Network. Accessed May 25, 2023.

16. Macnamara EF, D'Souza P, Tifft CJ. The undiagnosed diseases program: Approach to diagnosis. Transl Sci Rare Dis 2020;4(3–4):179–88.

17. Marwaha S, Knowles JW, Ashley EA. A guide for the diagnosis of rare and undiagnosed disease: beyond the exome. Genome Med 2022;14(1):23.

18. Schoch K, Esteves C, Bican A, et al. Clinical sites of the Undiagnosed Diseases Network: unique contributions to genomic medicine and science. Genet Med Off J Am Coll Med Genet 2021;23(2):259-71.

19. LeBlanc K, Kelley EG, Nagy A, et al. Rare disease patient matchmaking: development and outcomes of an internet case-finding strategy in the Undiagnosed Diseases Network. Orphanet J Rare Dis 2021;16(1):210.

20. Fishler KP, Euteneuer JC, Brunelli L. Ethical Considerations for Equitable Access to Genomic Sequencing for Critically Ill Neonates in the United States. Int J Neonatal Screen 2022;8(1):22.

21. Jacobsen JOB, Kelly C, Cipriani V, et al. Phenotype-driven approaches to enhance variant prioritization and diagnosis of rare disease. Hum Mutat 2022; 43(8):1071-81.

22. Cope H, Spillmann R, Rosenfeld JA, et al. Missed diagnoses: Clinically relevant lessons learned through medical mysteries solved by the Undiagnosed Diseases Network. Mol Genet Genomic Med 2020;8(10):e1397.

23. Thompson R, Papakonstantinou Ntalis A, Beltran S, et al. Increasing phenotypic annotation improves the diagnostic rate of exome sequencing in a rare neuromuscular disorder. Hum Mutat 2019;40(10):1797–812.

24. Bauskis A, Strange C, Molster C, et al. The diagnostic odyssey: insights from parents of children living with an undiagnosed condition. Orphanet J Rare Dis 2022; 17:233.
25. Zurynski Y, Deverell M, Dalkeith T, et al. Australian children living with rare diseases: experiences of diagnosis and perceived consequences of diagnostic delays. Orphanet J Rare Dis 2017;12:68.
26. Croskerry P. Bias: a normal operating characteristic of the diagnosing brain. Diagnosis 2014;1(1):23–7.
27. Berkwitt A, Grossman M. Cognitive Bias in Inpatient Pediatrics. Hosp Pediatr 2014;4(3):190–3.
28. Wolf M, Krause J, Carney PA, et al. Collective intelligence meets medical decision-making: the collective outperforms the best radiologist. PLoS One 2015;10(8):e0134269.
29. Barnett ML, Boddupalli D, Nundy S, et al. Comparative Accuracy of Diagnosis by Collective Intelligence of Multiple Physicians vs Individual Physicians. JAMA Netw Open 2019;2(3):e190096.
30. Kämmer JE, Hautz WE, Herzog SM, et al. The Potential of Collective Intelligence in Emergency Medicine: Pooling Medical Students' Independent Decisions Improves Diagnostic Performance. Med Decis Mak Int J Soc Med Decis Mak 2017;37(6):715–24.
31. Konersman CG, Bordini BJ, Scharer G, et al. BAG3 myofibrillar myopathy presenting with cardiomyopathy. Neuromuscul Disord NMD 2015;25(5):418–22.
32. Pasquini TLS, Goff SL, Whitehill JM. Navigating the U.S. health insurance landscape for children with rare diseases: a qualitative study of parents' experiences. Orphanet J Rare Dis 2021;16:313.

# Monogenetic Etiologies of Diabetes

Bethany Auble, MD, MEd[a],*, Justin Dey, MD[b]

## KEYWORDS

- Diabetes • MODY • Monogenic • Beta cell • Insulin

## KEY POINTS

- MODY should be considered in patients who do not have autoimmune markers for Type 1 Diabetes and who do not fit the typical body habitus or lack acanthosis nigricans seen with Type 2 Diabetes.
- A strong family history (3 or more generations) should clue the provider for potential MODY.
- Some forms of MODY respond to oral agents (eg, sulfonylureas), some require insulin, and others require monitoring without treatment.

## BACKGROUND

Diabetes Mellitus is a condition in which the body has a relative deficiency in insulin, leading to pathologic hyperglycemia. The underlying cause of this insulin deficiency characterizes the type of diabetes the patient has. In America, the prevalence of diabetes mellitus in children 0 to 19 years of age is 0.35%.[1]

There are multiple causes for diabetes mellitus, including polygenic and monogenic forms. Regardless of the cause, the diagnostic criteria[1] for diabetes mellitus remains the same:

A fasting plasma glucose of 126 mg/dL (7.0 mmol/L) or higher,

Oral glucose tolerance test with 2-h plasma glucose value of 200 mg/dL (11.1 mmol/L) or higher after the administration of a 1.75 g/kg (max to 75g) glucose load,

Hemoglobin A1C (HbA1C) value of 6.5% or higher on an assay that is NGSP-certified and standardized to the Diabetes Control and Complications Trial (DCCT) assay.

Random plasma glucose 200 mg/dL or higher with classic symptoms of hyperglycemia or hyperglycemic crisis.

[a] Medical College of Wisconsin, 9000 West Wisconsin Avenue, Milwaukee, WI 53226, USA;
[b] Medical College of Wisconsin Affiliated Hospitals, Inc., Graduate Medical Education, 8701 Watertown Plank Road, Milwaukee, WI 53226, USA
* Corresponding author.
*E-mail address:* bauble@mcw.edu

Med Clin N Am 108 (2024) 15–26
https://doi.org/10.1016/j.mcna.2023.05.013
0025-7125/24/© 2023 Elsevier Inc. All rights reserved.

Typically, the above tests should not be obtained during a time of illness to make the diagnosis. If hyperglycemia is equivocal, there must be 2 separate positive criteria from the same sample or two positive test results from separate samples.

In the pediatric population, Type 1 Diabetes is the most common form and is caused by the autoimmune destruction of beta cells in the Islets of Langerhans in the pancreas. This can be confirmed by measuring autoantibodies in the serum. The four most common autoantibodies are Zinc Transporter 8, anti-Insulin, Insulinoma-Antigen 2 (also known as IA-2, as well as Islet Cell 512), and Glutamic Acid Decarboxylase 65 (also known as GAD 65). These should be checked in all pediatric patients diagnosed with new-onset diabetes, as the presence of even one of these antibodies with diagnostic criteria for diabetes mellitus supports Type 1 Diabetes as the diagnosis. Type 1 Diabetes is primarily treated with insulin, although newer biologic agents are being developed (such as the newly FDA-approved teplizumab) to delay its onset and ultimately prevent its progression altogether. The term "LADA" refers to Latent Autoimmune Diabetes of Adulthood and is thought to represent slowly progressive autoimmune destruction of beta-cells. It can be considered Type 1 Diabetes with the clinical implication that its progression to insulin dependence is insidious and can vary greatly.

The population of pediatric patients with Type 2 Diabetes is increasing. This form of diabetes is characterized by tissue resistance to insulin and progressive beta-cell failure leading to a relative insulinopenic state and resultant hyperglycemia. Patients typically have an elevated BMI and thickening and darkening of the skin located in any skin folds called acanthosis nigricans, most often located on the neck.

Monogenic Diabetes refers to a collection of conditions in which one-gene mutations lead to altered beta-cell function, resulting in inappropriately decreased insulin secretion and hyperglycemia. This often progresses to clinical diabetes. Monogenic Diabetes encompasses Maturity Onset Diabetes of the Young (MODY) which include multiple types that present in childhood or older, and Neonatal Diabetes in which clinical disease onset typically occurs before 6 months of age due to mutations affecting the development of the pancreas (**Fig. 1**).[2]

Historically, Maturity Onset Diabetes of the Young, or MODY, was considered to be the presentation of Type 2 Diabetes in younger individuals with strong family history.[2]

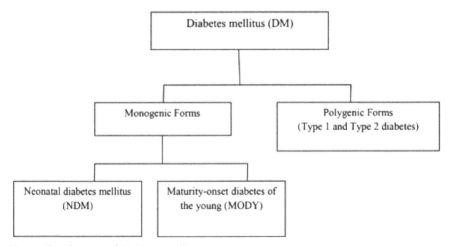

**Fig. 1.** Classification of diabetes mellitus.

With new understanding of beta-cell function and the dawn of genetic testing, it became evident that this group of diseases was distinct from Type 1 and Type 2 diabetes. Unfortunately, MODY often remains undiagnosed as patients are mislabeled as having Type 1 or Type 2 diabetes. Thus, it is imperative for the treating clinician to have a higher index of suspicion to pursue MODY testing when the clinical picture does not fit that of a typical Type 1 or Type 2 diagnosis.

## CASE

A 13-year-old white male had screening labs were performed that included a random blood glucose that resulted with value 167 mg/dL. Follow-up fasting labs were obtained with serum glucose 136 mg/dL and Hemoglobin A1C 6.6%. The patient is otherwise healthy and does not report increased thirst or urination. He is steadily gaining weight along his growth curve, weight consistently 75th percentile, length at the 90th percentile, and BMI 19.2 kg/m$^2$ (58th percentile). On physical exam, the patient does not have central obesity or acanthosis nigricans. There is a family history of Type 2 Diabetes in the patient's father (diagnosed 3 years ago, A1C 6%, briefly on metformin but did not tolerate due to side effects, A1C is steadily controlled on diet). The paternal aunt and paternal grandfather carry Type 2 Diabetes diagnoses as well.

The patient was seen at a Diabetes Clinic where serum autoantibody testing was performed for Highly Sensitive Insulin Antibodies, Zinc Transporter 8 Autoantibodies, Glutamic Acid Decarboxylase (GAD) 65 Antibodies, and Islet Cell Antibodies. Titers for all of these studies were unmeasurable. The patient had negative autoimmune thyroid and celiac screens as well.

The patient was not started on insulin and instructed to document fasting and 2-h postprandial blood glucoses. Once his autoantibody testing returned negative and the review of his blood glucose readings showed no further values above 150 mg/dL, genetic testing with 5-gene evaluation was sent to evaluate mutations in GCK, HNF1A, HNF1B, HNF4A, and IPF1 genes. Testing returned positive for heterozygous nonsense mutation associated with loss of function, corresponding with pathogenic autosomal dominant MODY 2. Counseling on the general healthy lifestyle was performed and the patient continues to follow in the diabetes clinic every 6 months, with HbA1C ranges 6.1% to 6.4%.

## BETA CELL PHYSIOLOGY

To fully understand the pathogenesis of each type of MODY, it is helpful to know the intracellular pathway that leads to insulin secretion in the pancreatic beta-cell. With this understanding, it becomes clear how mutations in various steps result in clinical diabetes. When there is an increase in extracellular glucose (eg, after carbohydrate ingestion and absorption), there is an increase in intracellular glucose transport through the Glucose Transporter Type 2 (GLUT2) located on the beta cell membrane. This is converted into glucose-6-phosphate (G6P) through the enzyme Glucokinase (GCK). The G6P then undergoes glycolysis and enters the citric acid cycle in the mitochondria, ultimately creating ATP. The increase in ATP relative to ADP triggers the closure of an ATP-sensitive potassium channel ($K_{ATP}$) on the beta cell membrane, leading to depolarization at the cell surface. This in turn activates via voltage-gated calcium receptor on the beta cell membrane, causing it to open with a resultant influx of calcium into the cell. The increased intracellular calcium induces insulin release by exocytosis of insulin-containing granules (**Fig. 2**).

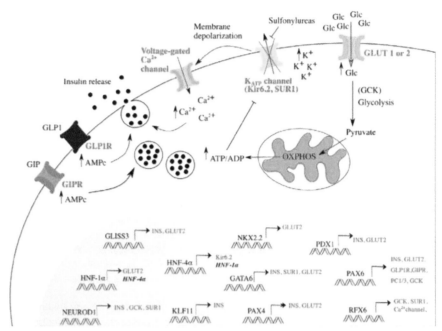

**Fig. 2.** Molecular mechanism of glucose-induced insulin secretion in pancreatic β-cells. In the nucleus, we show transcription factors controlling the expression of genes related to the insulin secretion machinery and whose mutations are associated with monogenic forms of diabetes. AMPc, cyclic AMP; GCK, glucokinase; GIP, glucose-dependent insulinotropic polypeptide; GIPR, GIP receptor; Glc, glucose; GLP1, glucagon-like peptide 1; GLP1R, GLP1 receptor, GLUT, glucose transporter; INS, insulin; OXPHOS, oxidative phosphorylation. (*From* Sanchez Caballero L, Gorgogietas V, Arroyo MN, Igoillo-Esteve M. Molecular mechanisms of β-cell dysfunction and death in monogenic forms of diabetes. Int Rev Cell Mol Biol (2021) 359:139–256. doi: 10.1016/bs.ircmb.2021.02.005.)

## THE MATURITY ONSET DIABETES OF THE YOUNG TYPES

The different types of monogenic diabetes are portrayed differently across literature; some resources bunch Neonatal Diabetes and MODY together and refer to each monogenic mutation as a MODY type, while other resources maintain the distinction by focusing on the age of typical clinical diabetes onset (**Table 1**). Neonatal diabetes is defined as onset before 6 months of age, and these mutations may occur from sporadic or inherited mutations in genes typically resulting in permanent diabetes although some forms have transient neonatal diabetes. For purposes of this review, both the gene mutation and its referenced MODY type will be introduced.

Also noteworthy is that some forms of MODY that were previously accepted are now being brought into question whether their associated genetic mutations are pathogenic and causative for the development of diabetes.[3] Specifically, mutations associated with MODY 7 (KLF11), MODY 9 (PAX4), and MODY 11 (BLK) are being brought into question due to their reports occurring greater than 10 years ago before larger scope population variant analysis was available. More recently, however, mutations in these genes are reported in population frequencies that are inconsistent with previously reported clinical significance.[4] This same concern has also been brought up for mutations associated with MODY 4 (PDX1), MODY 6 (NEUROD1), and MODY 14

**Table 1**
Mooogeneic forms of diabetes and their genetic cause classified according to the function or the subcellular localization of the causal protein

| Form of Diabetes | Mutated Gene | Encoded Protein | OMIM | Locus | Inheritance |
|---|---|---|---|---|---|
| Monogeneic forms of diabetes associated with mutations in transcription factors | | | | | |
| MODY I | HNF4A (HNF4, NR2A1, TCF14) | Hepatocyte nuclear factor 4-alpha (HNF-4α) | # 125850, *600281 | 20q13.12 | AD |
| MODY3 | HNF1A (TCF1) | Hepatocyte nuclear factor 1-alpha (HNF-Iα) | # 600496, *142410 | 12q24.31 | AD |
| MODY4 and NDM | PDX1 | Pancreas/duodenum homeobox protein 1 (PDX1) | # 606392, *600733 | 13q12.2 | AD/AR |
| MODY5 | HNF18 (TCF2) | Hepatocyte nuclear factor 1 -beta (HNF- 1β) | # 137920, *189907 | 17q I2 | AD |
| MODY6 | NEUROD1 (BHLHA3) | Neurogenic differentiation factor 1 (NEUROD I) | # 606394, *601724 | 2q31.3 | AD/AR |
| MODY7 | KLF11 (FKLF, TIEG2) | Kruppel-like factor 11 (KLF11) | # 610508, *603301 | 2p25.I | AD |
| MODY9 | PAX4 | Paired box protein Pax-4 | # 612225, *167413 | 7q32.I | AD |
| NDM | PTF1A (BHLHA29, PTF1P48) | Pancreas transcription factor 1 subunit alpha | * 607194 | 10pl2.2 | AR |
| Mitchell-Riley syndrome | RFX6 | DNA binding protein (RFX6) | * 612659 | 6q22.I | AR/AD |
| NDM | GATA4 | Transcription factor (GATA-4) | * 600576 | 8p23.I | AD |
| AOD | GATA6 | Transcription factor (GATA-6) | * 601656 | 18q I 1.2 | AD |
| NDM | GLIS3 | Zinc finger protein (GLIS3) | * 610192 | 9p24.2 | AR |
| NDM | MNX1 | Motor neuron and pancreas homeobox protein · 1 (MNX I) | * 142994 | 7q36.3 | AR |
| NDM, YOD | PAX6 | Paired box protein 6 (PAX6) | * 607108 | 11pl3 | AD/AR |
| NDM | NEUROG3, NGN3 | Neurogenin-3 (NGN3) | * 604882 | 10q22.I | AR |
| NDM | NKX2.2 | NK2 Homeobox 2 (NKX2.2) | * 604612 | 20pl 1.22 | AD |

(continued on next page)

**Table 1**
*(continued)*

| Form of Diabetes | Mutated Gene | Encoded Protein | OMIM | Locus | Inheritance |
|---|---|---|---|---|---|
| NDM | CNOT1 (CDC39, KIAA1007, NOT1) | CCR4-NOT transcription complex subunit 1 (CNOT1) | * 604917 | 16q21 | AD |
| TND | ZAG1/PLAGL1 | Pleiomorphic adenoma-like protein 1 (PLAGI) (ZAC1) | * 603044 | 6q24.2 | Imprinting disorder |
| Monogenic forms of diabetes associated with impaired glucose metabolism and iusulin secretiou | | | | | |
| MODY2, NDM | CCK | Glucokinase (GCK) | # 125851, *138079 | 7pl3 | AD/AR |
| MODY II, T2D | BLK | B-lymphocyte kinase (BLK) | # 613375, *191305 | 8p23.l | AD |
| MODY 12, NDM | ABCC8 (HRINS, SUR, SUR 1) | ATP-binding cassette Subfamily C member 8 | * 600509 | 11p15.1 | AD/AR/de novo |
| MODY I 3 | KCNJ11 | ATP-sensitive inward-rectifier potassium channel - 1 1 | # 616329, 600937 | 11p15.1 | AD/de novo |
| YOD | PCSK1 | Proprotein convertase I (PC1, PC1/3) | *162150 | 5q15 | AR |

*From Sanchez et al.[5]*

(APPL1).[4] The possibility remains that these genes may play a role in the polygenic development of Type 2 diabetes.

## MATURITY ONSET DIABETES OF THE YOUNG 1 – HEPATIC NUCLEAR FACTOR-4 ALPHA

MODY 1 is caused by mutations in the beta-cell transcription factor, Hepatic Nuclear Factor-4 alpha (HNF4A). MODY 1 accounts for 5% to 10% of all MODYs and is inherited in an autosomal dominant pattern.[5] This clinically presents as progressive insulin secretory defects until the onset of overt diabetes. Most patients present in adolescent or early adulthood, with a mean age presenting at 23 years.[5,6]

Up to 15% of patients with MODY 1 can have neonatal macrosomia and hypoglycemia from hyperinsulinism before later development of clinical diabetes.[7,8]

The initial treatment of choice includes oral agents, with patients responding to sulfonylureas or meglitinides.[4] After that, next-line treatments include insulin and GLP-1 Receptor Agonists, to which patients are known to respond with less hypoglycemia.[4,5] There is a regulatory loop between the HFN4A and HFN1A transcription factors, possibly explaining clinical similarities in presentation and treatment response between patients with mutations in HFN4A (MODY 1) and patients with mutations in HFN1A (MODY 3). However, patients with MODY 1 may have more significant beta-cell dysfunction and advance to additional treatments compared to patients with MODY 3.

## MATURITY ONSET DIABETES OF THE YOUNG 2 – GLUCOKINASE

MODY 2 is an autosomal dominant form caused by heterozygous inactivating mutations of the Glucokinase (GCK) gene. This leads to an altered glucokinase protein that requires a slightly higher glucose threshold before triggering its metabolism and proceeding toward normal insulin secretion. This manifests as stable, mild hyperglycemia and patients tend to have Hemoglobin A1C values of 5.6% to 7.6%.[4] MODY 2 accounts for 15% to 50% of all MODY types.[4] There are no differences in microvascular and macrovascular complications in patients receiving treatment or not, thus these patients do not require treatment if their glucoses remain stable.[4]

More rarely, homozygous mutations in the GCK mutation cause permanent neonatal diabetes.[5] Interestingly, activating mutations of GCK have been described in familial cases of hyperinsulinemic hypoglycemia.[5]

## MATURITY ONSET DIABETES OF THE YOUNG 3 – HEPATIC NUCLEAR FACTOR 1 ALPHA

MODY 3 is the most common form of MODY types, causing 30% to 65% of all MODY cases.[4] This autosomal-dominant form is caused by mutations in the Beta-cell transcription factor for Hepatic Nuclear Factor 1 alpha (HNF1A), which plays a role in the insulin gene. There are more than 1200 mutations that can affect the HNF1A gene,[5] and as such there is a variable expression of MODY 3 with appreciable differences in severity and onset,[6] with symptom onset anywhere from age 6 to 25 year old.[5] The HNF1A gene also plays a role in regulating the expression of the Sodium Glucose Cotransporter (SGLT2) which plays an important role in glycosuria; as such, the medication class of SGLT-2 inhibitors is not recommended in patients with MODY 3.[4,6] These patients have a similar risk of microvascular complications to those patients with Type 2 DM and should be screened annually.[4] There is a risk in a subset of HNF1A mutations associated with hepatocellular adenoma, as such these patients may receive screening liver ultrasound imaging annually.[5]

Patients with MODY 3 have good initial response to sulfonylureas and are typically started with a low dose before titration, similar to patients with MODY 1. Additional therapies include GLP-1 receptor agonists, Dipeptidyl peptidase-4 (DPP-4) inhibitors, and insulin.

## MATURITY ONSET DIABETES OF THE YOUNG 4 – PANCREAS/DUODENUM HOMEOBOX PROTEIN 1

MODY 4 refers to mutations in the gene, Pancreas/Duodenum homeobox protein 1 (PDX1), which encodes Insulin Promoter Factor 1 (IPF1), a transcription factor important for pancreatic and beta-cell development and function. Heterozygous mutations (often missense or frameshift) create the phenotype of diabetic onset in young adulthood, representing the autosomal dominant MODY 4. This condition may present in patients who are obese.[9] This accounts for less than 1% of all MODYs and is treated with oral hypoglycemic agents including sulfonylureas; second-line treatment is insulin.

Homozygous mutations lead to pancreatic agenesis with neonatal diabetes along with exocrine deficiency. There are reports of heterozygous mutations causing pancreatic development anomalies, diabetes, and pancreatic exocrine deficiency as well.[10]

## MATURITY ONSET DIABETES OF THE YOUNG 5 – HEPATIC NUCLEAR FACTOR 1 β

MODY 5 is a rarer form caused by mutation in the gene encoding the beta cell transcription factor, Hepatic Nuclear Factor 1 β (HNF1B). MODY 5 accounts for less than 5% of MODY types, although a prevalence study in Japan noted MODY 5 comprising 13.6%.[11] This form of autosomal dominant monogenic diabetes has a wide span of clinical heterogeneity that can exist within a family despite family members carrying the same genetic mutation.[12] Diabetes onset is typically between childhood and young adulthood.

Because the protein encoded by HNF1B spans multiple tissues including the liver, pancreas, kidney, urogenital tract, and intestine, its mutation can have multi-system effects. As a result, features of MODY 5 can include the malformation of the pancreas, exocrine pancreatic dysfunction, renal dysfunction, elevated liver enzymes, urogenital abnormalities, renal cysts, hypomagnesemia, hypokalemia, and neurodevelopmental disorders.[4,13] In addition, the chromosomal location of HNF1B, 17q12, contains 14 other genes, thus variable deletions correspond with different presentations based on which/how many neighboring genes might be effective. Indeed, with the advent of more accessible genetic testing, in this writer's experience there has been a referral and ultimately MODY 5 diagnosis given after genetic testing revealed a deletion for in chromosome 17q12 encompassing HNF1B gene during the evaluation of a completely independent reason. Again, a testament for the variable phenotype that can be expressed in this condition.

The mainstay for treatment in these patients remains insulin, although there are reports advocating for the effective use of GLP-1R Agonists in this population.[13]

## MATURITY ONSET DIABETES OF THE YOUNG 6 – NEUROGENIC DIFFERENTIATION FACTOR 1

Heterozygous mutations in Neurogenic differentiation factor 1 (NEUROD1), a transcription factor in the beta cell, cause MODY 6. This extremely rare form of autosomal dominant monogenic diabetes accounts for less than 1% of all MODY types. Patients with MODY 6 typically present with clinical diabetes in young adulthood. There is variable expression amongst family members of with the same mutation and even questions raising the possibility of variable penetrance of the disease, versus subclinical expression due to preserved beta-cell function in some family members.[5,11] First-line therapy includes dietary changes and oral hypoglycemic agents/sulfonylureas, while insulin is second-line therapy.

Like some of the other MODY conditions discussed, homozygous mutations in this gene cause a more significant phenotype with neonatal diabetes, cerebellar hypoplasia, sensorineural deafness, and visual impairment.[5,12]

## MATURITY ONSET DIABETES OF THE YOUNG 7 – KRUEPPEL-LIKE FACTOR 11

Heterozygous mutations in Krueppel-like factor 11 (KLF11) is thought to reflect the autosomal-dominant condition MODY 7. This affects beta cell growth and induces apoptosis, with clinical diabetes onset extremely variable. As such, KLF11 mutations can present as neonatal diabetes, or childhood- and adult-onset with MODY. Some mutations are associated with diabetes onset and obesity, often being diagnosed as Type 2 Diabetes. Treatment for this form of diabetes includes insulin.

## MATURITY ONSET DIABETES OF THE YOUNG 8 – CARBOXYL ESTER LIPASE

Mutations in the CEL gene, which encodes Carboxyl Ester Lipase, is referred to as MODY 8 which represents less than 1% of all MODY types.[4] This protein's function is to aid in digestion and is secreted by pancreatic apocrine cells. Mutations cause pancreatic atrophy and leads to progressive exocrine pancreatic insufficiency before the onset of diabetes. The onset of symptoms varies and can be as late as 40 years of age.[14] Initial therapy includes oral hypoglycemic agents including sulfonylureas, with second-line treatment being insulin.

## MATURITY ONSET DIABETES OF THE YOUNG 9 – PARED BOX 4

MODY 9 is due to mutations in the Pared Box 4 (PAX4) gene, which plays a role in the differentiation of beta cells. This is attributed to less than 1% of all MODY types, and patients typically present with diabetes in childhood or adolescence. There is a connection between PAX4 mutations and polymorphisms leading to Type 2 Diabetes as well.

Treatment for MODY 9 includes dietary changes and oral hypoglycemic agents (including sulfonylureas). Insulin is used as second-line treatment as well.[5]

## MATURITY ONSET DIABETES OF THE YOUNG 10 – INSULIN

Mutations in the Insulin gene, INS, can cause defects in the production of insulin or its action, causing MODY 10. This form of MODY is autosomal dominant. There are over 20 pathologic mutations in this gene that can cause diabetes, but the different mutations will confer different clinical significance. Some more severe forms can cause beta-cell apoptosis from the endoplasmic reticulum (ER) stress and present as neonatal diabetes. Less severe mutations may cause mild ER stress or partial insulin activity and can present as MODY in childhood or adulthood. Because of the variance, treatment options include diet changes alone to insulin replacement.

## MATURITY ONSET DIABETES OF THE YOUNG 11  B-LYMPHOCYTE KINASE (BLK)

Heterozygous mutations in B-Lymphocyte Kinase, BLK, cause the autosomal dominant MODY 11, responsible for less than 1% of all MODY types. This gene works to promote insulin synthesis and secretion in response to glucose by working through transcription factors. Treatment includes diet and oral hypoglycemic agents (including sulfonylureas, advancing to insulin as second-line 4).

### MATURITY ONSET DIABETES OF THE YOUNG 12  ATP-BINDING CASSETTE SUBFAMILY C MEMBER 8 (ABCC8)

Mutations in ATP-Binding Cassette ABCC8 commonly presents as neonatal diabetes before 6 months of age, but milder mutations can cause childhood onset and are referred to as MODY 12, which accounts for less than 1% of all MODY. The gene stands for ATP-Binding Casette subfamily C member 8, and encodes the $K_{ATP}$ subunit for the Sulfonylurea Receptor 1 (SUR1). Pathologic gain-of-function mutations in this gene typically are inherited in an autosomal dominant fashion, although autosomal recessive forms have been described as well.[5] Gain-of-function mutations lead to the $K_{ATP}$ channel remaining open, leading to less depolarization and thus less insulin release.

Patients with this mutation, as well as those with KCNJ11 mutations described later in discussion, can be treated with sulfonylureas, similar to those with MODY 1 and MODY 3. second-line therapies include insulin.

Patients with these mutations can have concurrent developmental delay and epilepsy, as a tried referred to as DEND syndrome.[4]

Inactivating mutations of the same gene have been implicated in dominant and recessive forms of congenital hyperinsulinism.

### MATURITY ONSET DIABETES OF THE YOUNG 13  POTASSIUM INWARDLY RECTIFYING CHANNEL SUBFAMILY J MEMBER 11 (KCNJ11)

MODY 13 refers to activating mutations in the KCNJ11 gene, which encodes a member of the inward rectifier potassium channel 11 called kir6.2. This is a subunit of the ATP-sensitive potassium channel. Thus, activating mutations of this gene will cause the $K_{ATP}$ channel to inappropriately remain open, preventing subsequent depolarization of the cell membrane, thus preventing calcium influx and no insulin would be released. These mutations may present as autosomal dominant or from de novo mutations.

The presentation of KCNJ11 can change based on the severity of the mutation. More severe KCNJ11 mutations are the most frequently identified cause for neonatal diabetes, accounting for ½ to 1/3 of cases. Milder forms causing childhood-onset or adult-onset diabetes. In these cases, MODY 13 represents less than 1% of all MODYs.

There is also documented variable expression in members of a family with the same genetic mutation. One multi-generation family was reported to have different disease presentations including transient neonatal diabetes, childhood-onset diabetes, and adult-onset diabetes.[15]

KCNJ11 mutations can be associated with developmental delay, muscle weakness, and epilepsy. A severe phenotype with severe delay, epilepsy, and neonatal diabetes is termed DEND syndrome.[6]

Because this mutation affects the $K_{ATP}$ channel, MODY 13 is sensitive to treatment with sulfonylurea treatment. Doses required can be relatively high but has been proven to be a safe and effective treatment.[6] Insulin can be used as a second-line agent.

Activating mutations of KCNJ11 are associated with congenital hyperinsulinism, as this causes more depolarization of the $K_{ATP}$ channel leading to downstream calcium influx and insulin release.

### MATURITY ONSET DIABETES OF THE YOUNG 14  ADAPTOR PROTEIN, PHOSPHOTYROSINE INTERACTION, PH DOMAIN, AND LEUCINE ZIPPER CONTAINING 1

MODY 14 refers to a rare form of autosomal dominant diabetes occurring from mutations in Adaptor Protein, Phosphotyrosine interaction, PH Domain, and Leucine zipper containing 1 (APPL1), accounting for less than 1% of MODY types. This gene codes for a protein that affects multiple steps in the insulin-signaling pathway such as the insulin signaling regulator AKT. This autosomal dominant condition is treated with diet and oral hypoglycemics such as sulfonylureas as first line, and insulin as second line.[4]

Having reviewed the types of MODY, the key message is that these represent a smaller portion of diabetes types but are often overlooked. Aspects of history and physical exam that should clue the provider to pursue further workup would be if the patient has negative antibodies and does not fit the typical body habitus or lacks acanthosis nigricans on exam. With the increase in obesity in pediatric patients, the clinician should be especially wary of overlapping features and should maintain a higher index of suspicion of the patient does not follow a typical treatment course while on standard therapy for type 2 diabetes. Additionally, since MODY tends to be autosomal dominant, if there is a strong family history (3 generations or more) then monogenic should be considered. Additionally, if a patient is very young at diagnosis (<6 month old), monogenic diabetes should be evaluated.

## CLINICS CARE POINTS

- Maturity Onset Diabetes of the Young (MODY) refers to monogenic forms of diabetes typically inherited in an autosomal dominant fashion.

- With the ongoing usage of MODY in the literature, the described monogenic mutations in adolescents as well as neonates have an associated MODY designation that is often tied to the specific genetic mutation.

- Factors that should prompt the clinical to consider genetic workup of MODY include: family history of 3 or more generations, onset in neonates or infants, other multi-system disease, or antibody-negative diabetes in a patient whose phenotype would be inconsistent with Type 2 Diabetes.

- The most common form of MODY presents as nonprogressive mild hyperglycemia due to mutation in the glucose-sensing glucokinase enzyme and does not require any treatment.

- Other forms of MODY are responsive to sulfonylureas, offering an oral medication alternative to insulin therapy.

## DISCLOSURE

The authors have no commercial or financial conflicts of interest.

## REFERENCES

1. American Diabetes Association Professional Practice Committee; 2. Classification and Diagnosis of Diabetes: Standards of Medical Care in Diabetes—2022. Diabetes Care 2022;45(Supplement_1):S17–38.
2. Siddiqui K, Musambil M, Nazir N. Maturity onset diabetes of the young (MODY)—History, first case reports and recent advances. Gene 2015;555(1):66–71.
3. Laver TW, Wakeling MN, Knox O, et al. Evaluation of Evidence for Pathogenicity Demonstrates That BLK, KLF11, and PAX4 Should Not Be Included in Diagnostic Testing for MODY. Diabetes 2022;71(5):1128–36.
4. Broome DT, Pantalone KM, Kashyap SR, et al. Approach to the Patient with MODY-Monogenic Diabetes. J Clin Endocrinol Metab 2021;106(1):237–50.

5. Sanchez Caballero L, Gorgogietas V, Arroyo MN, et al. Molecular mechanisms of β-cell dysfunction and death in monogenic forms of diabetes. Int Rev Cell Mol Biol 2021;359:139–256.

6. Steck AK, Winter WE. Review on monogenic diabetes. Curr Opin Endocrinol Diabetes Obes 2011;18(4):252–8.

7. Heuvel-Borsboom H, de Valk HW, Losekoot M, et al. Maturity onset diabetes of the young: Seek and you will find. Neth J Med 2016;74(5):193–200.

8. Tosur M, Philipson LH. Precision diabetes: Lessons learned from maturity-onset diabetes of the young (MODY). J Diabetes Investig 2022;13(9):1465–71.

9. Deng M, Xiao X, Zhou L, et al. First Case Report of Maturity-Onset Diabetes of the Young Type 4 Pedigree in a Chinese Family. Front Endocrinol 2019;10:406.

10. Caetano LA, Santana LS, Costa-Riquetto AD, et al. PDX1 -MODY and dorsal pancreatic agenesis: New phenotype of a rare disease. Clin Genet 2018;93(2):382–6.

11. Horikawa Y, Enya M, Mabe H, et al. NEUROD1-deficient diabetes (MODY6): Identification of the first cases in Japanese and the clinical features. Pediatr Diabetes 2018;19(2):236–42.

12. Zhang H, Colclough K, Gloyn AL, et al. Monogenic diabetes: a gateway to precision medicine in diabetes. J Clin Invest 2021;131(3):e142244.

13. Terakawa A, Chujo D, Yasuda K, et al. Maturity-Onset diabetes of the young type 5 treated with the glucagon-like peptide-1 receptor agonist: A case report. Medicine (Baltim) 2020;99(35):e21939.

14. Lombardo D, Silvy F, Crenon I, et al. Pancreatic adenocarcinoma, chronic pancreatitis, and MODY-8 diabetes: is bile salt-dependent lipase (or carboxyl ester lipase) at the crossroads of pancreatic pathologies? Oncotarget 2017;9(15):12513–33.

15. D'Amato E, Tammaro P, Craig TJ, et al. Variable phenotypic spectrum of diabetes mellitus in a family carrying a novel KCNJ11 gene mutation. Diabet Med 2008;25(6):651–6.

# Non-syndromic and Syndromic Severe Acne in Adolescent Patients

Hsi Yen, MD, MPH, Leah Lalor, MD*

## KEYWORDS

- Severe acne • Acne syndromes • Adolescent

## KEY POINTS

- Acne is a common skin disorder in adolescents. However, severe acne that is persistent and refractory to conventional treatment or has other associated symptoms should raise suspicion for non-syndromic or syndromic acne.
- Non-syndromic severe acne includes acne fulminans and acne conglobata. Syndromic severe acne encompasses both autoinflammatory syndromes as well as androgen-excess states.
- Drug-induced acne remains an important consideration, and when suspected a clear drug history and immediate cessation of trigger drug is essential.

## INTRODUCTION

Acne is a common inflammatory disorder of the skin pilosebaceous unit. While acne affects individuals of all ages, its prevalence peaks at around 15 - 20 year old and affects an estimated 36% - 93% of school-aged students.[1–3] The pathogenesis of acne involves a complex interplay of hair follicle epidermal hyperproliferation, increased sebum production due to androgen stimulation, bacterial involvement by *Cutibacterium acnes*, and inflammation.[4] Acne presents early as comedones, evolves into inflammatory papules or pustules, and can progress into inflamed nodules or cysts. Acne can result in scarring and detrimental psychosocial effects.[5]

## NON-SYNDROMIC SEVERE ACNE
### Acne Fulminans

Acne fulminans (AF) is a severe variant with explosive onset of ulcerative acne with or without systemic symptoms. It is most common in adolescent males between 13 and 22 year old.[6] While the pathogenesis is unknown, AF is thought to be an induced immune response causing systemic inflammation.[7] Clinically, there is a rapid exacerbation of

Department of Dermatology, Division of Pediatric Dermatology, Medical College of Wisconsin, 8701 Watertown Plank Road, TBRC 2nd Floor Suite C2010, Milwaukee, WI 53226, USA
* Corresponding author.
*E-mail address:* llalor@mcw.edu

Med Clin N Am 108 (2024) 27–42
https://doi.org/10.1016/j.mcna.2023.05.014
0025-7125/24/© 2023 Elsevier Inc. All rights reserved.

painful erosions and ulcers with hemorrhagic crusting of nodules on the face, chest, and back (**Fig. 1**).[6] Unlike acne conglobata, comedones are rare and not a defining feature. There is a predilection for lesions on the trunk with eventual severe scarring.[6,8] Systemic symptoms can include fever, malaise, weight loss, polyarthralgia, myalgia, hepatosplenomegaly, and bone pain especially of the sternum and clavicles.[9] Erythema nodosum is sometimes present.

Workup for AF includes complete blood cell count with differential and liver function tests.[6] Erythrocyte sedimentation rate (ESR) and C-reactive protein (CRP) should also be checked in patients with systemic findings, while women should undergo pregnancy screening. Lab abnormalities include anemia, leukocytosis, and elevated ESR and CRP.[6] If there is a concern for bone or joint involvement, plain radiographs may demonstrate osteolytic changes in areas of pain.[10]

First-line treatment involves systemic corticosteroids, which may start at 0.5 - 1 mg/kg/d for 2 to 4 weeks followed by a tapering course with halving of dose each week over 4 - 8 weeks.[6,11,12] When lesions have healed, isotretinoin should be initiated at low initial dosing of 0.1 mg/kg/d and slowly increased.[6] Corticosteroids should act as a bridge to isotretinoin therapy, and the two treatments should overlap for at least 4 weeks.[6] For patients where oral corticosteroids are not an option, high-potency topical corticosteroids can be applied one to two times daily.[6] Oral dapsone can also be considered if there is associated erythema nodosum.[13] For refractory cases of AF, successful treatment with tumor necrosis factor-$\alpha$ (TNF-$\alpha$) inhibitors such as adalimumab and infliximab has been reported.[14,15]

Isotretinoin can also induce AF, especially when initiated at high doses in patients with severe inflammatory acne and during the first month of therapy.[6] Isotretinoin-induced AF typically does not have systemic involvement, and can be prevented by lower initial dosing or concurrent use of systemic corticosteroid. Anabolic steroids, such as taken by bodybuilders to enhance muscle mass, can also induce AF.[16] For transgender individuals taking gender-affirming hormone therapy, AF has been reported with increased testosterone dosage.[17]

AF can also be associated with various syndromes involving severe acne, which will be discussed in greater detail in the sections on Syndromic Severe Acne.

### Acne Conglobata

Acne conglobata (AC) is a severe variant of nodulocystic acne that, unlike AF, does not typically have systemic involvement and presents with a chronic course.[18] It is more

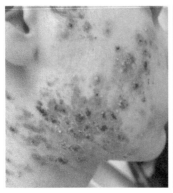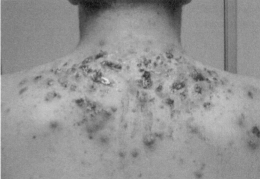

**Fig. 1.** Hemorrhagic crusting in a patient with acne fulminans (AF). (© American Acne & Rosacea Society. Printed with permission.)

common in young men in the second and third decades of life.[19] Clinically, there are widespread comedones and large, tender inflamed cysts and nodules, abscesses with purulent discharge, and draining sinus tracts.[19] This most commonly affects the face, shoulders, back, chest, and buttocks.

AC can occur in isolation or as part of the follicular occlusion tetrad, which includes hidradenitis suppurativa (HS), dissecting cellulitis of the scalp, and pilonidal cysts.

First-line treatment for AC is with isotretinoin dosed initially at 0.1 - 0.3 mg/kg/d with systemic corticosteroid concurrently.[20] AC resistant to conventional therapy may benefit from TNF-α inhibitors such as adalimumab or infliximab.[21–23]

## SYNDROMIC SEVERE ACNE: AUTOINFLAMMATORY
### Introduction

There are multiple autoinflammatory disorders in which acne presents as part of a clinical syndrome. Some have associated genetic changes but most are sporadic. Management of syndromic severe acne is best achieved with the care of a multi-disciplinary team.

### Synovitis, Acne, Pustulosis, Hyperostosis, Osteitis Syndrome

SAPHO syndrome is a rare autoinflammatory disorder with a spectrum of osteoarticular and dermatologic manifestations.[24] While it can occur at any age, SAPHO syndrome has been predominantly reported in adults during the third to fifth decades.[25–27] Most cases are sporadic, but some are familial. Pro-inflammatory cytokines such as TNF-α, interleukin (IL)-1, IL-8, IL-17, and IL-18 drive the disease.[28,29] SAPHO syndrome is usually a chronic disease with a relapsing-remitting or chronic indolent course.[25]

Onset is gradual and occurs in middle-aged adults, but can present earlier in childhood. The cardinal clinical manifestation in SAPHO syndrome is osteitis and hyperostosis, and can occur with or without dermatologic manifestations.[30] Osteoarticular involvement most prominently involves swelling or tenderness of the anterior chest wall, sternocostal, and sternoclavicular joints.[30] Timing of skin presentation is variable. In one study of 155 patients, skin lesions were found up to years before (54.2%),

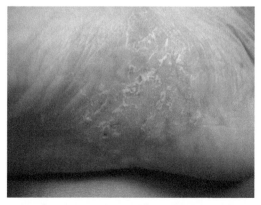

**Fig. 2.** Palmoplantar pustulosis in a patient with Synovitis, acne, pustulosis, hyperostosis, osteitis (SAPHO) syndrome. (Rena C. Zuo, Daniella M. Schwartz, Chyi-Chia Richard Lee, Milan J. Anadkat, Edward W. Cowen, Haley B. Naik, Palmoplantar pustules and osteoarticular pain in a 42-year-old woman, Journal of the American Academy of Dermatology, 72 (3), 2015, 550-553, https://doi.org/10.1016/j.jaad.2014.07.014.)

simultaneously (27.1%), or years after (18.7%) osteoarticular lesions.[31] The most common cutaneous presentation is exclusive palmoplantar pustulosis, occurring in 60% - 70% of patients (**Fig. 2**).[32] Acne, while less common, is usually severe and can present as AC or AF. Concurrent presentation with palmoplantar pustulosis and severe acne is exceptional.[32] Other skin findings include HS, pyoderma gangrenosum, and other subtypes of psoriasis such as psoriasis vulgaris or generalized pustular psoriasis.[32,33] Systemic symptoms such as fever or weight loss are uncommon.

No laboratory test is diagnostic for SAPHO syndrome, though elevated ESR and CRP, as well as mild leukocytosis and anemia may be observed.[25] Work-up involves imaging studies to assess for osteoarticular involvement.

Treatment with non-steroidal anti-inflammatory drugs (NSAIDs) is first-line for pain relief, while intra-articular and systemic corticosteroids are rapidly effective for most patients and can be a bridge to other therapeutic modalities.[29] Topical corticosteroid and psoralen and UVA therapy are effective options for palmoplantar pustulosis. Bisphosphonates and methotrexate can be helpful for bone lesions and pain.[34,35] Biologics have been used for refractory cases: TNF-$\alpha$ inhibitors such as infliximab, etanercept, and adalimumab have the most extensive evidence and should be first choice; IL-1 inhibition with anakinra; and IL-23/IL-17 blockade with ustekinumab or secukinumab.[36] However, paradoxic skin flares can occur in the setting of TNF-$\alpha$ inhibitor use, and mainly presents as psoriasiform lesions on the limbs and trunk.[37] There has also been a report of successful treatment of refractory SAPHO syndrome by Janus kinase (JAK) inhibition with tofacitinib.[38]

Pyogenic arthritis, pyoderma gangrenosum, acne (PAPA) syndrome
Pyoderma gangrenosum, acne, suppurative hidradenitis (PASH) syndrome
Pyogenic arthritis, pyoderma gangrenosum, acne, suppurative hidradenitis (PA-PASH) syndrome

PAPA syndrome, PASH syndrome, and PAPASH syndrome are a group of rare, hereditary autoinflammatory diseases that share the common hallmark of excessive activation of the immune system, presenting with diverse clinical features such as recurrent fevers, neutrophilic dermatoses (commonly pyoderma gangrenosum [PG] and HS), and acne.[39,40] PG manifests as skin ulcers with undermined violaceous borders. HS is characterized by painful draining papulonodules and sinus tracts involving the intertriginous skin, and usually results in scarring. Laboratory testing is non-specific and typically reveals leukocytosis and elevated acute-phase reactants secondary to systemic inflammation.[39]

### Pyogenic Arthritis, Pyoderma Gangrenosum, Acne Syndrome

PAPA syndrome is associated with autosomal dominant pathogenic variant in *PSTPIP1* on chromosome 15q that encodes PSTPIP1, which binds with pyrin and regulates inflammasome.[41] The pathogenic variant results in increased binding to pyrin and overproduction of IL-1$\beta$ and IL-18, causing release of proinflammatory cytokines IL-1, IL-17, and TNF-$\alpha$.[39,42]

PAPA syndrome often presents in the first decade with fever and recurrent spontaneous aseptic purulent synovial inflammation leading to progressively destructive joint involvement.[40] Joint involvement is usually pauci-articular and non-axial, commonly affecting the ankles, knees, elbows, and wrists.[39,43] Joint symptoms initially predominate but improve after puberty, which is when acne begins.[43] In one study of 49 cases of PAPA syndrome, the average age of acne onset was 13 years and most were nodulocystic.[40] PG is less common and manifests later in adolescence or adulthood, typically involving the lower extremities and can vary in severity.[18]

Leukocytosis and elevated acute phase reactants are common but non-diagnostic.[39] Plain radiographs demonstrate pauciarticular, erosive arthritis. MRI findings are non-specific.[43]

Treatment of arthritis includes aspiration, drainage, and intra-articular corticosteroids to relieve joint pain during flares.[43] High-dose systemic corticosteroids dosed at 0.5 - 1 mg/kg/d are also effective for arthritis and PG.[44] The most consistent responses to biologic treatment are with TNF-$\alpha$ inhibitors, including etanercept, adalimumab, and infliximab.[45–47] IL-1 receptor antagonist anakinra and anti-IL-1$\beta$ monoclonal antibody canakinumab have demonstrated efficacy for cutaneous manifestations and spondyloarthropathy, and may be an alternative for non-responders to TNF-$\alpha$ inhibition.[48] Topical retinoids and isotretinoin are helpful for acne.[40]

### Pyoderma Gangrenosum, Acne, Suppurative Hidradenitis Syndrome

PASH syndrome is characterized by PG, acne, and HS. Unlike PAPA syndrome, there is a characteristic absence of pyogenic sterile arthritis. Increased number of CCTG microsatellite repeats in the *PSTPIP1* promoter region, as well as *PSTPIP1* and *NCSTN* pathogenic variants have been associated with this syndrome.[49–51]

The onset of PASH syndrome typically occurs in young adulthood, initially presenting with acne on average at 17 years old.[40] The acne can be mild to severe. Other skin lesions include PG and HS (**Fig. 3**). One review of 43 cases identified 23% of patients presenting concurrently with acne and HS.[40]

Due to the extensive cutaneous involvement of PASH, patients typically have a severe impact on their quality of life. Treatment considerations are similar to PAPA syndrome. Sustained improvement of skin lesions have been noted in patients treated with anakinra and canakinumab.[48]

### Pyogenic Arthritis, Pyoderma Gangrenosum, Acne, Suppurative Hidradenitis Syndrome

PAPASH syndrome is defined as a constellation of pyogenic sterile arthritis, PG, acne, and HS. It is associated with the *E277D* pathogenic variant in *PSTPIP1* gene.[52]

Like PASH syndrome, the average age of onset for PAPASH syndrome is young adulthood at around 31 years old, while acne typically presents around 15 years old.[40]

## SYNDROMIC SEVERE ACNE: ANDROGEN-EXCESS STATES
### Introduction

Both ovarian and adrenal etiologies can result in hyperandrogenism in females.[53] Polycystic ovary syndrome (PCOS) accounts for the majority of androgen-excess states in females.

### Polycystic Ovary Syndrome

PCOS is a complex multigenic endocrine disorder characterized by androgen excess and ovarian dysfunction.[54] While it remains without definitively established diagnostic criteria in adolescents, the classic presentation includes anovulation, clinical or biochemical signs of hyperandrogenism, and polycystic ovaries.[55] The syndrome is a result of hormonal imbalances, with an increased ratio of luteinizing hormone (LH) to follicle-stimulating hormone (FSH) stimulating the ovarian theca cells and leading to excess androgen production.[56] Insulin resistance and obesity also play important roles in PCOS.[57]

Hyperandrogenism has multiple cutaneous manifestations which include acne, hirsutism, and androgenetic alopecia (**Fig. 4**).[56] Insulin resistance presents on the skin as acanthosis nigricans (AN). This manifests as a velvety darkening and thickening of the

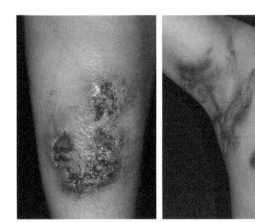
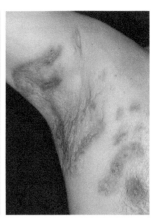

**Fig. 3.** Multilocular pyoderma gangrenosum and suppurative hidradenitis of axillae in a patient with Pyoderma gangrenosum, acne, suppurative hidradenitis (PASH) syndrome. (Markus Braun-Falco, Oleksandr Kovnerystyy, Peter Lohse, Thomas Ruzicka, Pyoderma gangrenosum, acne, and suppurative hidradenitis (PASH)-a new autoinflammatory syndrome distinct from PAPA syndrome, Journal of the American Academy of Dermatology, 66 (3), 2012, 409-415, https://doi.org/10.1016/j.jaad.2010.12.025.)

flexural skin such as the neck, axillae, and antecubital fossae. Hirsutism presents as excessive terminal body hair in a male distribution involving the upper lip, chin, areola, chest, back, or lower abdomen.[56]

Obese females with severe, treatment-resistant acne and other signs of hyperandrogenism such as hirsutism and/or AN should prompt consideration for PCOS. PCOS-associated acne is often moderate or severe inflammatory type and typically persists into adulthood.[56] The prevalence of acne, hirsutism, and androgenetic alopecia in PCOS patients is 15% - 95%, 8.1% - 77.5%, and 22% - 35%, respectively.[58] Of note, some females with "lean PCOS" may present with normal or low body mass index and without overt signs of virilization.[59]

Common workup includes serum androgens (dehydroepiandrosterone sulfate [DHEAS], total testosterone, and free testosterone), LH, FSH, 17-hydroxyprogesterone, and prolactin, though protocols vary.[58]

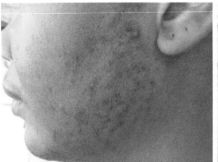
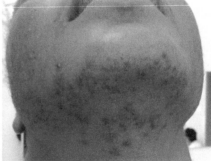

**Fig. 4.** Hirsutism and acne are signs of hyperandrogenism in a patient with polycystic ovary syndrome (PCOS). (Elizabeth Housman, Rachel V. Reynolds, Polycystic ovary syndrome: A review for dermatologists: Part I. Diagnosis and manifestations, Journal of the American Academy of Dermatology, 71 (5), 2014, 847.e1-847.e10, https://doi.org/10.1016/j.jaad.2014.05.007.)

First-line treatment for PCOS-associated acne that have failed topical therapies is combined oral contraceptives (COCs), while the addition of the antiandrogen medication spironolactone starting at 50 mg daily can be considered if there is a poor response.[60] Second-line therapy involves a short course of oral antibiotics as adjunctive therapy to hormonal treatment. In patients with severe acne that have failed other treatments, isotretinoin would be reasonable.[60]

### Hyperandrogenism, Insulin Resistance, Acanthosis Nigricans Syndrome

HAIR-AN syndrome occurs in a subset of PCOS patients and represents about 5% of women with hyperandrogenism.[61] Insulin resistance with compensatory hyperinsulinemia plays an important role in the pathogenesis of disease.[62]

Clinically, HAIR-AN presents in early adolescence with prominent cutaneous manifestations of AN and hyperandrogenism, including hirsutism, acne, alopecia, and oily skin.[63] There may also be signs of virilization which include deepening of voice, increased libido, clitoromegaly, and changes in muscle mass.

Workup typically demonstrates elevated levels of insulin, testosterone, and androstenedione.[64]

COCs, antiandrogenic agents, and metformin are first-line therapy.[63]

### Seborrhea, acne, hirsutism, alopecia (SAHA) syndrome

SAHA syndrome is a cause of post-adolescent hyperandrogenism in young females that is defined by the tetrad of seborrhea, acne, hirsutism, and alopecia.[65] It can be associated with insulin resistance and hyperprolactinemia.[66] The androgen excess of SAHA is due to either high levels of androgens or increased sensitivity of pilosebaceous units to normal levels of androgens, both which result in increase in sebum production by sebaceous glands.[66,67]

Onset of SAHA syndrome occurs after puberty, and about 20% of patients have all four major cutaneous manifestations.[68] Seborrhea is the most common clinical manifestation of SAHA syndrome, and occurs in all patients. Androgenetic alopecia occurs in 21% of cases, acne in 10%, and hirsutism in 6%.[68] Management is similar to that of PCOS.

## DRUG-INDUCED ACNE

There are many drugs which can induce acne (**Box 1**). It is therefore important to elucidate a clear drug history in patients who have sudden onset of acne at an unusual age, presenting with monomorphous papulopustular eruption beyond the typical seborrheic areas, or with persistent severe acne refractory to conventional treatment.[69] Identifying and discontinuation of the trigger drug will result in dramatic improvement. While not all medications will be discussed in this section, a few key considerations for adolescents are mentioned.

### Testosterone

For transgender individuals undergoing gender-affirming hormone therapy with testosterone, acne is a common side effect (**Fig. 5**). Treatment is guided by acne type and severity. Specific considerations include: contraception counseling for teratogenic medications in transmasculine patients with childbearing potential, discussing potential feminizing effects of COCs, and discussing topical clascoterone as a potential treatment option that targets androgen receptors on the skin.[70]

---

**Box 1**
**Causes of drug-induced acne**

Testosterone

Anabolic steroids

High-dose vitamin B6 and B12

Corticosteroids

Halogenated compounds: iodines, chlorides, bromides

Phenytoin

Lithium

Isoniazid

Epidermal growth factor receptor (EGFR) inhibitors

MEK inhibitors

Serine–threonine protein kinase B-RAF (BRAF) inhibitors

Cystic fibrosis transmembrane conductance regulator (CTFR) modulators

---

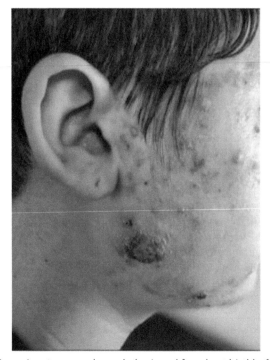

**Fig. 5.** Acne fulminans in a transgender male (assigned female at birth) after starting testosterone injections for gender-affirming hormone therapy. (Gayin Lee, Rita Ferri-Huerta, Katherine B. Greenberg, Kathryn E. Somers, Acne fulminans in a transgender boy after an increase in testosterone dosage, JAAD Case Reports, 21, 2022, 32-34, https://doi.org/10.1016/j.jdcr.2021.11.029.)

**Table 1**
**Summary of uncommon causes of severe adolescent acne**

**Non-syndrome severe acne**

| | |
|---|---|
| Acne fulminans (AF) | • Adolescent males.<br>• Explosive onset of ulcerative acne that forms hemorrhagic crusting.<br>• Can have systemic symptoms.<br>• First-line treatment with systemic corticosteroids as a bridge to isotretinoin. |
| Acne conglobata (AC) | • Adults in the second and third decades of life.<br>• Chronic course with widespread comedones. Large nodulocystic acne, abscesses, and draining sinus tracts.<br>• Typically without systemic symptoms.<br>• First-line treatment with systemic corticosteroid and concurrent isotretinoin. |

**Syndromic severe acne: autoinflammatory**

| | |
|---|---|
| Synovitis, acne, pustulosis, hyperostosis, osteitis (SAPHO) syndrome | • Adults in the third to fifth decades of life.<br>• Presents with osteitis and hyperostosis, most prominently with swelling and tenderness of the anterior chest wall.<br>• Most common cutaneous presentation is palmoplantar pustulosis.<br>• Acne is less common but is usually severe.<br>• Non-steroidal anti-inflammatory drugs (NSAIDs) are first-line for pain relief.<br>• Topical corticosteroid and psoralen and UVA therapy effective for palmoplantar pustulosis. |
| Pyogenic arthritis, pyoderma gangrenosum, acne (PAPA) syndrome | • Autosomal dominant pathogenic variant in *PSTPIP1*.<br>• Childhood in the first decade.<br>• Presents with recurrent fever and progressively destructive joint inflammation.<br>• Acne begins after puberty, while PG varies in occurrence and severity.<br>• Treatment of arthritis and PG with high-dose systemic corticosteroid. TNF-α inhibitors have demonstrated efficacy. |
| Pyoderma gangrenosum, acne, suppurative hidradenitis (PASH) syndrome | • Pathogenic variant in *PSTPIP1* and *NCSTN*.<br>• Onset in young adulthood.<br>• Characteristic absence of arthritis.<br>• Variable acne, can have other skin lesions such as PG and HS.<br>• Treatment similar to PAPA syndrome. |
| Pyogenic arthritis, pyoderma gangrenosum, acne, suppurative hidradenitis (PAPASH) syndrome | • *E277*D pathogenic variant in *PSTPIP1* gene<br>• Onset in young adulthood. |

**Syndromic severe acne: androgen-excess states**

| | |
|---|---|
| Polycystic ovary syndrome (PCOS) | • Accounts for the majority of androgen excess states in females<br>• Hyperandrogenism presents as acne, hirsutism in male distribution, and androgenetic alopecia.<br>• Insulin resistance presents as AN. |

*(continued on next page)*

| Table 1 (continued) | |
|---|---|
| Hyperandrogenism, insulin resistance, acanthosis nigricans (HAIR-AN) syndrome | • Presents in early adolescence.<br>• Prominent AN and hyperandrogenism.<br>• May also have signs of virilization.<br>• First-line treatment includes oral contraceptives, antiandrogenic agents, and metformin. |
| Seborrhea, acne, hirsutism, alopecia (SAHA) syndrome | • Onset after puberty in young females.<br>• Seborrhea most common.<br>• Management similar to PCOS. |
| **Drug-induced acne** | |
| Testosterone | • Transgender individuals receiving gender-affirming hormone therapy with testosterone.<br>• Topical clascoterone potential treatment option. |
| Anabolic steroids | • Adolescents using performance-enhancing drugs.<br>• Discontinue administration of anabolic steroids. |
| Molecular targeted therapies | • Patients using epidermal growth factor receptor (EGFR) inhibitors.<br>• Unlike true acne, this is predominantly inflammation-driven.<br>• Treat with topical corticosteroids and oral tetracycline antibiotics for anti-inflammatory properties. |
| Cystic fibrosis transmembrane conductance regulator (CFTR) modulators | • Cystic fibrosis patients taking newer combination CFTR modulators. |

### Anabolic Steroids

The use of performance-enhancing drugs such as anabolic steroids is of special concern in adolescent athletes. It is estimated that 1% - 12% of high school boys and 0.5% - 3% of high school girls report the use of anabolic steroids, with the highest rate in male athletes in football, wresting, and weight lifting.[71] Acne is one of the most common side effects from anabolic steroid use, with an estimated 43% of users affected.[72] In these cases, the most important step in management is to immediately discontinue anabolic steroids.[73] If AF is present, treatment with isotretinoin and concurrent systemic corticosteroid should be initiated.

### Molecular Targeted Therapies

Epidermal growth factor receptor (EGFR) inhibitors can cause an acneiform papulopustular eruption. Unlike true acne, this is predominantly secondary to inflammation, presenting as pruritic papules and pustules without comedones.[74] It is one of the earliest and most common adverse effects of EGFR inhibitors, and occurs as early as the first few weeks of treatment.[69] Treatment is guided by severity, and includes topical corticosteroid or oral tetracycline antibiotics for their anti-inflammatory properties.[75] Importantly, the presence and severity of the acneiform eruption is often predictive of treatment response to EGFR inhibitors, and therefore it is advisable to continue

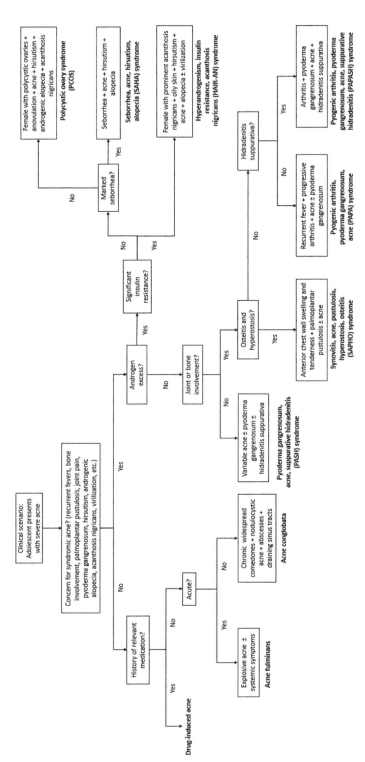

**Fig. 6.** Diagnostic approach to adolescent with severe acne.

treatment and manage the acneiform eruption separately. Similar acneiform papulopustular eruptions are seen with MEK inhibitors and serine–threonine protein kinase B-RAF (BRAF) inhibitors.[76,77]

### Cystic Fibrosis Transmembrane Conductance Regulator Modulators

Cystic fibrosis patients taking newer combination CFTR modulators such as elexacaftor-tezacaftor-ivacaftor (ELX/TEZ/IVA) are at increased risk of acneiform eruptions. In two case series of 35 patients, new-onset or worsening acne was noted, typically within the first 2 to 3 months of therapy.[78,79] Most of these patients reported improvement with topical or oral acne treatments. Due to potential malabsorption of isotretinoin secondary to pancreatic insufficiency common in cystic fibrosis patients, taking pancreatic enzymes concurrently with isotretinoin may be helpful for cases refractory to isotretinoin alone.

### SUMMARY

While acne is a common skin disorder in adolescents, providers should have increased awareness when there are clinical signs and symptoms that may indicate the patient may not have "typical teenage acne." Uncommon causes of severe adolescent acne are summarized in **Table 1**. A simplified diagnostic approach is presented in **Fig. 6**. Two common non-syndromic entities associated with severe acne are AF and AC. Explosive ulcerative acne with systemic symptoms should raise suspicion for AF, and concurrent treatment with systemic corticosteroids and isotretinoin is key to management. The presence of widespread comedones, cysts, abscesses, and draining sinus tracts with a more chronic course is suggestive for AC. Rarer autoinflammatory syndromic causes of acne include SAPHO, PAPA, PASH, and PAPASH syndromes. These are characterized by features such as recurrent febrile outbreaks, osteoarticular involvement, and neutrophilic dermatoses. PCOS accounts for the majority of acne associated with excess androgen states, while HAIR-AN and SAHA syndromes are less common. Finally, drug-induced acne should be considered in unique adolescent populations such as transgender individuals on gender-affirming medications, athletes using anabolic steroids, patients receiving molecular targeted therapies, and cystic fibrosis patients using newer combination CFTR modulators.

### CLINICS CARE POINTS

- Treatment of acne fulminans is with systemic corticosteroids which should act as a bridge to isotretinoin.
- TNF-α inhibitors have been used successfully to treat autoinflammatory syndromic acne.
- Oral contraceptives and spironolactone are helpful for PCOS-associated acne.
- Reviewing drug history and discontinuing trigger drug when possible are key to managing drug-induced acne.

### REFERENCES

1. Tan JKL, Bhate K. A global perspective on the epidemiology of acne. Br J Dermatol 2015;172(S1):3–12.
2. Lynn DD, Umari T, Dunnick CA, et al. The epidemiology of acne vulgaris in late adolescence. Adolesc Health Med Ther 2016;7:13–25.

3. Layton AM, Thiboutot D, Tan J. Reviewing the global burden of acne: how could we improve care to reduce the burden? Br J Dermatol 2021;184(2):219–25.
4. Tuchayi SM, Makrantonaki E, Ganceviciene R, et al. Acne vulgaris. Nat Rev Dis Prim 2015;1(1):15029.
5. Sachdeva M, Tan J, Lim J, et al. The prevalence, risk factors, and psychosocial impacts of acne vulgaris in medical students: a literature review. Int J Dermatol 2021;60(7):792–8.
6. Greywal T, Zaenglein AL, Baldwin HE, et al. Evidence-based recommendations for the management of acne fulminans and its variants. J Am Acad Dermatol 2017;77(1):109–17.
7. Zito PM, Badri T. Acne fulminans. StatPearls. Treasure Island, FL: StatPearls Publishing Copyright © 2022. StatPearls Publishing LLC.; 2022.
8. Alakeel A, Ferneiny M, Auffret N, et al. Acne Fulminans: Case Series and Review of the Literature. Pediatr Dermatol 2016;33(6):e388–92.
9. Zaba R, Schwartz R, Jarmuda S, et al. Acne fulminans: explosive systemic form of acne. J Eur Acad Dermatol Venereol 2011;25(5):501–7.
10. Laasonen LS, Karvonen SL, Reunala TL. Bone disease in adolescents with acne fulminans and severe cystic acne: radiologic and scintigraphic findings. AJR Am J Roentgenol 1994;162(5):1161–5.
11. Seukeran DC, Cunliffe WJ. The treatment of acne fulminans: a review of 25 cases. Br J Dermatol 1999;141(2):307–9.
12. Karvonen SL. Acne fulminans: report of clinical findings and treatment of twenty-four patients. J Am Acad Dermatol 1993;28(4):572–9.
13. Tan BB, Lear JT, Smith AG. Acne fulminans and erythema nodosum during isotretinoin therapy responding to dapsone. Clin Exp Dermatol 1997;22(1):26–7.
14. Marasca C, Fabbrocini G, Abategiovanni L, et al. Adalimumab in the Management of Isotretinoin-Induced Acne Fulminans: Report of a Case. Skin Appendage Disord 2021;7(2):115–9.
15. Iqbal M, Kolodney MS. Acne fulminans with synovitis-acne-pustulosis-hyperostosis-osteitis (SAPHO) syndrome treated with infliximab. J Am Acad Dermatol 2005;52(5 Suppl 1):S118–20.
16. Kraus SL, Emmert S, Schön MP, et al. The Dark Side of Beauty: Acne Fulminans Induced by Anabolic Steroids in a Male Bodybuilder. Arch Dermatol 2012; 148(10):1210–2.
17. Lee G, Ferri-Huerta R, Greenberg KB, et al. Acne fulminans in a transgender boy after an increase in testosterone dosage. JAAD Case Rep 2022;21:32–4.
18. Dessinioti C, Katsambas A. Difficult and rare forms of acne. Clin Dermatol 2017; 35(2):138–46.
19. Hafsi W, Arnold DL, Kassardjian M. Acne conglobata. StatPearls. Treasure Island, FL: StatPearls Publishing Copyright © 2022. StatPearls Publishing LLC.; 2022.
20. Mehra T, Borelli C, Burgdorf W, et al. Treatment of severe acne with low-dose isotretinoin. Acta Derm Venereol 2012;92(3):247–8.
21. Sand FL, Thomsen SF. Adalimumab for the Treatment of Refractory Acne Conglobata. JAMA Dermatology 2013;149(11):1306–7.
22. Shirakawa M, Uramoto K, Harada FA. Treatment of acne conglobata with infliximab. J Am Acad Dermatol 2006;55(2):344–6.
23. Yiu ZZN, Madan V, Griffiths CEM. Acne conglobata and adalimumab: use of tumour necrosis factor-α antagonists in treatment-resistant acne conglobata, and review of the literature. Clin Exp Dermatol 2015;40(4):383–6.
24. Kahn MF, Khan MA. The SAPHO syndrome. Bailliere's Clin Rheumatol 1994;8(2): 333–62.

25. Rukavina I. SAPHO syndrome: A review. Journal of Children's Orthopaedics 2015;9(1):19–27.
26. Colina M, Govoni M, Orzincolo C, et al. Clinical and radiologic evolution of synovitis, acne, pustulosis, hyperostosis, and osteitis syndrome: a single center study of a cohort of 71 subjects. Arthritis Rheum 2009;61(6):813–21.
27. Hayem G, Bouchaud-Chabot A, Benali K, et al. SAPHO syndrome: a long-term follow-up study of 120 cases. Semin Arthritis Rheum 1999;29(3):159–71.
28. Hurtado-Nedelec M, Chollet-Martin S, Nicaise-Roland P, et al. Characterization of the immune response in the synovitis, acne, pustulosis, hyperostosis, osteitis (SAPHO) syndrome. Rheumatology 2008;47(8):1160–7.
29. Liu S, Tang M, Cao Y, et al. Synovitis, acne, pustulosis, hyperostosis, and osteitis syndrome: review and update. Therapeutic Advances in Musculoskeletal Disease 2020;12. 1759720X20912865.
30. Nguyen MT, Borchers A, Selmi C, et al. The SAPHO Syndrome. Semin Arthritis Rheum 2012;42(3):254–65.
31. Li C, Zuo Y, Wu N, et al. Synovitis, acne, pustulosis, hyperostosis and osteitis syndrome: a single centre study of a cohort of 164 patients. Rheumatology 2016; 55(6):1023–30.
32. Chen W, Ito T, Lin SH, et al. Does SAPHO syndrome exist in dermatology? J Eur Acad Dermatol Venereol 2022;36(9):1501–6.
33. Marzano AV, Borghi A, Meroni PL, et al. Pyoderma gangrenosum and its syndromic forms: evidence for a link with autoinflammation. Br J Dermatol 2016; 175(5):882–91.
34. Zwaenepoel T, Vlam K. SAPHO: Treatment options including bisphosphonates. Semin Arthritis Rheum 2016;46(2):168–73.
35. Akçaboy M, Bakkaloğlu-Ezgü SA, Büyükkaragöz B, et al. Successful treatment of a childhood synovitis, acne, pustulosis, hyperostosis and osteitis (SAPHO) syndrome with subcutaneous methotrexate: A case report. Turk J Pediatr 2017; 59(2):184–8.
36. Daoussis D, Konstantopoulou G, Kraniotis P, et al. Biologics in SAPHO syndrome: A systematic review. Semin Arthritis Rheum 2019;48(4):618–25.
37. Li C, Wu X, Cao Y, et al. Paradoxical skin lesions induced by anti-TNF-α agents in SAPHO syndrome. Clin Rheumatol 2019/01/01 2019;38(1):53–61.
38. Yang Q, Zhao Y, Li C, et al. Case report: successful treatment of refractory SAPHO syndrome with the JAK inhibitor tofacitinib. Medicine (Baltim) 2018;97(25): e11149.
39. Cugno M, Borghi A, Marzano AV. PAPA, PASH and PAPASH Syndromes: Pathophysiology, Presentation and Treatment. Am J Clin Dermatol 2017;18(4):555–62.
40. Maitrepierre F, Marzano AV, Lipsker D. A Unified Concept of Acne in the PAPA Spectrum Disorders. Dermatology 2021;237(5):827–34.
41. Holzinger D and Roth J. PAPA syndrome and the spectrum of PSTPIP1-associated inflammatory diseases, In: Efthimiou P., Auto-inflammatory syndromes: pathophysiology, diagnosis, and management, 2019, Springer International Publishing; Cham Switzerland, 39–59.
42. Stone DL, Ombrello A, Arostegui JI, et al. Excess Serum Interleukin-18 Distinguishes Patients With Pathogenic Mutations in PSTPIP1. Arthritis Rheumatol 2022;74(2):353–7.
43. Martinez-Rios C, Jariwala MP, Highmore K, et al. Imaging findings of sterile pyogenic arthritis, pyoderma gangrenosum and acne (PAPA) syndrome: differential diagnosis and review of the literature. Pediatr Radiol 2019;49(1):23–36.

44. George C, Deroide F, Rustin M. Pyoderma gangrenosum - a guide to diagnosis and management. Clin Med 2019;19(3):224–8.
45. Tofteland ND, Shaver TS. Clinical efficacy of etanercept for treatment of PAPA syndrome. J Clin Rheumatol 2010;16(5):244–5.
46. Sood AK, McShane DB, Googe PB, et al. Successful Treatment of PAPA Syndrome with Dual Adalimumab and Tacrolimus Therapy. J Clin Immunol 2019; 39(8):832–5.
47. Staub J, Pfannschmidt N, Strohal R, et al. Successful treatment of PASH syndrome with infliximab, cyclosporine and dapsone. J Eur Acad Dermatol Venereol 2015;29(11):2243–7.
48. Challamel C, Girard C, Misery L, et al. The efficacy of anti-IL-1 targeted therapy in PAPA and PASH syndrome. JEADV Clinical Practice 2022;1(3):275–80.
49. Braun-Falco M, Kovnerystyy O, Lohse P, et al. Pyoderma gangrenosum, acne, and suppurative hidradenitis (PASH)–a new autoinflammatory syndrome distinct from PAPA syndrome. J Am Acad Dermatol 2012;66(3):409–15.
50. Calderón-Castrat X, Bancalari-Díaz D, Román-Curto C, et al. PSTPIP1 gene mutation in a pyoderma gangrenosum, acne and suppurative hidradenitis (PASH) syndrome. Br J Dermatol 2016;175(1):194–8.
51. Faraji Zonooz M, Sabbagh-Kermani F, Fattahi Z, et al. Whole Genome Linkage Analysis Followed by Whole Exome Sequencing Identifies Nicastrin (NCSTN) as a Causative Gene in a Multiplex Family with γ-Secretase Spectrum of Autoinflammatory Skin Phenotypes. J Invest Dermatol 2016;136(6):1283–6.
52. Marzano AV, Trevisan V, Gattorno M, et al. Pyogenic arthritis, pyoderma gangrenosum, acne, and hidradenitis suppurativa (PAPASH): a new autoinflammatory syndrome associated with a novel mutation of the PSTPIP1 gene. JAMA Dermatol 2013;149(6):762–4.
53. Ghosh S, Chaudhuri S, Jain VK, et al. Profiling and hormonal therapy for acne in women. Indian J Dermatol 2014;59(2):107–15.
54. Escobar-Morreale HF. Polycystic ovary syndrome: definition, aetiology, diagnosis and treatment. Nat Rev Endocrinol 2018/05/01 2018;14(5):270–84.
55. Revised 2003 consensus on diagnostic criteria and long-term health risks related to polycystic ovary syndrome (PCOS). Hum Reprod 2004;19(1):41–7.
56. Housman E, Reynolds RV. Polycystic ovary syndrome: a review for dermatologists: Part I. Diagnosis and manifestations. J Am Acad Dermatol 2014;71(5): 847.e1-e10 [quiz: 857-8].
57. Rosenfield RL. The Diagnosis of Polycystic Ovary Syndrome in Adolescents. Pediatrics 2015;136(6):1154–65.
58. Schmidt TH, Shinkai K. Evidence-based approach to cutaneous hyperandrogenism in women. J Am Acad Dermatol 2015;73(4):672–90.
59. Toosy S, Sodi R, Pappachan JM. Lean polycystic ovary syndrome (PCOS): an evidence-based practical approach. J Diabetes Metab Disord 2018;17(2):277–85.
60. Buzney E, Sheu J, Buzney C, et al. Polycystic ovary syndrome: a review for dermatologists: Part II. Treatment. J Am Acad Dermatol 2014;71(5):859.e1-15 [quiz: 873-4].
61. Omar HA, Logsdon S, Richards J. Clinical profiles, occurrence, and management of adolescent patients with HAIR-AN syndrome. Sci World J 2004;4:507–11.
62. Barbieri RL, Ryan KJ. Hyperandrogenism, insulin resistance, and acanthosis nigricans syndrome: a common endocrinopathy with distinct pathophysiologic features. Am J Obstet Gynecol 1983;147(1):90–101.
63. Elmer KB, George RM. HAIR-AN syndrome: a multisystem challenge. Am Fam Physician 2001;63(12):2385–90.

64. O'Brien B, Dahiya R, Kimble R. Hyperandrogenism, insulin resistance and acanthosis nigricans (HAIR-AN syndrome): an extreme subphenotype of polycystic ovary syndrome. BMJ Case Rep 2020;13(4). https://doi.org/10.1136/bcr-2019-231749.

65. Orfanos CE, Adler YD, Zouboulis CC. The SAHA syndrome. Horm Res 2000; 54(5–6):251–8.

66. Dalamaga M, Papadavid E, Basios G, et al. Ovarian SAHA syndrome is associated with a more insulin-resistant profile and represents an independent risk factor for glucose abnormalities in women with polycystic ovary syndrome: a prospective controlled study. J Am Acad Dermatol 2013;69(6):922–30.

67. Carmina E, Dreno B, Lucky WA, et al. Female Adult Acne and Androgen Excess: A Report From the Multidisciplinary Androgen Excess and PCOS Committee. Journal of the Endocrine Society 2022;6(3). https://doi.org/10.1210/jendso/bvac003.

68. Chen W, Obermayer-Pietsch B, Hong JB, et al. Acne-associated syndromes: models for better understanding of acne pathogenesis. J Eur Acad Dermatol Venereol 2011;25(6):637–46.

69. Kazandjieva J, Tsankov N. Drug-induced acne. Clin Dermatol 2017;35(2):156–62.

70. Radi R, Gold S, Acosta JP, et al. Treating Acne in Transgender Persons Receiving Testosterone: A Practical Guide. Am J Clin Dermatol 2022;23(2):219–29.

71. White ND, Noeun J. Performance-Enhancing Drug Use in Adolescence. Am J Lifestyle Med 2017;11(2):122–4.

72. O'Sullivan AJ, Kennedy MC, Casey JH, et al. Anabolic-androgenic steroids: medical assessment of present, past and potential users. Med J Aust 2000;173(6): 323–7.

73. Melnik B, Jansen T, Grabbe S. Abuse of anabolic-androgenic steroids and bodybuilding acne: an underestimated health problem. J Dtsch Dermatol Ges 2007; 5(2):110–7.

74. Lacouture ME. Mechanisms of cutaneous toxicities to EGFR inhibitors. Nat Rev Cancer 2006;6(10):803–12.

75. Melosky B, Burkes R, Rayson D, et al. Management of skin rash during EGFR-targeted monoclonal antibody treatment for gastrointestinal malignancies: Canadian recommendations. Curr Oncol 2009;16(1):16–26.

76. Anforth R, Liu M, Nguyen B, et al. Acneiform eruptions: a common cutaneous toxicity of the MEK inhibitor trametinib. Australas J Dermatol 2014;55(4):250–4.

77. Anforth RM, Blumetti TC, Kefford RF, et al. Cutaneous manifestations of dabrafenib (GSK2118436): a selective inhibitor of mutant BRAF in patients with metastatic melanoma. Br J Dermatol 2012;167(5):1153–60.

78. Hudson BN, Jacobs HR, Philbrick A, et al. Drug-induced acne with elexacaftor/tezacaftor/ivacaftor in people with cystic fibrosis. J Cyst Fibros 2022;21(6): 1066–9.

79. Okroglic L, Sohier P, Martin C, et al. Acneiform Eruption Following Elexacaftor-Tezacaftor-Ivacaftor Treatment in Patients With Cystic Fibrosis. JAMA Dermatol 2023;159(1):68–72.

# Unusual Presentations of Systemic Lupus Erythematosus

Kaitlin V. Kirkpatrick, MD, James J. Nocton, MD*

## KEYWORDS

- Systemic lupus erythematosus • Adolescence • Lupus • Pediatrics

## KEY POINTS

- Adolescents with systemic lupus erythematosus (SLE) may present with unusual signs and symptoms.
- Understanding and recognition of uncommon SLE presentations allow prompt diagnosis and management.
- Specific histologic, laboratory, and imaging findings in the appropriate clinical context will lead to a diagnosis of SLE.
- SLE during adolescence may mimic other diseases, leading to delays in diagnosis and treatment.
- SLE should be considered in the differential diagnosis of a wide variety of signs and symptoms.

Systemic lupus erythematosus (SLE) is a chronic multisystem autoimmune disease that most commonly begins in adolescence and early adulthood and can involve nearly any organ system in the body.[1] The diagnosis is clinical, primarily based on signs and symptoms and supported by characteristic laboratory test results. Several classification criteria for SLE have been developed,[2–4] and the European League Against Rheumatism/American College of Rheumatology 2019 criteria[4] is the most recent (**Box 1**). Although SLE will often present with the characteristic clinical and laboratory abnormalities emphasized in these criteria, unusual manifestations may sometimes be the first to appear. This review discusses several of the less common presenting manifestations of SLE, focusing on clinical, laboratory, and imaging features. This discussion of the treatment of SLE is limited to specific therapies targeting unusual manifestations. Further information regarding the overall management of SLE can be found in several references,[1,5] and a comprehensive list of unusual

Pediatric Rheumatology, Medical College of Wisconsin, Children's Corporate Center, 999 North 92nd Street Suite C465, Milwaukee, WI 53226, USA
* Corresponding author.
*E-mail address:* jnocton@mcw.edu

Med Clin N Am 108 (2024) 43–57
https://doi.org/10.1016/j.mcna.2023.05.015
0025-7125/24/© 2023 Elsevier Inc. All rights reserved.

---

**Box 1**
**EULAR/ACR criteria for classification of systemic lupus erythematosus**

| Entry Criterion | ANA titer >/ = 1:80 | |
|---|---|---|
| Clinical Domains | | Points |
| Constitutional | Fever | 2 |
| Hematological | Leukopenia | 3 |
| | Thrombocytopenia | 4 |
| | Coombs + Autoimmune hemolytic anemia | 4 |
| Neuropsychiatric | Delirium | 2 |
| | Psychosis | 3 |
| | Seizure | 5 |
| Mucocutaneous | Nonscarring alopecia | 2 |
| | Oral ulcers | 2 |
| | Subacute cutaneous or discoid lupus | 4 |
| | Acute cutaneous lupus | 6 |
| Serosal | Pleural or pericardial effusion | 5 |
| | Acute pericarditis | 6 |
| Musculoskeletal | Joint involvement | 6 |
| Renal | Proteinuria > 0.5 g/24 h | 4 |
| | Renal biopsy class II or V nephritis | 8 |
| | Renal biopsy class III or IV nephritis | 10 |
| Immunologic Domains | | |
| Antiphospholipid antibodies | Anticardiolipin | 2 |
| | Anti-β2-glycoprotein 1 lupus anticoagulant | |
| Complement | Low C3 or C4 | |
| | Low C3 AND C4 | |
| SLE-specific antibodies | Anti-dsDNA | |
| | Anti-Smith | |

Requires presence of entry criterion, ≥1 clinical criterion, and ≥10 points. Within each domain only the highest weighted criterion is counted toward the total score. Occurrence of criterion on at least one occasion is sufficient; criteria need not occur simultaneously.

*Adapted from* Petty RE et al, editors: *Textbook of Pediatric Rheumatology*, ed 8, Philadelphia, 2021, Elsevier (Table 23.2, p 296), with permission.

---

presentations of SLE is listed in **Box 2**, including additional manifestations not specifically discussed here.

## HEMATOLOGIC MANIFESTATIONS
### Lupus Anticoagulant Hypoprothrombinemia Syndrome

Lupus anticoagulant hypoprothrombinemia syndrome (LAHS) is caused by an acquired factor II (prothrombin) inhibitor in combination with a lupus anticoagulant. Despite the presence of the prothrombotic lupus anticoagulant, nonneutralizing antiprothrombin antibodies result in the rapid clearance of prothrombin-antibody complexes from the serum, leading to hypoprothrombinemia and subsequent bleeding.[6,7] LAHS occurs in all ages with SLE and seems to be more frequent in children and adolescents.[7] Symptoms may range from mild mucocutaneous bleeding including epistaxis, gum bleeding, menorrhagia, ecchymoses (**Fig. 1**), and hematochezia to severe life-threatening bleeding.[8] Additional signs and symptoms of SLE are not always present, and the evidence of associated SLE may be restricted to laboratory test findings. Laboratory testing will reveal a prolonged prothrombin time and activated partial thromboplastin time, an elevated lupus anticoagulant, and factor II

| **Box 2** | |
|---|---|
| **Uncommon systemic lupus erythematosus manifestations in adolescence** | |
| Musculoskeletal | Myositis |
| | Tenosynovitis |
| Vascular | Leukocytoclastic vasculitis |
| | Cryoglobulinemia |
| | Livedo reticularis |
| Hematologic | Hypoprothrombinemia |
| | Catastrophic antiphospholipid syndrome |
| | Thrombotic microangiopathy |
| Neuropsychiatric | Aseptic meningitis |
| | Cognitive dysfunction |
| | Mood disorders/psychiatric disease |
| | Pseudotumor cerebri |
| | Acute inflammatory demyelinating polyradiculoneuropathy |
| | Cranial neuropathy |
| | Neuromyelitis optica |
| | Mononeuropathy multiplex |
| | Myasthenia gravis |
| | Chorea |
| | Transverse myelitis |
| Cardiovascular | Coronary artery disease/myocardial infarction |
| | Libman-Sacks endocarditis |
| Pulmonary | Pneumonitis |
| | Pulmonary hypertension |
| | Diffuse alveolar hemorrhage |
| | Shrinking lung syndrome |
| Gastrointestinal | Enteritis |
| | Pancreatitis |
| | Protein-losing enteropathy |
| Ocular | Keratoconjunctivitis sicca |
| | Orbital pseudotumor |
| | Ulcerative keratitis |
| | Uveitis |
| | Episcleritis scleritis |
| | Optic nerve disease |
| | Ocular motor abnormalities |
| | Retinopathy |
| Dermatologic | Panniculitis |
| | Bullous lupus |

*Modified from* Petty RE et al, editors: *Textbook of Pediatric Rheumatology*, ed 8, Philadelphia, 2021, Elsevier (Table 23.4, p 301), with permission.

deficiency.[7,8] Hypocomplementemia, elevated anticardiolipin antibodies, and additional autoantibodies characteristic of SLE may also be present. Treatment includes controlling bleeding, when necessary, with fresh frozen plasma, red blood cell transfusions, and factor concentrate as well as immunomodulators to decrease antibody and inhibitor formation.[6,8] Rituximab may be particularly effective, and plasmapheresis has been used in severe cases.[7]

### Catastrophic Antiphospholipid Syndrome

Catastrophic antiphospholipid syndrome (CAPS) is a rare life-threatening variant of antiphospholipid syndrome (APS) (<1% of all patients with APS), characterized by multiple small vessel occlusions resulting in multiorgan failure associated with elevated

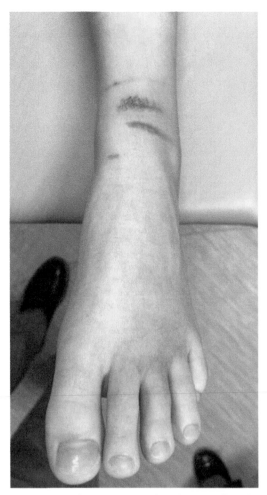

**Fig. 1.** Soft tissue hemorrhage in lupus anticoagulant hypoprothrombinemia syndrome.

serum antiphospholipid antibodies.[9] Although it can occur in isolation, up to 30% of pediatric patients with CAPS are also diagnosed with SLE.[9,10] Diagnostic criteria for CAPS are listed in **Box 3**. In children and adolescents, the most commonly affected organs include the kidneys and lungs, with many additional organ systems potentially affected by both APS and CAPS (**Box 4**).[11] Other associated signs and symptoms may include livedo reticularis, arthritis, leukopenia, and thrombocytopenia.[9,11] The mortality rate is high (24%–50%), and therefore, prompt recognition and treatment of CAPS is critical.[9,11] Therapy targets the elimination of precipitating factors, treatment of ongoing thrombotic processes with anticoagulation, and suppression of commonly associated cytokine storm.[9] Immunomodulators such as cyclophosphamide or rituximab have been demonstrated to be effective in improving survival.[9,11,12]

### Thrombotic Microangiopathy

Thrombotic microangiopathy (TMA) has been reported in 2% to 3% of those with SLE, with 15% to 60% of childhood and adolescent SLE–associated TMA occurring at the

---

**Box 3**
**Criteria for the classification of catastrophic antiphospholipid syndrome**

1. Evidence of involvement of 3 or more organs, systems, and/or tissues

2. Development of manifestations simultaneously or in less than 1 week

3. Confirmation by histopathology of small vessel occlusion in 1 or more organs/tissues

4. Laboratory confirmation of the presence of antiphospholipid antibodies (APLA)

Definite CAPS
  All 4 criteria present

Probable CAPS
- All 4 criteria except only 2 organs, systems, and/or tissue involvement
- All 4 criteria except for absence of laboratory confirmation more than or equal to 6 weeks apart because of early death of patient or never tested for APLA before CAPS
- 1, 2, and 4 criteria present
- 1, 3, and 4 criteria present + development of third event in more than 1 week but less than 1 month despite anticoagulation.

*Adapted from* Petty RE et al, editors: *Textbook of Pediatric Rheumatology*, ed 8, Philadelphia, 2021, Elsevier (Table 24.1, p 331), with permission.

---

**Box 4**
**Venous and arterial thrombosis manifestations of antiphospholipid syndrome in children and adolescents**

| Site of Vessel Involvement | Clinical Manifestations |
| --- | --- |
| Limbs | Deep vein thrombosis |
| | Ischemia/gangrene |
| Skin | Livedo reticularis, chronic leg ulcers, superficial thrombophlebitis |
| Large veins | SVC or IVC thrombosis |
| Lungs | Pulmonary embolus, pulmonary hypertension |
| Brain | Cerebral venous sinus thrombosis |
| | Cerebral infarction, transient ischemic attack, acute ischemic encephalopathy |
| Eyes | Retinal vein thrombosis |
| | Retinal artery thrombosis |
| Liver | Budd-Chiari syndrome, portal vein thrombosis |
| | Hepatic infarction |
| Kidney | Renal vein thrombosis |
| | Renal artery thrombosis, renal thrombotic microangiopathy |
| Adrenal glands | Hypoadrenalism, Addison disease |
| Heart | Myocardial infarction |
| Spleen | Splenic infarction |
| Gut | Mesenteric artery thrombosis |
| Bones | Bone infarction |

*Abbreviations:* IVC, inferior vena cava; SVC, superior vena cava.

*Adapted from* Petty RE et al, editors: *Textbook of Pediatric Rheumatology*, ed 8, Philadelphia, 2021, Elsevier (Table 24.2, p 336), with permission.

onset of SLE.[13] TMA can occur as the result of an inhibitor of a disintegrin and metalloprotease with thrombospondin-type motif (ADAMTS13), equivalent to thrombotic thrombocytopenic purpura[14]; however, some instances of TMA are hypothesized to be complement mediated with a normal or only minimally reduced ADAMTS13.[15] The diagnosis should be suspected in patients with SLE with the combination of acute thrombocytopenia and hemolytic anemia, fevers, rapidly worsening renal insufficiency, and/or neurologic involvement.[16] A peripheral smear will reveal abundant schistocytes characteristic of a microangiopathy. Plasmapheresis is an effective treatment of TMA in addition to glucocorticoids and immunomodulation, and prognosis is favorable when recognized and treated early.[14] Eculizumab, a terminal complement inhibitor, has also demonstrated efficacy when ADAMTS13 levels are not severely reduced.[15,17,18]

## DERMATOLOGIC MANIFESTATIONS
### Lupus Panniculitis

In 2% to 5% of patients with SLE, the first skin finding may be panniculitis.[19,20] Lesions appear as recurrent tender erythematous indurated nodules and plaques in the deep dermis and subcutaneous tissues with initial local swelling followed by subsequent scarring and lipoatrophy[20] (**Fig. 2**). In children and adolescents, the face is the most common affected location, with areas of higher fat composition such as the breasts, upper thighs, and buttocks also frequently affected.[21] Histopathology reveals lobular

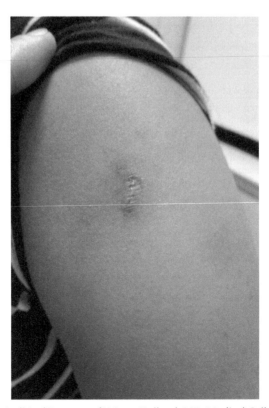

**Fig. 2.** Lupus panniculitis. (*Courtesy of* Kristen Holland, MD, Medical College of Wisconsin.)

dense lymphoplasmacytic and histiocytic patchy infiltrates, hyaline fat necrosis, mucin deposition, and lymphocytic vasculitis in fat lobules.[20] Specific findings that are suggestive of SLE-associated panniculitis include vacuolar changes at the dermal-epidermal interface, periadnexal lymphocytic infiltrates, interstitial deposition of mucin in the reticular dermis, and lymphoid follicles with reactive germinal centers in the subcutis.[19] Direct immunofluorescence may reveal immunoglobulin (Ig) G, IgM, and complement 3 (C3) deposition in the basal membrane of overlying skin.[22] Lupus panniculitis may occur in isolation or in association with SLE, and when associated with SLE, treatment with hydroxychloroquine and glucocorticoids is often effective.[21] For refractory cases, additional immunomodulators are used. If left untreated, profound lipoatrophy can lead to severe disfigurement.[23,24]

### Bullous Lupus

Vesiculobullous lesions are exceedingly rare manifestations of SLE, occurring in less than 5% of patients.[25] Bullous lupus (BSLE) represents only 2% to 3% of all subepidermal autoimmune bullous skin diseases.[25] Antibodies targeting type VII collagen result in weakened basement membrane-dermal adhesion with subsequent subepidermal blistering.[25] Widespread blistering lesions appear that can resemble large burns (**Fig. 3**). These are most commonly present on the upper trunk, neck, and other sun-exposed areas.[22] Mucosal surfaces can be affected, particularly the oropharynx, and can potentially compromise the airway. Biopsy reveals a neutrophil predominant infiltrate and multiple immunoglobulins and immune complexes along the basement membrane zone.[22] Direct immunofluorescence characteristically reveals IgG, IgM, IgA, and C3 at the dermal-epidermal junction and the absence of eosinophils, differentiating BSLE from other bullous diseases.[22] Treatment with dapsone is effective, with a dramatic response in the first 24 to 48 hours of use.[25] In contrast to other cutaneous manifestations of SLE, glucocorticoids and hydroxychloroquine have limited efficacy for BSLE, and methotrexate, cyclophosphamide, and mycophenolate mofetil all have modest efficacy.[25] In refractory cases, rituximab has had promising results.[22] Lesions typically heal with residual hyperpigmentation, scarring, or milia, and recurrences are common.[22]

## CENTRAL NERVOUS SYSTEM MANIFESTATIONS
### Chorea

Chorea as an initial manifestation of SLE is unusual (incidence 0.6%–2.3%).[26,27] It is defined as involuntary purposeless rapid, jerky, forceful movements. Patients may

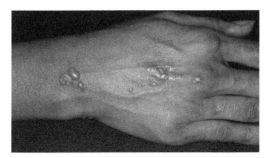

**Fig. 3.** Bullous lupus. (*From* Lee, Lela A.; Werth, Victoria P. Lupus Erythematosus. In: Bolognia JL, Schaffer JV, Cerroni L, eds. *Dermatology*. 4th ed. Elsevier; 2018: Fig 41.16 p 671. with permission.)

have difficulty walking or remaining upright. Loss of coordination of tongue or hand muscles may result in dysarthria and difficulties grasping objects or writing.[26] Movements are typically discrete but can sometimes seem to flow more consistently and resemble athetosis and often worsen with stress and excitement.[28,29] The exact pathogenesis in those with SLE remains unclear, but possible explanations include direct antineural antibody–mediated damage to phospholipid-containing structures in the basal ganglia and reversible ischemia.[26,28] MRI may demonstrate focal findings such as vasculopathy or demyelination, particularly hyperintensities in the basal ganglia on T1-weighted images.[26,28] PET may reveal hypermetabolism in the contralateral striatum.[29] However, in most of the cases neuroimaging studies are typically normal or nonspecific.[28] Cerebrospinal fluid (CSF) analysis is nonspecific, typically disclosing findings characteristic of inflammation within the CNS, including pleocytosis, elevated protein, elevated IgG and IgG index, and oligoclonal bands.[26,29] SLE-associated chorea usually responds very well to treatment with glucocorticoids and hydroxychloroquine, and when refractory, immunomodulators such as azathioprine, cyclophosphamide, and intravenous immunoglobulin have been effective.[29–31] Prognosis is favorable with rapid resolution of symptoms often within days of starting therapy.[30]

### Acute Transverse Myelitis

Acute transverse myelitis (ATM) occurs in approximately 1% to 2% of those with SLE and can be an initial manifestation (39% of all SLE-associated ATM).[32–34] The peak incidence among pediatric patients occurs in adolescence, and the severity of symptoms varies depending on the number of spinal cord segments involved.[35] Weakness, sensory changes, and bowel and bladder dysfunction are common.[32,35] Symptoms may progress within a few hours or may gradually develop over a few weeks. The specific pathologic mechanism of transverse myelitis in SLE remains unknown. An increased incidence of antiphospholipid antibodies (APLAs) has been reported, suggesting thrombosis as a possible explanation.[36] The small longitudinal arterial blood vessels in the thoracic spine may be more vulnerable to thrombosis and ischemia, a possible explanation for the predominance of involvement of this area in patients with SLE.[32] Demyelinating lesions visualized on MRI and high IgG levels in the CSF may be present.[35] Treatment is predominantly anticoagulation if APLAs are present in addition to immunomodulators such as cyclophosphamide and glucocorticoids.[33] Recurrences within the first several months are common, with 21% to 55% of patients reporting at least one recurrence.[35]

### Systemic Lupus Erythematosus–Associated Psychosis

Acute psychosis is present in 2% to 24% of patients with SLE with neuropsychiatric disease and typically occurs within a year after the onset of SLE.[37,38] The pathogenesis is unclear and postulated to be secondary to autoantibody-mediated cerebral vasculopathy and/or direct neuronal damage.[37–39] Symptoms of SLE-associated psychosis are not unique to SLE and include auditory and visual hallucinations, delusions, and acute confusional states.[38,40] The presence of visual distortions, such as objects moving or changing shape and color, and retained insight earlier on in disease course have been reported to be more suggestive of SLE-associated psychosis than other causes.[40] Psychosis is also more likely to occur in the setting of other systemic manifestations of SLE. CSF analysis may reveal pleocytosis, elevated protein, and oligoclonal bands.[39,41] MRI may demonstrate hyperintensities in the white matter, particularly the frontal cortex, and/or diffuse cortical atrophy.[39,41] The diagnosis may be challenging because these findings are nonspecific, and patients with SLE may have coincidental psychiatric illnesses that are not directly secondary to SLE. The exclusion of infectious, metabolic, and thrombotic causes and the presence of additional clinical and laboratory features of active SLE will be most suggestive of SLE-associated psychosis. Treatment includes antipsychotics, glucocorticoids, and cyclophosphamide acutely followed by maintenance treatment, most often with mycophenolate mofetil or azathioprine.[37] Intravenous Ig, plasmapheresis, and rituximab have been reported to be effective in refractory cases.[37,38] Prognosis is typically good with recurrences uncommon.[39]

## GASTROINTESTINAL MANIFESTATIONS
### Lupus Enteritis

Although relatively unusual, acute abdominal pain in children and adolescents as a manifestation of SLE is most commonly caused by lupus enteritis.[42–45] It is thought to occur secondary to immune complex deposition and inflammation and/or thrombosis of intestinal blood vessels. The clinical manifestations vary widely from mild nonspecific abdominal pain, nausea, vomiting, and diarrhea to severe gastrointestinal (GI) bleeding, peritonitis, and ascites.[44] Laboratory test results and radiographs are often nonspecific. Computed tomography (CT) may be useful diagnostically with the identification of (1) engorgement of mesenteric vessels (comb sign), (2) diffuse thickened bowel wall with peripheral rim enhancement (target sign), and/or (3) increased attenuation of mesenteric fat[44] (**Fig. 4**). The jejunum is most frequently involved followed by the ileum.[45] Glucocorticoids, bowel rest, and hydration are often effective with immunomodulators used for refractory disease.[44,45] Surgical interventions are necessary for those with the rare complications of intestinal necrosis or perforation. Overall prognosis is good; however, mortality rates increase when recognition is delayed.[44,45]

### Pancreatitis

Pancreatitis occurs in approximately 5% to 6% of children and adolescents with SLE, often early in the course of disease.[46–48] Possible pathologic mechanisms of

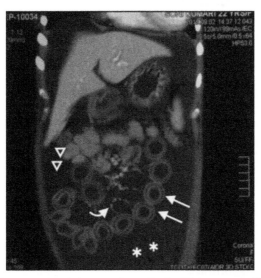

**Fig. 4.** Computed tomography abdomen of a patient with lupus enteritis showing "target sign" of small intestinal loops with circumferential wall thickening (*straight arrows*) compared with normal bowel loops (*open arrowheads*). Also noted are mesenteric vasculature leading to loops (*curved arrows*) and massive ascites (*asterisks*). (*From* Patro PS et al. "Presumptive Lupus Enteritis." The American Journal of Medicine 2016; 129(11):278; with permission.)

SLE-related pancreatitis include vascular ischemia and damage secondary to vasculitis, immune complex deposition, and microthrombi secondary to APLAs and antipancreas autoantibodies.[49–51] Children with pancreatitis present with generalized abdominal pain, fevers, and nausea or vomiting. CT or MRI may reveal pancreatic edema, necrosis, or peripancreatic fluid collections.[48] Acute pancreatitis typically occurs in patients with increased overall lupus activity; therefore, additional clinical findings and abnormal laboratory test results such as low complements and cytopenias are often present.[48] The mortality rate of pancreatitis in children has been reported to be 2% to 21%,[46,50] and early treatment with glucocorticoids, immunomodulators for severe or refractory disease, nutritional support, and pain management are essential.[48]

### Systemic Lupus Erythematosus–Related Protein-Losing Enteropathy

Protein-losing enteropathy (PLE) presents with peripheral edema, ascites, diarrhea, and hypoalbuminemia.[52] Differentiation from other more common causes of protein loss in SLE such as nephrotic syndrome may be challenging. Laboratory test results such as hypocomplementemia, elevated stool alpha-1-antitrypsin, and the absence of proteinuria may be most helpful in confirming the presence of PLE associated with SLE.[43,53] CT of the abdomen often reveals prominent mucosal patterns due to edema, spiculation, or thickened folds/nodules indicative of lymphangiectasia.[53] Technetium-labeled serum albumin scintigraphy may also reveal leakage of albumin into the intestine.[53] Small bowel biopsies are typically normal. The pathogenesis is unclear and possibly due to increased vascular permeability due to complement-/cytokine-mediated damage and intestinal vessel vasculitis or intestinal lymphangiectasia.[53] Relapse is common when treated with glucocorticoids alone; therefore, additional immunomodulators are often necessary.[43,53]

## OPHTHALMOLOGIC MANIFESTATIONS
### Systemic Lupus Erythematosus Retinopathy

Nearly one-third of the patients with SLE develop ophthalmic symptoms, and retinal involvement is the second most common ophthalmologic manifestation (incidence 3%–29% of adult lupus patients).[54,55] Retinopathy may present with acute painless vision loss or visual field defects as an initial manifestation of SLE; however, it may also occur silently; therefore, routine funduscopic examination is prudent for all patients with SLE.[54,56] Pathogenesis is theorized to be the result of immune complex deposition, leading to occlusion of the retinal vessels and localized inflammatory vasculitis.[56] Cotton wool spots, macular edema, perivascular exudates, retinal hemorrhages, or microaneurysms may be seen on funduscopic examination (**Fig. 5**).[55] As with other SLE manifestations, management of retinopathy includes glucocorticoids and immunosuppression.[54] Rituximab has resulted in rapid improvement in several patients.[54,57,58] Adjunctive periocular and intraocular glucocorticoids, panretinal photocoagulation, intravitreal antivascular endothelial growth factor injections, and vitrectomy have also been used to halt neovascularization.[54,57,58] Although retinal involvement is uncommon in children and adolescents with lupus, it poses a severe threat to vision and thus prompt recognition and treatment is critical.

## PULMONARY MANIFESTATIONS
### Shrinking Lung Syndrome

Shrinking lung syndrome (SLS) has a prevalence in SLE of 0.5% to 1.1%.[59–61] Despite typically occurring as a later complication, it has been documented at initial diagnosis in 9% of children and adolescents with SLE.[61] The pathogenesis remains unknown,

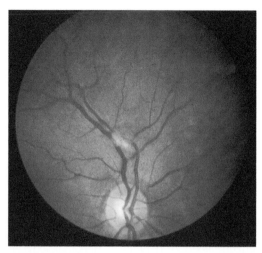

**Fig. 5.** Lupus retinitis cotton wool spot in the posterior retinal pole. (*Adapted from* Petty RE et al, editors: *Textbook of Pediatric Rheumatology*, ed 8, Philadelphia, 2021, Elsevier (Fig 23.20, p 320), with permission.)

and it is hypothesized that chronic pleural inflammation results in pain, with deep breathing leading to inhibition of diaphragmatic activation and ultimately chronic lung hypoinflation and decreased lung compliance.[61] Patients will develop progressive exertional dyspnea of variable severity and/or pleuritic chest pain. Because of the nonspecific nature of these symptoms, diagnosis of SLS is often delayed.[59,61,62] Hypoinflation may be evident on chest radiograph, and high-resolution CT may reveal elevated hemidiaphragms and reduced lung volumes in the absence of parenchymal lung disease or vascular pathology.[59,61] Pulmonary function tests (PFTs) reveal a restrictive ventilatory defect with reduced total lung capacity and diffusion capacity of the lungs for carbon monoxide.[60] Glucocorticoids and immunomodulators such as cyclophosphamide, rituximab, or belimumab have been effective.[61,63] Prognosis is favorable, with patients showing significant clinical improvement and stabilization or improvement in PFTs, although a persistent chronic restrictive defect is common.[62] Progression to respiratory failure or death is very uncommon.[59]

## SUMMARY

SLE commonly presents during adolescence and may present with unusual clinical features in potentially any organ system. SLE should therefore be considered as part of the differential diagnosis for a wide variety of signs and symptoms. Early recognition allows appropriate treatment and ultimately decreased morbidity and mortality.

## CLINICS CARE POINTS

- Children and adolescents with SLE may not present with characteristic signs and symptoms.
- Unusual SLE manifestations may mimic many other diseases, leading to delays in diagnosis and treatment.
- Specific laboratory, histologic, and imaging findings can help to diagnose SLE.

- Recognition of unusual SLE presentations allows for prompt diagnosis and better long-term outcomes.
- SLE should be considered in the differential diagnosis of a wide variety of signs and symptoms.

## DISCLOSURE

The authors have nothing to disclose.

## REFERENCES

1. Klein-Gitelman MS, Beresford MW. Systemic Lupus Erythematosus, Mixed Connective Tissue Disease, and Undifferentiated Connective Tissue Disease. In: Petty RE, et al, editors. Textbook of pediatric Rheumatology. 8th edition. Philadelphia: Elsevier; 2021. p. 295–329.
2. Hochberg MC. Updating the American College of Rheumatology revised criteria for the classification of systemic lupus erythematosus. Arthritis Rheum 1997; 40(9):1725.
3. Petri M, Orbai AM, Alarcon GS, et al. Derivation and validation of the Systemic Lupus International Collaborating Clinics classification criteria for systemic lupus erythematosus. Arthritis Rheum 2012;64(8):2677–86.
4. Aringer M., Costenbader K., Daikh D., et al., 2019 European League against Rheumatism/American College of Rheumatology classification criteria for systemic lupus erythematosus. Arthritis Rheum, 2019, 1, 1400-1412.
5. Sadun RE, Ardoin SP, Schanberg LE. Systemic Lupus Erythematosus. In: Kliegman RM, et al, editors. Textbook of pediatrics. 21st edition. Philadelphia: Elsevier; 2020. p. 1274–9.
6. Galland J, Mohamed S, Revuz S, et al. Lupus anticoagulant-hypoprothrombinemia syndrome and catastrophic antiphospholipid syndrome in a patient with anti-domain I antibodies. Blood Coagul Fibrinolysis 2016;27(5):580–2.
7. Kocheril AP, Vettiyil GI, George AS, et al. Pediatric systemic lupus erythematosus with lupus anticoagulant hypoprothrombinemia syndrome—A case series with review of literature. Lupus 2021;30(4):641–8.
8. Pilania RK, Suri D, Jindal AK, et al. Lupus anticoagulant hypoprothrombinemia syndrome associated with systemic lupus erythematosus in children: report of two cases and systematic review of the literature. Rheumatol Int 2018;38(10): 1933–40.
9. Bayraktar UD, Erkan D, Bucciarelli S, et al. The clinical spectrum of catastrophic antiphospholipid syndrome in the absence and presence of lupus. J Rheumatol 2007;34(2):346–52.
10. Senken B, Whitehead A. Catastrophic Antiphospholipid Syndrome Presenting as a Stroke in an 11-Year-Old with Lupus. Case Reports in Pediatrics 2022;2022:1–4.
11. Cervera R, Rodríguez-Pintó I, Espinosa G. The diagnosis and clinical management of the catastrophic antiphospholipid syndrome: a comprehensive review. J Autoimmun 2018;92:1–11.
12. Elagib E.M., Ibrahim N., Essa M.E., et al., Catastrophic antiphospholipid syndrome in combination with SLE treated by Rituximab: a case report and literature review, *Lupus: Open Access*, 4 (1), 2019, 1–6.

13. Orbe Jaramillo IA, De Lucas Collantes C, Martínez de Azagra A, et al. Systemic lupus erythematosus presenting as thrombotic thrombocytopaenic purpura in a child: a diagnostic challenge. BMJ Case Rep 2020;13(9):1–4.

14. Yue C., Su J., Gao R., et al., Characteristics and outcomes of patients with systemic lupus erythematosus–associated thrombotic microangiopathy, and their acquired ADAMTS13 inhibitor profiles, *J Rheumatol*, 45 (11), 2018, 1549–1556.

15. Wright R.D., Bannerman F., Beresford M., et al., A systematic review of the role of eculizumab in systemic lupus erythematosus-associated thrombotic microangiopathy, *BMC Nephrol*, 21 (1), 2020, 1–8.

16. Li J, Jiang JJ, Wang CY, et al. Clinical features and prognosis of patients with thrombotic thrombocytopenic purpura associated with systemic lupus erythematosus: a review of 25 cases. Ital J Pediatr 2019;45(1):1–6.

17. El-Husseini A., Hannan S., Awad A., et al., Thrombotic microangiopathy in systemic lupus erythematosus: efficacy of eculizumab, *Am J Kidney Dis*, 65 (1), 2015, 127–130.

18. Kello N., El Khoury L., Marder G., et al., Secondary thrombotic microangiopathy in systemic lupus erythematosus and antiphospholipid syndrome, the role of complement and use of eculizumab: case series and review of literature, Semin Arthritis Rheum, 49 (1), 2019, 74–83.

19. Weingartner JS, Zedek DC, Burkhart CN, et al. Lupus erythematosus panniculitis in children: report of three cases and review of previously reported cases. Pediatr Dermatol 2012;29(2):169–76.

20. Zhang R., Dang X., Shuai L., et al., Lupus erythematosus panniculitis in a 10-year-old female child with severe systemic lupus erythematosus: A case report, *Medicine*, 97 (3), 2018, 1–4.

21. Guissa V.R., Trudes G., Jesus A.A., et al., Lupus erythematosus panniculitis in children and adolescents, *Acta Reumatol Port*, 37 (1), 2012, 82–85.

22. Herzum A., Gasparini G., Cozzani E., et al., Atypical and rare forms of cutaneous lupus erythematosus: the importance of the diagnosis for the best management of patients, *Dermatology*, 238 (2), 2022, 195–204.

23. Zhao Y.K., Wang F., Chen W.N., et al., Lupus panniculitis as an initial manifestation of systemic lupus erythematosus: A case report, *Medicine*, 95 (16), 2016, 1–5.

24. Rangel L.K., Villa-Ruiz C., Lo K., et al., Clinical characteristics of lupus erythematosus panniculitis/profundus: a retrospective review of 61 patients, *JAMA dermatology*, 156 (11), 2020, 1264–1266.

25. Chanprapaph K, Sawatwarakul S, Vachiramon V. A 12-year retrospective review of bullous systemic lupus erythematosus in cutaneous and systemic lupus erythematosus patients. Lupus 2017;26(12):1278–84.

26. Athanasopoulos E, Kalaitzidou I, Vlachaki G, et al. Chorea revealing systemic lupus erythematosus in a 13-year old boy: A case report and short review of the literature. Int Rev Immunol 2018;37(4):177–82.

27. Mrabet S, Benrhouma H, Kraoua I, et al. Mixed movements disorders as an initial feature of pediatric lupus. Brain and Development 2015;37(9):904–6.

28. Baizabal-Carvallo JF, Bonnet C, Jankovic J. Movement disorders in systemic lupus erythematosus and the antiphospholipid syndrome. J Neural Transm 2013;120(11):1579–89.

29. Torreggiani S, Torcoletti M, Cuoco F, et al. Chorea, a little-known manifestation in systemic lupus erythematosus: short literature review and four case reports. Pediatr Rheumatol Online J 2013;11(36):1–7.

30. Herd J.K., Medhi M., Uzendoski D., et al., Chorea associated with systemic lupus erythematosus: report of two cases and review of the literature, *Pediatrics*, 61 (2), 1978, 308–315.

31. Lazurova I, Macejova Z, Benhatchi K, et al. Efficacy of Intravenous Immunoglobulin treatment in lupus erythematosus chorea. Clin Rheumatol 2007;26:2145–7.

32. Katsiari CG, Giavri I, Mitsikostas DD, et al. Acute transverse myelitis and antiphospholipid antibodies in lupus. No evidence for anticoagulation. Eur J Neurol 2011;18(4):556–63.

33. Kovacs B, Lafferty TL, Brent LH, et al. Transverse myelopathy in systemic lupus erythematosus: an analysis of 14 cases and review of the literature. Ann Rheum Dis 2000;59(2):120–4.

34. Shivamurthy VM, Ganesan S, Khan A, et al. Acute longitudinal myelitis as the first presentation in child with systemic lupus erythematosus. J Pediatr Neurosci 2013; 8(2):150–3.

35. Schulz SW, Shenin M, Mehta A, et al. Initial presentation of acute transverse myelitis in systemic lupus erythematosus: demographics, diagnosis, management and comparison to idiopathic cases. Rheumatol Int 2012;32(9):2623–7.

36. Zhang S., Wang Z., Zhao J., et al., Clinical features of transverse myelitis associated with systemic lupus erythematosus, *Lupus*, 29 (4), 2020, 389–397.

37. Kumar P., Kumar A., Thakur V., et al., Acute psychosis as the presenting manifestation of lupus, *J Fam Med Prim Care*, 10 (2), 2021, 1050–1053.

38. Johnson M.C., Sathappan A., Hanly J.G., et al., From the blood-brain barrier to childhood development: a case of acute-onset psychosis and cognitive impairment attributed to systemic lupus erythematosus in an adolescent female, *Harv Rev Psychiatr*, 30 (1), 2022, 71–82.

39. Muscal E, Nadeem T, Li X, et al. Evaluation and treatment of acute psychosis in children with systemic lupus erythematosus (SLE): consultation–liaison service experiences at a tertiary-care pediatric institution. Psychosomatics 2010;51(6): 508–14.

40. Lim L, Lefebvre A, Benseler S, et al. Psychiatric illness of systemic lupus erythematosus in childhood: spectrum of clinically important manifestations. J Rheumatol 2013;40(4):506–12.

41. Sharma S, Lerman MA, Fitzgerald MP, et al. Acute psychosis presenting in a patient with systemic lupus erythematosus: Answers. Pediatr Nephrol 2016;31: 229–31.

42. Chowichian M., Aanpreung P., Pongpaibul A., et al., Lupus enteritis as the sole presenting feature of systemic lupus erythematosus: case report and review of the literature, *Paediatr Int Child Health*, 39 (4), 2019, 294–298.

43. Sönmez HE, Karhan AN, Batu ED, et al. Gastrointestinal system manifestations in juvenile systemic lupus erythematosus. Clin Rheumatol 2017;36(7):1521–6.

44. Bodh V, Kalwar R, Sharma R, et al. Lupus enteritis: An uncommon manifestation of systemic lupus erythematosus as an initial presentation. J Dig Endosc 2017; 8(3):134–6.

45. Smith LW, Petri M. Lupus enteritis: an uncommon manifestation of systemic lupus erythematosus. J Clin Rheumatol 2013;19(2):84–6.

46. Wang CH, Yao TC, Huang YL, et al. Acute pancreatitis in pediatric and adult-onset systemic lupus erythematosus: a comparison and review of the literature. Lupus 2011;20(5):443–52.

47. Limwattana S, Dissaneewate P, Kritsaneepaiboon S, et al. Systemic lupus erythematosus-related pancreatitis in children. Clin Rheumatol 2013;32(6):913–8.

48. Marques VL, Gormezano NW, Bonfa E, et al. Pancreatitis subtypes survey in 852 childhood-onset systemic lupus erythematosus patients. J Pediatr Gastroenterol Nutr 2016;62(2):328–34.
49. Makol A, Petri M. Pancreatitis in systemic lupus erythematosus: frequency and associated factors—a review of the Hopkins Lupus Cohort. J Rheumatol 2010; 37(2):341–5.
50. Nesher G, Breuer GS, Temprano K, et al. Lupus-associated pancreatitis. Semin Arthritis Rheum 2006;35(4):260–7.
51. Wang F, Wang NS, Zhao BH, et al. Acute pancreatitis as an initial symptom of systemic lupus erythematosus: a case report and review of the literature. World J Gastroenterol: WJG 2005;11(30):4766–8.
52. Tahernia L, Alimadadi H, Tahghighi F, et al. Frequency and type of hepatic and gastrointestinal involvement in juvenile systemic lupus erythematosus. Autoimmune Dis 2017;2017:1–5.
53. Al-Mogairen, Sultan M. Lupus protein-losing enteropathy (LUPLE): a systematic review. Rheumatol Int 2011;31(8):995–1001.
54. Alhassan E, Gendelman HK, Sabha MM, et al. Bilateral Retinal Vasculitis as the First Presentation of Systemic Lupus Erythematosus. Am J Case Rep 2021; 22:1–4.
55. Dammacco R. Systemic lupus erythematosus and ocular involvement: an overview. Clin Exp Med 2018;18(2):135–49.
56. Guleria S, Kumar Jindal A, Bhattarai D, et al. Retinal vasculopathy in children with systemic lupus erythematosus: report of two cases. Lupus 2020;29(12):1633–7.
57. Donnithorne KJ, Read RW, Lowe R, et al. Retinal vasculitis in two pediatric patients with systemic lupus erythematosus: a case report. Pediatr Rheumatol Online J 2013;11(25):1–6.
58. Huang G, Shen H, Zhao J, et al. Severe vaso-occlusive lupus retinopathy in the early stage of a pediatric patient with systemic lupus erythematosus: a case report. Medicine 2020;99(16):1–5.
59. Borrell H, Narváez J, Alegre JJ, et al. Shrinking lung syndrome in systemic lupus erythematosus: A case series and review of the literature. Medicine 2016; 95(33):1–9.
60. Pillai S, Mehta J, Levin T, et al. Shrinking lung syndrome presenting as an initial pulmonary manifestation of SLE. Lupus 2014;23(11):1201–3.
61. Torres Jimenez AR, Ruiz Vela N, Cespedes Cruz AI, et al. Shrinking lung syndrome in pediatric systemic lupus erythematosus. Lupus 2021;30(7):1175–9.
62. Delgado EA, Malleson PN, Pirie GE, et al. The pulmonary manifestations of childhood onset systemic lupus erythematosus. Semin Arthritis Rheum 1990;19(5): 285–93.
63. DeCoste C, Mateos-Corral D, Lang B. Shrinking lung syndrome treated with rituximab in pediatric systemic lupus erythematosus: a case report and review of the literature. Pediatr Rheumatol Online J 2021;19(7):1–7.

# Adolescent Onset of Acute Heart Failure

Tracey Thompson, MD, Ashley Phimister, MD,
Alexander Raskin, MD*

## KEYWORDS

- Heart failure • Myocarditis • Cardiomyopathy • Arrhythmia
- Congenital heart disease

## KEY POINTS

- Causes of acute heart failure in the adolescent include myocarditis, cardiomyopathies, metabolic disorders, congenital heart disease, and renal disease, among others.
- The presentation of heart failure can be extremely variable ranging from asymptomatic to acute cardiogenic shock or sudden cardiac arrest.
- A thorough assessment and family history are vital for guiding the evaluation and diagnostic work up.

## INTRODUCTION

Heart failure is a well recognized condition in adults, largely secondary to hypertension and coronary artery disease.[1] Causes in the adolescent are broad and can include myocarditis, cardiomyopathies, structural heart disease, nutritional deficiencies, metabolic disorders, hypertensive crises, and arrhythmias, among others.[2] In developed countries, congenital heart disease and cardiomyopathies are the 2 leading causes of heart failure in children, whereas in developing countries, leading causes include infections and severe anemia.[3] Although causes differ, the presentation of heart failure in the adolescent is similar to that of an adult. Common presenting symptoms include dyspnea, peripheral edema, orthopnea, cough, wheezing, and paroxysmal nocturnal dyspnea secondary to developing edema but can also include nonspecific symptoms such as fatigue, nausea, anorexia, or weight gain due to fluid retention.[4] The spectrum of presentation is highly variable ranging from no discernible symptoms, signs of congestive heart failure, and in extreme cases presenting in cardiogenic shock. Similarly, the physical examination can be highly variable. If patients are in compensated heart failure, they can have a relatively benign examination.

Pediatrics, Medical College of Wisconsin, Milwaukee, WI, USA
* Attn: Pediatric Cardiology Department, 9000 W. Wisconsin Avenue, Milwaukee, WI 53226.
*E-mail address:* araskin@mcw.edu

Med Clin N Am 108 (2024) 59–77
https://doi.org/10.1016/j.mcna.2023.06.016
medical.theclinics.com

Subtle but highly relevant examination findings suggestive of heart failure include tachycardia, abnormal heart sounds (gallop, diastolic murmur, or pathologic systolic murmur), tachypnea, and hepatomegaly. Chest radiograph and electrocardiography (ECG) may show nonspecific findings. A chest radiograph can demonstrate cardiomegaly with pulmonary congestion. ECG findings are commonly nonspecific.[5] This article provides an overview and insight into both rare and common causes of heart failure in the adolescent.

## MYOCARDITIS
### Background

Myocarditis is defined as inflammation of the heart muscle, which can cause cardiac dysfunction and decompensated heart failure. This disease can be diagnostically challenging due to the wide spectrum of clinical presentations that varies from mild, with recovery in a few days, to fulminant, requiring mechanical circulatory support (MCS).[6] The true incidence is difficult to ascertain due to high frequency of subclinical disease, but it is estimated to be in the range of 0.15% and 0.6% based on postmortem studies.[7] Furthermore, it accounts for a significant proportion of sudden cardiac death (SCD) in the young, with rates from 8.6% to 12% and is also a frequent cause of dilated cardiomyopathy.[6]

### Evaluation

The causes of myocarditis are broad (**Table 1**) and include infectious, autoimmune diseases, hypersensitivity reactions, and toxins.[6–9] In North America, viral infections are the predominant cause of pediatric myocarditis, with enteroviruses and adenovirus being the most common.[9]

The spectrum of presentation of myocarditis is wide. The classic presentation of acute myocarditis includes chest pain, tachypnea, tachycardia, and orthopnea after a viral prodrome in the preceding days to weeks.[7] Fulminant myocarditis can present

| Table 1 Causes of myocarditis[6–8] | | |
|---|---|---|
| Infectious | Viral | Adenoviruses, echoviruses, enteroviruses, herpesviruses (cytomegalovirus, Epstein-Barr virus), hepatitis C, HIV, influenza A, parvovirus B19, novel coronavirus (COVID-19) |
| | Bacterial | Mycobacterial, streptococcal species, pneumococcal species, *Mycoplasma pneumonia*, *Treponema pallidum*, *Klebsiella*, *Salmonella*, *Legionella*, *Toxoplasma gondii*, *Leptospirosis*, *Listeria*, *Coxiella*, *Borrelia* |
| | Fungal | *Aspergillus*, *Candida*, *Coccidioides*, *Cryptococcus*, *Histoplasma*, *Actinomyces*, |
| | Parasitic | Schistosomiasis, Larva Migrans, *Trypanosoma cruzi* |
| Autoimmune | | Churg-Strauss, inflammatory bowel disease, diabetes mellitus, sarcoidosis, systemic lupus erythematosus, thyrotoxicosis, Takayasu arteritis, granulomatosis with polyangiitis, MIS-C (COVID-19) |
| Toxicity | | Anthracyclines, cocaine, interleukin-2, sulfonamides, amphetamines, cyclophosphamide, t-fluorouracil, phenytoin, lead |
| Hypersensitivity reactions | | Sulfonamides, cephalosporins, loop and thiazide diuretics, digoxin, tricyclic antidepressants, benzodiazepines, clozapine, venoms (including bee, wasp, black widow spider, scorpion) |

*Abbreviations:* HIV, human immunodeficiency virus; MIS-C, multisystem inflammatory syndrome in children.

similarly but usually with rapid and acute decompensation in the setting of dysrhythmias and hemodynamic collapse, necessitating induction of inotropic support or MCS.[10,11] The acute phase of myocarditis is largely driven by active viral entry and replication. Inflammation persists in the subacute stage secondary to inflammatory cell infiltration. Some individuals can show complete resolution, whereas others progress to a chronic myocarditis marked by myocardial remodeling and fibrosis presenting as dilated cardiomyopathy.[12]

In endemic areas, Lyme disease–associated carditis should be considered as part of the differential diagnosis, especially in individuals presenting with conduction abnormalities. The infection is caused by *Borrelia burgdorferi* and is the most common tick-borne illness in the United States. Lyme carditis occurs in 4% to 10% of adult patients with Lyme disease, although the incidence in children is likely less.[13] Lyme carditis usually occurs within weeks to months of the initial infection and is commonly accompanied by skin and joint symptoms. Lyme carditis is more likely to occur in the months of June to December. The first phase of the disease is characterized by localized infection, which includes erythema migrans. Patients may then progress to develop systemic symptoms including headache, myalgias, arthralgias, and dizziness. During this time, cardiac involvement may occur. Patients with Lyme carditis often present with dyspnea, chest pain, palpitations, and lightheadedness.[14] If Lyme disease is suspected, serologic testing should be performed. During the initial phase of the disease, patients will have both immunoglobulin (Ig) M and IgG seropositivity against *B burgdorferi*. However, by the time carditis occurs, IgM may be negative and IgG will be positive. When there is concern for Lyme carditis, an ECG and Holter monitor must be performed. Conduction abnormalities are seen in 4% to 10% of adults, but this is likely less in the pediatric patient population. The most common manifestation of Lyme carditis is atrioventricular (AV) block, which can range from first-degree to third-degree AV block. Less often, patients will demonstrate more significant global myocardial inflammation with evidence of endocarditis, myocarditis, or pericarditis. Echocardiogram should be considered for patients with advanced heart block or signs and symptoms of heart failure.[13] Echocardiogram may show ventricular dilation or dysfunction that can be perpetuated by heart block. Most often though, the echocardiogram is normal.[14] Although Lyme carditis can resolve spontaneously, antibiotics are recommended to decrease the duration of disease and prevent complications.[13,14] For patients with high-grade AV block, more than 90% will have resolution to normal conduction within 1 week of antibiotic treatment.[14]

Traditionally, the diagnostic gold standard for myocarditis was histopathology from tissue biopsy samples demonstrating lymphocytic infiltration.[10] However, the heterogeneous nature of myocarditis coupled with random sampling of specimens results in a high false-negative rate.[15] Cardiac magnetic resonance (CMR) imaging using the Lake Louise criteria has become the primary diagnostic modality for identifying acute myocarditis.[10,16] Other imaging modalities such as transthoracic echocardiography are readily available but have significantly lower sensitivity and specificity. Echocardiographic findings may be normal or can demonstrate left ventricular enlargement, valvular regurgitation, pericardial effusion, or systolic dysfunction.[17] Inflammation of the conduction system may manifest as arrhythmias such as AV block and ventricular tachycardia. ECG can be normal but can also show variable features such as sinus tachycardia, ST–T-wave changes, ST-segment elevation, or low-voltage QRS. Laboratory evaluation may show elevated C-reactive protein (CRP), erythrocyte sedimentation rate, troponin, and B-type natriuretic. Chest radiograph may show pulmonary edema or pleural effusions.[7,10,18]

### Discussion

The mainstay of treatment of myocarditis is supportive care. Given the possibility of rapid deterioration, early recognition is paramount in order to facilitate transport to a regional center that can provide MCS and advanced cardiac therapies, if necessary. Development of arrhythmias is an important prognostic factor associated with increased disease severity and adverse outcomes.[19,20] Milrinone is considered first-line inotropic support, with other agents such as epinephrine reserved for refractory hypotension and cardiogenic shock. If the patient is not adequately supported with conventional medical therapies, MCS may be needed as a bridge to recovery or transplantation.[10,18] Immunomodulators, such as intravenous immunoglobulin, corticosteroids, cyclosporine, azathioprine, and biologics targeting cytokine/complement activation have been proposed as treatments of myocarditis. Currently there is insufficient evidence for broad evidence-based recommendations regarding immunomodulators.[10] However, emerging understanding of pathophysiology suggests improved survival in fulminant myocarditis with early diagnosis and timely initiation of MCS and immunomodulators.[11]

### Summary

The hallmark of myocarditis is inflammation of the myocardium most commonly due to an acute viral infection. The presentation of acute myocarditis can be quite variable and ranges from little clinical symptoms to severe hemodynamic compromise with cardiogenic shock. Standard evaluation includes cardiac imaging, rhythm assessment with ECG, and laboratory evaluation to assess end-organ function, inflammation, and evidence of myocardial injury. Treatment ranges from supportive care to inotropes, immunomodulators, and MCS in more severe cases.

### Clinics Care Points

- Presenting symptoms of myocarditis can vary broadly.
- Treatment can be variable and include supportive care, immunomodulators, inotropes, and MCS.
- Patients can deteriorate rapidly, and early recognition is critical to improving outcomes.

## DILATED CARDIOMYOPATHY
### Background

Dilated cardiomyopathy (DCM) is characterized by left ventricular dilation and systolic dysfunction; it is the most common cardiomyopathy in children. There are a wide variety of causes of DCM including primary and secondary causes. Primary causes include idiopathic, familial sarcomeric, mitochondrial, and neuromuscular diseases. Idiopathic DCM makes up to 50% of pediatric cardiomyopathies, and most cases likely have an underlying genetic cause that has not been identified by current testing. Secondary causes include inflammatory, endocrine, toxic, metabolic disorders, nutritional, structural heart disease, myocardial ischemia, and pulmonary disease.[21]

The pathophysiology of DCM is driven by reduced sarcomeric contractility due to either a primary or a secondary insult. Myocardial dysfunction triggers compensatory neurohormonal activation of the sympathetic nervous system and the renin-angiotensin aldosterone system. Initially this maintains cardiac output and organ perfusion by increasing preload, heart rate, and afterload. However, chronic activation of these compensatory mechanisms leads to deleterious cardiac remodeling including fibrosis and further sarcomeric dysfunction. In addition, sustained increased preload leads to progressive dilation and thinning of the left ventricle, which results in poorly coapting and insufficient atrioventricular valves, further impairing cardiac output.[22,23] Symptoms, as in other types of heart failure, can vary widely depending on acuity and level of compensation.

### Evaluation

Echocardiography is essential to making the diagnosis of DCM. It provides information about ventricular size, function, and valvular abnormalities.[21] CMR can help identify underlying causes of dilated cardiomyopathy such as inflammatory and iron overload. In addition, CMR can provide additional data regarding ventricular volumes, calculated function, and degree of myocardial fibrosis.[24]

Finally, laboratory workup is important both to evaluate for end-organ dysfunction and to identify potential causes of DCM such as thyroid disorders, anemia, iron overload, acute toxicities, or genetic disorders as indicated by clinical presentation, family history, and previous diagnostic workup.[21,23]

### Familial/Sarcomeric Dilated Cardiomyopathy

DCM can appear as an inherited trait or a sporadic gene variant encoding structural and functional genes affecting cardiac myocytes. A family history of SCD, cardiomyopathy, or other features such as valvular abnormalities should increase suspicion of an underlying genetic cause for DCM.[25] There are more than 100 genes that have been implicated in DCM, with the majority inherited in an autosomal-dominant pattern, although autosomal-recessive, X-linked recessive, and mitochondrial inheritance have also been described.[26] Diagnosis requires careful assessment of clinical presentation, morphologic cardiac findings on imaging, genetic evaluation, and extensive family history. The diagnosis of familial DCM can still be established in the absence of positive genetic testing.[21]

### Metabolic/Mitochondrial/Storage Diseases

Mitochondria are responsible for energy production in the cell. Tissues with high aerobic metabolism, such as the myocardium, are highly susceptible in mitochondrial diseases and can present with various forms of cardiomyopathy including DCM, hypertrophic cardiomyopathy (HCM), and left ventricular noncompaction (LVNC).[27,28] Storage disorders involve a deficiency of enzymes, membrane transporters, or other proteins, resulting in an accumulation of macromolecules that are normally broken down by lysosomes. Symptoms and organ involvement are based on the accumulation of these molecules.[29] Other metabolic disorders such as primary carnitine deficiency, fatty acid oxidation disorders, and congenital disorders of glycosylation can also affect cardiac morphology and function. The clinical presentations of mitochondrial, metabolic, and storage disorders are broad and can affect nearly every organ system (**Table 2**).[21,30]

### Neuromuscular Disorders

Cardiomyopathies are frequently associated with neuromuscular disorders and are the leading cause of morbidity and mortality in this population. Neuromuscular disorders are extremely diverse in their presentation, onset, associated comorbidities, cardiac morphology, and mode of inheritance. The development of DCM is well described in X-linked recessive Duchenne and Becker muscular dystrophies. Dysrhythmias and conduction abnormalities are commonly seen in LMNA associated autosomal-dominant form of Emery-Dreifuss syndrome. Although DCM

**Table 2**
Metabolic, mitochondrial, and storage disease associated with cardiomyopathy[21,27–41]

| | Disorders | Cause | Clinical Features | Cardiac Manifestations |
|---|---|---|---|---|
| Mitochondrial disorders | Kearns Sayre syndrome | Large deletions in mitochondrial DNA involved in oxidative phosphorylation | Retinopathy, ophthalmoplegia | Conduction abnormalities (heart block), rare cases of dilated cardiomyopathy |
| | Leigh syndrome | Genetic variants in mitochondrial or nuclear DNA (more than 60 described) | Gliosis, demyelination, respiratory failure, optic atrophy, hypotonia, ataxia | Hypertrophic cardiomyopathy (predominantly) Dilated cardiomyopathy, Wolff-Parkinson-White (WPW syndrome) |
| | Sengers syndrome | Autosomal-recessive variant in acylglycerol kinase (AGK) | Cataracts, skeletal myopathy, lactic acidosis | Hypertrophic cardiomyopathy |
| | Myoclonic epilepsy with ragged red fibers (MERRF syndrome) | Genetic variant in mitochondrial DNA A8344G | Myoclonus, seizures, lactic acidosis, ataxia, ragged red fibers on muscle biopsy, dementia | Dilated cardiomyopathy, hypertrophic cardiomyopathy, WPW |
| | Barth syndrome | X-linked recessive TAZ gene variant causing defect in cardiolipin, a component of mitochondrial inner membrane | Abnormal urine organic acid screen with elevated 3-methylglutaconic acid, cyclic neutropenia, growth failure, skeletal myopathy | Dilated cardiomyopathy (predominantly) and left ventricular noncompaction cardiomyopathy |
| Storage disorders | Pompe disease (glycogen storage disease type IIA) | Deficiency in enzyme acid α-glucosidase | Hypotonia, hepatomegaly | Hypertrophic cardiomyopathy |
| | Hurler-Scheie syndrome Mucopolysaccharidosis (MPS1) | Deficiency of enzyme alpha-L-iduronidase | Spinal abnormalities, course facial features, corneal opacities | Valvulopathy, conduction abnormalities, coronary vasculopathy |
| | Gaucher disease Sphingolipidosis | Deficiency of β-glucocerebrosidase | Anemia, thrombocytopenia, hepatosplenomegaly, skeletal abnormalities | Calcific mitral and aortic valve disease, hypertrophic cardiomyopathy |
| | Niemann-Pick disease (type B) Sphingolipidosis | Deficiency in acid sphingomyelinase | Hepatosplenomegaly, growth restriction delayed puberty, osteopenia, thrombocytopenia, leukopenia | Coronary heart disease, valvular disease |

| | | | |
|---|---|---|---|
| | Fabry disease | X-linked, deficiency of lysosomal α-galactosidase A | Angiokeratosis, corneal opacities, renal failure | Hypertrophic cardiomyopathy |
| | Danon disease | Glycogen storage disorder, X-linked dominant LAMP2 variant | Skeletal myopathy, developmental delays, visual acuity abnormality | Hypertrophic cardiomyopathy progressing to dilated cardiomyopathy, WPW, conduction abnormalities |
| Metabolic disorders | Congenital disorders of glycosylation | Deficiency of PGM1 | Hepatopathy, bifid uvula, growth restriction, myopathy, hypoglycemia | Dilated cardiomyopathy, sudden cardiac arrest |
| | Fatty acid oxidation disorders | Very long-chain acyl-CoA dehydrogenase deficiency | Hypoglycemia, hepatomegaly, myopathy, episodic rhabdomyolysis | Dilated and hypertrophic (predominant) cardiomyopathy, arrhythmias, and sudden death |
| | Primary carnitine deficiency | Autosomal-recessive variant in SLC22A5 encoding cation transported type 2 | Hypoketotic hypoglycemia, hepatomegaly, and muscle weakness | Dilated and hypertrophic cardiomyopathy, arrhythmias |

is the predominant form of cardiomyopathy of neuromuscular disorders, some neuromuscular disorders, such as Friedreich ataxia, present with an HCM phenotype.[21,42]

### Endocrinopathies

Endocrine disorders are a rare but potentially readily identifiable and reversible cause of cardiac dysfunction. Based on presenting features, evaluation of patients presenting with cardiac dysfunction should consider workup of thyroid disease, parathyroid disorders, and catecholamine-secreting tumors, as these conditions can adversely affect cardiac energetics and loading conditions.[21]

### Oncological Cardiomyopathies

Chemotherapeutic agents have been linked to many adverse cardiotoxic effects including ventricular dysfunction, pericarditis, and arrhythmias. Anthracyclines are the most well-known causative agents, although monoclonal antibodies, such as trastuzumab, alkylating agents, CAR-T, and protein kinase inhibitors have also been implicated.[43] *Anthracyclines* can cause heart failure in the acute setting (within 1 year), as well as late-onset (months or years after completing treatment).[44] The incidence of heart failure is dose dependent based on cumulative dosing, with doses greater than a doxorubicin equivalent of 250 mg/m$^2$ considered high dose.[45] Concomitant exposure to anthracyclines and radiation therapy has an additive cardiotoxic effect. Thoracic radiation has been linked with a significantly increased risk of nonischemic cardiomyopathy due to direct fibrosis, development of valvular disease, and constrictive pericarditis. In general, no known dose of radiation is considered safe, but generally greater than 30 Gy of total exposure and greater than 15 Gy for direct cardiac exposure is considered high risk.[46,47] Alkylating agents such as cyclophosphamide and ifosfamide have also been implicated in ventricular dysfunction in a dose-dependent fashion. Commonly, dysfunction is seen acutely following treatment with alkylating agents.[43,45]

### Recreational Drugs

Recreational alcohol and drug use can have both acute and chronic cardiac implications. Alcohol abuse has been noted to impair myocardial contractility and has also been associated with the development of cardiac arrhythmias, most commonly atrial fibrillation.[48,49] Acute and chronic abuse of recreational stimulants such as methamphetamines and cocaine have also been shown to have deleterious cardiac affects.[21,50] Chronic cocaine abuse can lead to irreversible damage of the myocardium due to overstimulation of the adrenergic system. Stimulant abuse can also cause acute coronary vasoconstriction and arrhythmogenesis.[49]

### Tachycardia Induced Cardiomyopathy

Prolonged periods of unrecognized and unmanaged tachycardia can produce cardiac dysfunction with a DCM phenotype. The dysfunction is often reversible once the arrhythmia is controlled. Tachycardia-induced cardiomyopathy usually occurs in patients without underlying structural heart disease. The most common causes in children include ectopic atrial tachycardia, orthodromic reentrant tachycardia (including Wolff-Parkinson-White syndrome), and permanent junctional reciprocating tachycardia. Other arrhythmias such as atrial fibrillation, atrial flutter, and ventricular tachycardia can also lead to tachycardia-induced cardiomyopathy but are rare in the pediatric population.[51] Adolescents may complain of palpitations and can present with heart failure symptoms weeks to months after the onset of the tachycardia.[52]

Establishing the diagnosis requires a high index of suspicion. An ECG should be performed, which may demonstrate a pathologic tachyarrhythmia or preexcitation suggestive of Wolff-Parkinson-White syndrome.

### Anemia and Nutritional Impact on Cardiomyopathy

Severe anemia has been noted to cause myocardial disease and subsequently heart failure, particularly in developing countries due to nutritional deficiencies or infectious diseases such as malaria.[53,54] Chronic anemia can cause a sustained increase in cardiac output at levels less than 7 gm/100 mL due to decreased oxygen-carrying capacity, and levels less than 5 gm/100 mL can cause circulatory congestion and symptoms consistent with congestive heart failure.[55] Patients with chronic anemia requiring recurrent transfusions are at risk of developing iron overload cardiomyopathy, which initially demonstrates a restrictive phenotype but progresses to DCM with restrictive physiology.[21]

Significant nutritional deficits including hypocalcemia, thiamine deficiency, selenium deficiency, and severe malnutrition are associated with development of heart failure. Calcium plays an important role in myocyte excitation-contraction coupling, and severe hypocalcemia can lead to diminished ventricular function and QT prolongation.[56,57] Thiamine plays a vital role in the generation of adenosine triphosphate in the citric acid cycle, and its deficiency is a well-known cause of heart failure termed "wet beriberi."[58] Selenium deficiency leads to increased production of free radicals and direct cardiac injury that can cause DCM.[21]

### Discussion

A thorough history and diagnostic workup for patients presenting with DCM is paramount because reversible causes of heart failure can be identified and mitigated. Treatment of DCM is multifaceted and can include specific therapies based on an established diagnosis. For diseases states associated with reversible dysfunction, recovery may take weeks to months. Other forms of DCM such as familial or neuromuscular disease can be irreversible and progressive in nature. Common medical management includes heart failure treatment with diuretics, β-blockers, angiotensin-converting enzyme (ACE) inhibitors, and more recently angiotensin receptor-neprilysin inhibitors. Heart failure refractory to medical management may require advanced cardiac therapies in the form of inotropic support, ventricular assist device, and consideration for cardiac transplantation.[25,31,59]

### Summary

Dilated cardiomyopathy has many causes, including genetic, metabolic, toxic, nutritional, and rhythm-induced. The clinical presentation can vary depending on degree of compensation. Evaluation should include a thorough history and physical examination to determine what further evaluation is needed. Treatment is usually guided toward the underlying cause. If no underlying cause is found, supportive care and general heart failure treatment is recommended.

### Clinics Care Points

- Genetic evaluation should be pursued in cases with concerning familial history including SCD or cardiomyopathy.
- A through and thoughtful evaluation of a patient presenting in heart failure can identify reversible causes.

## HYPERTROPHIC CARDIOMYOPATHY

### Background

HCM is defined as unexplained LVH in the absence of another cardiac or systemic disease that could lead to LVH. The prevalence is about 1:500 in the general population.[21,60] In almost all cases, HCM is a genetic disease with autosomal dominant inheritance and more than 50 identified genetic variants.60,61[,62] Most HCM is related to variants in sarcomeric proteins. Other causes of HCM can be related to RASopathies, neurodegenerative disorders (Friedreich ataxia), metabolic disease, storage disorders, and mitochondrial disorders (see **Table 2**).[21,63] RASopathies refer to abnormalities in the RAS/MAPK signaling pathway and include disorders such as Noonan and Costello syndromes. The prevalence of HCM in RASopathies ranges from 20% to 80%, depending on the specific gene variant involved.[64]

Adolescents with HCM have highly variable presenting features, including many that are asymptomatic. The most common symptoms are exertional dyspnea and chest pain. History suggestive of exertional arrhythmias and syncope should also raise concern for HCM. Pathologic LVH in HCM leads to dynamic left ventricular outflow tract (LVOT) obstruction and is largely responsible for exertional symptoms. In addition, hypertrophy creates disruption of the normal myocyte architecture, promotes myocardial ischemia, and ultimately leads to fibrosis. Myocardial fibrosis is a trigger for ventricular arrhythmias and SCD. HCM is the leading cause of SCD in the young.[62,65,66]

### Evaluation

When evaluating a patient for HCM, initial diagnostic workup includes a through physical examination, 12-lead ECG, and echocardiogram. A systolic ejection murmur increasing in intensity with Valsalva maneuver or standing is pathognomonic for HCM. ECG can demonstrate LVH with strain pattern. There is no consistent correlation between the severity of ECG findings and the severity of ventricular hypertrophy. Echocardiogram can assess for ventricular hypertrophy, function, and detect LVOT gradient. There is a growing role for advanced imaging such as cardiac CMR, which provides more precise cardiac measurements and quantifies the degree of myocardial fibrosis.[60,65]

### Discussion

Management of patients with HCM is focused on relieving symptoms and preventing SCD. The major risk factors for SCD in patients with HCM include family history of SCD, unexplained syncope, documented nonsustained ventricular tachycardia, maximal left ventricular wall thickness greater than 30 mm, and amount of myocardial fibrosis.[60] Pharmacologic therapy is first-line treatment and often includes β-blockers and nondihydropyridine calcium channel blockers. Nonpharmacologic treatments include surgical myomectomy and ultimately cardiac transplant if patients have failed other medical and surgical options. Implantable cardioverter defibrillators (ICD) are used for primary and secondary prevention of SCD. Generally, ICDs are not recommended when the 5-year risk of SCD is less than 4% based on validated risk calculators for patient aged 16 years and older. Adolescents with HCM are advised to refrain from competitive sports.[60,62,65]

### Summary

Hypertrophic cardiomyopathy has several different underlying causes including sarcomeric, RASopathies, and metabolic disorders. The clinical presentation can vary depending on the underlying cause. The first steps of evaluation include echocardiogram and ECG. Treatment is focused on relieving symptoms and preventing SCD.

### Clinics Care Points

- HCM is the leading cause of SCD in the young.
- Adolescents with HCM are advised to refrain from competitive sports.

## LEFT VENTRICULAR NONCOMPACTION
### Background

LVNC is the third most common cardiomyopathy in the pediatric population after DCM and HCM, and it is characterized by prominent trabeculations and deep intertrabecular recesses in the myocardium. The LV apex and free wall are commonly the most affected. LVNC can have overlapping features with other cardiomyopathies and structural heart disease. Many structural myocyte gene variants have been implicated in the development of LVNC, most commonly Titin (TTN) and Myosin Heavy Chain 7 (MYH7). Clinical presentation is highly variable, ranging from asymptomatic to heart failure symptoms and even SCD.[21,30,67–69] This wide overlap of clinical features and outcomes poses significant challenges to diagnosis, prognostication, and management.

### Evaluation

Diagnosis of LVNC is made by cardiac imaging. Because of availability and cost, echocardiography is most frequently used to measure the ratio of noncompacted to compacted layers of myocardium, for which diagnostic criteria have been established. CMR can provide further tissue characterization analysis and improved imaging resolution when echocardiography is equivocal. Familial screening is indicated in first-degree family members, and genetic testing is recommended if a pathogenic variant is identified.[30,67,68]

### Discussion

LVNC-specific guidelines do not currently exist, and management is directed toward heart failure symptoms and SCD prevention, as primarily seen with DCM and HCM. Additional consideration is also given toward anticoagulation to reduce the risk of stroke associated with potential LV trabecular thrombosis.[21,30,66–68]

### Summary

LVNC is a rare cause of heart failure. Clinical presentation can vary from asymptomatic to severe. There is no known specific therapy for LVNC, and management is largely driven by phenotypic overlap with other cardiomyopathies.

### Clinics Care Points

- Familial screening is recommended in first-degree family members of index cases of LVNC.
- LVNC overlaps with DCM, HCM, and structural heart disease.

## RESTRICTIVE CARDIOMYOPATHY
### Background

Restrictive cardiomyopathy (RCM) is characterized by restrictive filling and decreased diastolic volume of one or both ventricles with near-normal systolic function and wall thickness. Restrictive cardiomyopathy makes up 2.5% to 5% of cardiomyopathies.[70] RCM is often a rapidly progressive disease manifesting as congestive heart failure complicated by conduction abnormalities, SCD, and thromboembolic complications.[21,71–73]

The most common causes of RCM in adolescents are idiopathic, familial, and sarcomeric. Other causes include storage disease, infiltrative, endomyocardial diseases, and heart transplant graft dysfunction. Pediatric infiltrative diseases, such as amyloidosis, are exceptionally rare. The hallmark pathophysiology of RCM is abnormal ventricular compliance, leading to marked biatrial enlargement with pulmonary and systemic venous congestion.[21,71]

### Evaluation

Patients with RCM often present with pulmonary symptoms of dyspnea and exercise intolerance. History of "asthma" and "lower respiratory tract infections" is frequently reported. A chest radiograph is a useful screening modality and typically shows cardiomegaly with pulmonary venous congestion. Approximately 10% of patients will present with syncope.[72] ECGs in patients with RCM are usually abnormal with atrial enlargement and ST segment–T-wave abnormalities. Cardiac catheterization provides direct hemodynamic data and helps distinguish RCM from constrictive pericarditis. On physical examination, patients often have a gallop, loud P2, hepatomegaly, ascites, and edema. Echocardiogram is typically diagnostic with marked biatrial enlargement and normal systolic function.[21,70,71]

### Discussion

Medical management of RCM is challenging. Diuretics provide symptomatic relief but have to be used judicially in order to maintain preload-dependent cardiac output. Pediatric RCM has significantly worse outcomes compared with other cardiomyopathies with 20% to 30% mortality at 5 years. Once symptoms develop, they can be rapidly progressive and difficult to manage. Heart transplantation offers improved survival with posttransplant outcomes that are comparative to other cardiomyopathies.[70–73]

### Summary

Restrictive cardiomyopathy is characterized by restrictive filling and decreased diastolic volume with near-normal systolic function. Chest radiograph and ECG are useful screening tests, and echocardiography is diagnostic. RCM has significant risk of morbidity and mortality, and early transplant evaluation should be considered.

### Clinical Care Points

- Recurrent respiratory symptoms with cardiomegaly on radiograph are common manifestation of RCM.
- RCM carries a significant risk of mortality with limited therapeutic options requiring early referral and consideration of transplantation.

## ARRHYTHMOGENIC VENTRICULAR CARDIOMYOPATHY
### Background

Arrhythmogenic ventricular cardiomyopathy (AVC) is a disorder of the myocardium that results in fibro-fatty infiltration and ventricular tachyarrhythmias. Classically, the right ventricle was thought to be most affected, but current understanding implicates biventricular involvement.[21,74] AVC makes up ~4% of SCD in young competitive athletes.[75] It has an estimated prevalence of 1:2500 to 1:5000. The presentation of AVC varies widely from asymptomatic to palpitations, fatigue, syncope, and SCD.[21,75]

Majority of AVC cases stem from autosomal-dominant pathogenic variant genes encoding desmosomes and other components of cardiac intercalated discs, leading to myocyte apoptosis with fibro-fatty infiltration. Clinically, this manifests as conduction system abnormalities, ventricular arrhythmias, and systolic dysfunction.[21,74]

### Evaluation

The diagnosis of AVC is established on family history, genetic testing, cardiac imaging, ECG, and ambulatory rhythm monitoring based on specified Task Force criteria, which are beyond the scope of this review.[21,74,76]

### Discussion

Patients with AVC should be counseled on the risks of SCD with exercise, and they should be activity restricted. Medical management involves arrhythmia suppression and prevention of SCD. Catheter ablation for incessant ventricular tachycardia is sometimes required. In addition, ICD placement is considered for either primary or secondary prevention of SCD. Finally, cardiac transplant may be required for uncontrolled arrhythmias or end-stage heart failure.[21,74]

### Summary

AVC is an arrhythmogenic cardiomyopathy that has variable presentation but carries a significant risk of SCD. Treatment is focused on suppressions of arrhythmias and prevention of SCD.

### Clinics Care Points

- AVC can have wide spectrum of presentation but should be considered when patients present with exertional arrhythmias, syncope, or aborted cardiac arrest.

## CARDIO-RENAL INTERACTION
### Background

Cardiorenal syndrome is a disorder that involves the heart and kidney, where dysfunction in one organ leads to dysfunction in the other. Type 3 (acute) and type 4 (chronic) cardiorenal syndromes describe renal disease causing heart failure.[77] The pathogenesis of cardiorenal syndrome is not completely understood. However, cardiovascular disease is a major cause of morbidity and mortality in children with chronic kidney disease. Cardiomyopathy is reported in 9.6% of chronic kidney disease patients.[78–80] Hypertension is a major cardiac comorbidity of renal disease, and hypertensive crisis (independent of chronic kidney disease) can manifest with acute cardiac dysfunction.[81]

### Discussion

Hypertensive crises require immediate intervention in order to lower the blood pressure, both safely and effectively. Treatment should aim to lower blood pressure by no more than 25% in the first 6 to 8 hours, with a gradual return to a normal blood pressure in 24 to 72 hours.[81] Heart failure management in the setting of chronic kidney disease primarily revolves around medical management and multidisciplinary cooperation between nephrologists and cardiologists to optimize volume status and hemodynamics. Ultimately, for patients with end-stage renal disease, renal transplantation can provide recovery of cardiac function and offers survival benefit over chronic dialysis.[77,79,80]

## Summary

Children with acute and chronic kidney disease can develop heart failure. Additionally, hypertensive crisis, an acute period of severely elevated blood pressure, can cause cardiac dysfunction.

### Clinics Care Points

- Complex cardio-renal interactions impact function of both organ systems.
- There is a 9.6% prevalence of cardiomyopathy with chronic kidney disease.

## STRUCTURAL HEART DISEASE

### Background

Congenital and acquired structural heart disease can lead to heart failure due to adverse pressure and volume loading conditions (**Table 3**). Significant left to right shunting creates overcirculation (volume loading) and eventual congestive heart failure even in patients with preserved systolic function. Pressure overload initially triggers compensatory ventricular hypertrophy but overtime can lead to systolic dysfunction.[82] Acquired heart disease due to rheumatic heart disease, systemic lupus erythematosus (SLE), and Kawasaki disease are associated with valvular disease. Adolescents with SLE are at high risk for cardiac disease, including pericarditis, valvular insufficiency, endocarditis, and myocarditis.[83]

Rheumatic heart disease (RHD) is an entity that is caused by an abnormal immune response to group A streptococcal infection (GAS), causing valvular damage in the heart.[84] The global prevalence of the disease has come down significantly due to preventative measures such as antibiotic treatment directed against GAS. However, RHD remains persistent, especially in developing nations.[85] Acute rheumatic fever (ARF) typically occurs in children aged 5 to 14 year around 3 weeks after GAS pharyngitis. Clinical features include fever, polyarthritis, chorea, and erythema marginatum.[84] The diagnosis of ARF is established using the modified Jones criteria.[86] ARF typically affects the left-sided valves, in particular the mitral valve, characteristically causing mitral regurgitation (MR) and sometimes chordal rupture.[87] Over time, persistent valve damage with or without recurrent episodes of ARF can result in chronic RHD. Persistent MR can cause progressive left-sided heart dilation, which may further worsen MR.[88] Mitral stenosis may develop later in the course due to persistent valvular inflammation. Cardiac signs and symptoms can include sinus tachycardia, a pansystolic murmur consistent with MR, PR prolongation on ECG, or clinical signs of heart failure. Echocardiography is the hallmark diagnostic test to identify valvular pathology and may also show a pericardial effusion or ventricular dilation. Often, chronic RHD may be diagnosed in patients who were asymptomatic or do not remember their ARF

| Table 3 | |
|---|---|
| **Structural heart disease associated with heart failure** | |
| **Volume Overload** | **Pressure Overload** |
| • Ventricular septal defect (VSD) | • Subaortic stenosis |
| • Atrial septal defect (ASD) | • Aortic stenosis |
| • Patent ductus arteriosus (PDA) | • Supra-aortic stenosis |
| • Atrioventricular (AV) canal defect | • Coarctation of the aorta |
| • Partial anomalous pulmonary venous connection | • Pulmonary stenosis |
| • Significant atrioventricular and/or semilunar valve regurgitation | • Distal branch pulmonary artery hypoplasia and stenosis |

symptoms.[84] Treatment of ARF is largely supportive, with little evidence to show treatment with anti-inflammatory agents improves outcome. Standard heart failure treatment including diuretics and ACE inhibitors can be used for severe carditis, and refractory cases may require surgical valvular intervention.[86] Secondary prevention against repeated ARF includes penicillin prophylaxis, with duration depending on patient age and severity of RHD.[84]

## Discussion

Management of heart failure secondary to structural heart disease varies widely depending on the cause. ECG and echocardiography are the main diagnostic and surveillance tools. Medical management includes diuretics and heart failure medications. Often surgery will be required to correct a specific cardiac lesion. Diagnosis of acute rheumatic heart disease is established by the Jones criteria, and management largely revolves around antibiotic prophylaxis for recurrent GAS infection and heart failure medications if significant cardiac lesions persist.[89,90] Management of SLE often requires anti-inflammatory and immune modulatory therapy.[91]

## Summary

Heart failure occurs with congenital and acquired heart disease due to pressure or volume overload. Management is incredibly heterogeneous and depends on the underlying cause.

## Clinics Care Points

- Volume overload causes congestive heart failure, and pressure overload may progress to systolic dysfunction.
- Rheumatic heart disease most commonly involves the mitral and aortic valves.
- Cardiac manifestations are common in adolescents presenting with new-onset SLE.

## REFERENCES

1. Bui AL, Horwich TB, Fonarow GC. Epidemiology and risk profile of heart failure. Nat Rev Cardiol 2011;8(1):30–41.
2. Price JF. Congestive Heart Failure in Children. Pediatr Rev 2019;40(2):60–70.
3. Shaddy RE, George AT, Jaecklin T, et al. Systematic Literature Review on the Incidence and Prevalence of Heart Failure in Children and Adolescents. Pediatr Cardiol 2018;39(3):415–36.
4. Chen J, Aronowitz P. Congestive Heart Failure. Med Clin North Am 2022;106(3): 447–58.
5. Lin K, Rossano JW. Moss and Adams' heart disease in Infants, children and adolescents. 9th edition. Philadelphia, PA: Wolters Kluwer; 2016.
6. Magnani JW, Dec GW. Myocarditis: current trends in diagnosis and treatment. Circulation 2006;113(6):876–90.
7. Bejiqi R, Retkoceri R, Maloku A, et al. The Diagnostic and Clinical Approach to Pediatric Myocarditis: A Review of the Current Literature. Open Access Maced J Med Sci 2019;7(1):162–73.
8. Tunuguntla H, Jeewa A, Denfield SW. Acute Myocarditis and Pericarditis in Children. Pediatr Rev 2019;40(1):14–25.
9. Kühl U, Schultheiss HP. Myocarditis in children. Heart Fail Clin 2010;6(4):483–96, viii-ix.

10. Law YM, Lal AK, Chen S, et al. Diagnosis and Management of Myocarditis in Children: A Scientific Statement From the American Heart Association. Circulation 2021;144(6):e123–35.
11. Hang W, Chen C, Seubert JM, et al. Fulminant myocarditis: a comprehensive review from etiology to treatments and outcomes. Signal Transduct Target Ther 2020;5:287.
12. Fung G, Luo H, Qiu Y, et al. Myocarditis. Circ Res 2016;118(3):496–514.
13. Costello JM, Alexander ME, Greco KM, et al. Lyme carditis in children: presentation, predictive factors, and clinical course. Pediatrics 2009;123(5):e835–41.
14. Radesich C, Del Mestre E, Medo K, et al. Lyme Carditis: From Pathophysiology to Clinical Management. Pathogens 2022;11(5):582.
15. Chow LH, Radio SJ, Sears TD, et al. Insensitivity of right ventricular endomyocardial biopsy in the diagnosis of myocarditis. J Am Coll Cardiol 1989;14(4):915–20.
16. Friedrich MG, Sechtem U, Schulz-Menger J, et al. Cardiovascular magnetic resonance in myocarditis: A JACC White Paper. J Am Coll Cardiol 2009;53(17):1475–87.
17. Skouri HN, Dec GW, Friedrich MG, et al. Noninvasive imaging in myocarditis. J Am Coll Cardiol 2006;48(10):2085–93.
18. Dasgupta S, Iannucci G, Mao C, et al. Myocarditis in the pediatric population: A review. Congenit Heart Dis 2019;14(5):868–77.
19. Al-Khatib SM, Stevenson WG, Ackerman MJ, et al. 2017 AHA/ACC/HRS Guideline for Management of Patients With Ventricular Arrhythmias and the Prevention of Sudden Cardiac Death: Executive Summary: A Report of the American College of Cardiology/American Heart Association Task Force on Clinical Practice Guidelines and the Heart Rhythm Society. Circulation 2018;138(13):e210–71.
20. Ogunbayo GO, Elayi SC, Ha LD, et al. Outcomes of Heart Block in Myocarditis: A Review of 31,760 Patients. Heart Lung Circ 2019;28(2):272–6.
21. Lipshultz SE, Law YM, Asante-Korang A, et al. Cardiomyopathy in Children: Classification and Diagnosis: A Scientific Statement From the American Heart Association. Circulation 2019;140(1):e9–68.
22. De Paris V, Biondi F, Stolfo D, et al. Pathophysiology. In: Sinagra G, Merlo M, Pinamonti B, editors. Dilated cardiomyopathy: from genetics to clinical management. Springer; 2019. Available at: http://www.ncbi.nlm.nih.gov/books/NBK553848/. Accessed April 25, 2023.
23. Mahmaljy H, Yelamanchili VS, Singhal M. Dilated Cardiomyopathy. In: StatPearls. StatPearls Publishing; 2023. Available at: http://www.ncbi.nlm.nih.gov/books/NBK441911/. Accessed April 25, 2023.
24. Francone M. Role of Cardiac Magnetic Resonance in the Evaluation of Dilated Cardiomyopathy: Diagnostic Contribution and Prognostic Significance. Int Sch Res Not 2014;2014:e365404.
25. Peters S, Johnson R, Birch S, et al. Familial Dilated Cardiomyopathy. Heart Lung Circ 2020;29(4):566–74.
26. McNally EM, Mestroni L. Dilated Cardiomyopathy: Genetic Determinants and Mechanisms. Circ Res 2017;121(7):731–48.
27. Holmgren D, Wåhlander H, Eriksson BO, et al. Cardiomyopathy in children with mitochondrial disease; clinical course and cardiological findings. Eur Heart J 2003;24(3):280–8.
28. Meyers DE, Basha HI, Koenig MK. Mitochondrial cardiomyopathy: pathophysiology, diagnosis, and management. Tex Heart Inst J 2013;40(4):385–94.
29. Nair V, Belanger EC, Veinot JP. Lysosomal storage disorders affecting the heart: a review. Cardiovasc Pathol Off J Soc Cardiovasc Pathol 2019;39:12–24.

30. Towbin JA, Jefferies JL. Cardiomyopathies Due to Left Ventricular Noncompaction, Mitochondrial and Storage Diseases, and Inborn Errors of Metabolism. Circ Res 2017;121(7):838–54.
31. Towbin JA, Lowe AM, Colan SD, et al. Incidence, Causes, and Outcomes of Dilated Cardiomyopathy in Children. JAMA 2006;296(15):1867–76.
32. Goldstein A, Falk MJ. Mitochondrial DNA Deletion Syndromes. In: Adam MP, Mirzaa GM, Pagon RA, et al, editors. GeneReviews®. Seattle, WA: University of Washington, Seattle; 1993. Available at: http://www.ncbi.nlm.nih.gov/books/NBK1203/. Accessed April 26, 2023.
33. Di Nora C, Paldino A, Miani D, et al. Heart Transplantation in Kearns-Sayre Syndrome. Transplantation 2019;103(12):e393–4.
34. Duran J, Martinez A, Adler E. Cardiovascular Manifestations of Mitochondrial Disease. Biology 2019;8(2):34.
35. Lorenzoni PJ, Scola RH, Kay CSK, et al. MERRF: Clinical features, muscle biopsy and molecular genetics in Brazilian patients. Mitochondrion 2011;11(3):528–32.
36. Kubaski F, de Oliveira Poswar F, Michelin-Tirelli K, et al. Mucopolysaccharidosis Type I. Diagn Basel Switz 2020;10(3):161.
37. del Carmen García del Rey M, Castrodeza J, Pinto Á, et al. Heart valve disease in Hurler-Scheie syndrome. Cardiol J 2022;29(5):875–7.
38. Eh S, Rj D. Types A and B Niemann-Pick disease. Mol Genet Metab 2017;120(1–2). https://doi.org/10.1016/j.ymgme.2016.12.008.
39. Tegtmeyer LC, Rust S, van Scherpenzeel M, et al. Multiple phenotypes in phosphoglucomutase 1 deficiency. N Engl J Med 2014;370(6):533–42.
40. Mayr JA, Haack TB, Graf E, et al. Lack of the mitochondrial protein acylglycerol kinase causes Sengers syndrome. Am J Hum Genet 2012;90(2):314–20.
41. Haghighi A, Haack TB, Atiq M, et al. Sengers syndrome: six novel AGK mutations in seven new families and review of the phenotypic and mutational spectrum of 29 patients. Orphanet J Rare Dis 2014;9(1):119.
42. Feingold B, Mahle WT, Auerbach S, et al. Management of Cardiac Involvement Associated With Neuromuscular Diseases: A Scientific Statement From the American Heart Association. Circulation 2017;136(13):e200–31.
43. Higgins AY, O'Halloran TD, Chang JD. Chemotherapy-induced cardiomyopathy. Heart Fail Rev 2015;20(6):721–30.
44. Robinson EL, Azodi M, Heymans S, et al. Anthracycline-Related Heart Failure: Certain Knowledge and Open Questions. Curr Heart Fail Rep 2020;17(6):357–64.
45. Brickler M, Raskin A, Ryan TD. Current State of Pediatric Cardio-Oncology: A Review. Child Basel Switz 2022;9(2):127.
46. Belzile-Dugas E, Eisenberg MJ. Radiation-Induced Cardiovascular Disease: Review of an Underrecognized Pathology. J Am Heart Assoc 2021;10(18):e021686.
47. Darby SC, Cutter DJ, Boerma M, et al. Radiation-related heart disease: current knowledge and future prospects. Int J Radiat Oncol Biol Phys 2010;76(3):656–65.
48. Day E, Rudd JHF. Alcohol use disorders and the heart. Addict Abingdon Engl 2019;114(9):1670–8.
49. Varga ZV, Ferdinandy P, Liaudet L, et al. Drug-induced mitochondrial dysfunction and cardiotoxicity. Am J Physiol Heart Circ Physiol 2015;309(9):H1453–67.
50. Elkattawy S, Alyacoub R, Al-Nassarei A, et al. Cocaine induced heart failure: report and literature review. J Community Hosp Intern Med Perspect 2021;11(4):547–50.
51. Umana E, Solares CA, Alpert MA. Tachycardia-induced cardiomyopathy. Am J Med 2003;114(1):51–5.

52. Khasnis A, Jongnarangsin K, Abela G, et al. Tachycardia-induced cardiomyopathy: a review of literature. Pacing Clin Electrophysiol PACE 2005;28(7):710–21.
53. Sadoh WE, Uduebor JO. Electrocardiographic changes and troponin T levels in children with severe malaria anemia and heart failure. Niger J Clin Pract 2017; 20(5):552–6.
54. Varat MA, Adolph RJ, Fowler NO. Cardiovascular effects of anemia. Am Heart J 1972;83(3):415–26.
55. Lopez A, Cacoub P, Macdougall IC, et al. Iron deficiency anaemia. Lancet Lond Engl 2016;387(10021):907–16.
56. Newman DB, Fidahussein SS, Kashiwagi DT, et al. Reversible cardiac dysfunction associated with hypocalcemia: a systematic review and meta-analysis of individual patient data. Heart Fail Rev 2014;19(2):199–205.
57. Baqi DH, Ahmed SF, Baba HO, et al. Hypocalcemia as a cause of reversible heart failure: A case report and review of the literature. Ann Med Surg 2022;77:103572.
58. Roman-Campos D, Cruz JS. Current aspects of thiamine deficiency on heart function. Life Sci 2014;98(1):1–5.
59. Rath A, Weintraub R. Overview of Cardiomyopathies in Childhood. Front Pediatr 2021;9. Available at: https://www.frontiersin.org/article/10.3389/fped.2021. 708732. Accessed June 30, 2022.
60. Ommen SR, Mital S, Burke MA, et al. 2020 AHA/ACC Guideline for the Diagnosis and Treatment of Patients With Hypertrophic Cardiomyopathy: Executive Summary: A Report of the American College of Cardiology/American Heart Association Joint Committee on Clinical Practice Guidelines. J Am Coll Cardiol 2020; 76(25):3022–55.
61. Basit H, Brito D, Sharma S. Hypertrophic Cardiomyopathy. [Updated 2023 Apr 7]. In: StatPearls [Internet]. Treasure Island (FL): StatPearls Publishing; 2023 Jan-. Available at: https://www.ncbi.nlm.nih.gov/books/NBK430788/. Accessed April 27, 2023.
62. Nguyen MB, Mital S, Mertens L, et al. Pediatric Hypertrophic Cardiomyopathy: Exploring the Genotype-Phenotype Association. J Am Heart Assoc 2022;11(5): e024220.
63. Monda E, Rubino M, Lioncino M, et al. Hypertrophic Cardiomyopathy in Children: Pathophysiology, Diagnosis, and Treatment of Non-sarcomeric Causes. Front Pediatr 2021;9. Available at: https://www.frontiersin.org/articles/10.3389/fped.2021. 632293. Accessed April 27, 2023.
64. Lioncino M, Monda E, Verrillo F, et al. Hypertrophic Cardiomyopathy in RASopathies. Heart Fail Clin 2022;18(1):19–29.
65. Arghami A, Dearani JA, Said SM, et al. Hypertrophic cardiomyopathy in children. Ann Cardiothorac Surg 2017;6(4):376–85.
66. Gajewski KK, Saul JP. Sudden cardiac death in children and adolescents (excluding Sudden Infant Death Syndrome). Ann Pediatr Cardiol 2010;3(2):107–12.
67. Towbin JA, Lorts A, Jefferies JL. Left ventricular non-compaction cardiomyopathy. Lancet Lond Engl 2015;386(9995):813–25.
68. Srivastava S, Yavari M, Al-Abcha A, et al. Ventricular non-compaction review. Heart Fail Rev 2022;27(4):1063–76.
69. Richard P, Ader F, Roux M, et al. Targeted panel sequencing in adult patients with left ventricular non-compaction reveals a large genetic heterogeneity. Clin Genet 2019;95(3):356–67.
70. Denfield SW, Rosenthal G, Gajarski RJ, et al. Restrictive cardiomyopathies in childhood. Etiologies and natural history. Tex Heart Inst J 1997;24(1):38–44.
71. Webber SA, Lipshultz SE, Sleeper LA, et al. Outcomes of Restrictive Cardiomyopathy in Childhood and the Influence of Phenotype. Circulation 2012;126(10):1237–44.

72. Rivenes SM, Kearney DL, Smith EO, et al. Sudden death and cardiovascular collapse in children with restrictive cardiomyopathy. Circulation 2000;102(8): 876–82.
73. Russo LM, Webber SA. Idiopathic restrictive cardiomyopathy in children. Heart 2005;91(9):1199–202.
74. Krahn AD, Wilde AAM, Calkins H, et al. Arrhythmogenic Right Ventricular Cardiomyopathy. JACC Clin Electrophysiol 2022;8(4):533–53.
75. Maron BJ, Doerer JJ, Haas TS, et al. Sudden deaths in young competitive athletes: analysis of 1866 deaths in the United States, 1980-2006. Circulation 2009;119(8):1085–92.
76. Marcus FI, McKenna WJ, Sherrill D, et al. Diagnosis of Arrhythmogenic Right Ventricular Cardiomyopathy/Dysplasia (ARVC/D). Circulation 2010;121(13):1533–41.
77. Rangaswami J, Bhalla V, Blair JEA, et al. Cardiorenal Syndrome: Classification, Pathophysiology, Diagnosis, and Treatment Strategies: A Scientific Statement From the American Heart Association. Circulation 2019;139(16):e840–78.
78. Mitsnefes MM. Cardiovascular Disease in Children with Chronic Kidney Disease. J Am Soc Nephrol JASN 2012;23(4):578–85.
79. Pradhan SK, Adnani H, Safadi R, et al. Cardiorenal syndrome in the pediatric population: A systematic review. Ann Pediatr Cardiol 2022;15(5 & 6):493.
80. Ceravolo G, Macchia TL, Cuppari C, et al. Update on the Classification and Pathophysiological Mechanisms of Pediatric Cardiorenal Syndromes. Children 2021; 8(7):528.
81. Raina R, Mahajan Z, Sharma A, et al. Hypertensive Crisis in Pediatric Patients: An Overview. Front Pediatr 2020;8:588911.
82. Hsu DT, Pearson GD. Heart failure in children: part I: history, etiology, and pathophysiology. Circ Heart Fail 2009;2(1):63–70.
83. Chang JC, Xiao R, Mercer-Rosa L, et al. Child-onset systemic lupus erythematosus is associated with a higher incidence of myopericardial manifestations compared to adult-onset disease. Lupus 2018;27(13):2146–54.
84. Marijon E, Mirabel M, Celermajer DS, et al. Rheumatic heart disease. Lancet Lond Engl 2012;379(9819):953–64.
85. Watkins DA, Johnson CO, Colquhoun SM, et al. Global, Regional, and National Burden of Rheumatic Heart Disease, 1990-2015. N Engl J Med 2017;377(8): 713–22.
86. Lahiri S, Sanyahumbi A. Acute Rheumatic Fever. Pediatr Rev 2021;42(5):221–32.
87. Kumar RK, Antunes MJ, Beaton A, et al. Contemporary Diagnosis and Management of Rheumatic Heart Disease: Implications for Closing the Gap: A Scientific Statement From the American Heart Association. Circulation 2020;142(20): e337–57.
88. Arvind B, Ramakrishnan S. Rheumatic Fever and Rheumatic Heart Disease in Children. Indian J Pediatr 2020;87(4):305–11.
89. Gewitz MH, Baltimore RS, Tani LY, et al. Revision of the Jones Criteria for the diagnosis of acute rheumatic fever in the era of Doppler echocardiography: a scientific statement from the American Heart Association. Circulation 2015;131(20): 1806–18.
90. Beaton A, Okello E, Rwebembera J, et al. Secondary Antibiotic Prophylaxis for Latent Rheumatic Heart Disease. N Engl J Med 2022;386(3):230–40.
91. Zagelbaum Ward NK, Linares-Koloffon C, Posligua A, et al. Cardiac Manifestations of Systemic Lupus Erythematous: An Overview of the Incidence, Risk Factors, Diagnostic Criteria, Pathophysiology and Treatment Options. Cardiol Rev 2022;30(1):38.

# Fever of Unknown Origin

Kathleen Ryan, MD, MPH*

## KEYWORDS

- FUO • Fever of unknown origin • PUO • Prolonged fever

## KEY POINTS

- A thorough history and physical examination is critical for identifying etiology of a fever of unknown origin (FUO).
- Causes of FUO in adolescents are broad and most commonly include infectious etiology, although autoimmune, connective tissue disorders, other inflammatory processes and malignancy are among the more than 200 etiologies.
- Connective tissue disorders and autoimmune disorders are more frequent causes of FUO in adolescents than in children.
- Classic FUO occuring in healthy adolescents without "red flag" symptoms with a normal physical exam and initial lab work up, and a negative diagnostic work up is reassuring for eventual resolution without sequel.

## INTRODUCTION
### Definition

Fever of unknown origin (FUO) has been recognized as a disease state for over 100 years. The first commonly accepted definition of FUO was published in 1961 and included (1) fever greater than 101° F (38.3° C) on multiple occasions (2) at least 3 week duration of fever (3) without identifiable cause despite at least a 1 week inpatient evaluation.[1] Overtime, this definition was considered both too rigid and too ill defined. Given the impracticality of prolonged hospitalizations and advancing technology for diagnosis, the duration of work up was shortened to 3 days inpatient evaluation and/or 3 outpatient clinic visits.[2]

Multiple sources suggest that all time requirements regarding the duration of evaluation be eliminated and instead FUO should be defined as a fever lacking known etiology after completing a minimum work up.[3–5] Additionally, the recommended minimum duration of fever to meet the definition of "FUO" has been decreased. Some studies suggest a minimum duration of 14 days of fevers to be considered in evaluations of FUO.[6–8] Other studies suggested that evaluation for "FUO" can begin in as little as 5 to 7 days of fever in pediatric patients.[8–10] Starting evaluation at shorter

Infectious Disease, Department of Pediatric, Medical College of Wisconsin & Children's Hospital of Wisconsin, Suite C450, 999 North 92 nd Street, Wauwatosa, WI 53226, USA
* Corresponding author.
*E-mail address:* ktryan@mcw.edu

duration is also appropriate in certain patient populations (see Considerations later in discussion).

Given the heterogeneity of the etiology of FUO, individualized approach to patients with FUO has always been recommended. Although this personalized approach allows for more tailored care, the lack of consistency in diagnostic criteria does present problems when attempting to define the prevalence, shifting dynamics of etiology, and following outcomes for FUO on a population level.

## Incidence

Fevers of unknown origin occur worldwide to people of all ages. As noted above, inconsistencies in inclusion criteria over time and geographic location limits the generalizability of any study results. The limited data that exists demonstrated FUO accounts for almost 3% of hospital admissions in adults.[11] Additional data suggests an incidence of 0.5% to 3% of hospital admission in pediatric patients are a result of FUOs.[8,12] Studies demonstrate adolescents make up approximately 20% to 25% of all pediatric patients with FUO.[6,10]

Although different studies have shown varying incidence of gender predominance, two different systemic reviews of adults with FUO have indicated there may be, at most, a slight increase incidence of male over females (55% males and 50% females).[13,14] Single site studies from both US and Korea also found an increase incidence in males (53%–65%) overall in the pediatric population as well.[6,10,15] The subset of patients ultimately found to have connective tissue disorders are predominantly female.[6]

## Nature of The Problem

Fevers of unknown origin (FUO) are caused by over 200 different etiologies.[16] (**Table 1**). The etiology of FUO can be subdivided into four major etiologic subcategories including (1) infectious, (2) non-infectious inflammatory or autoimmune disorders (sometimes only including connective tissue disorders) (3) malignancy and (4) other. Overall, an increasing proportion of FUO fall into a fifth category in which no etiology is ever found.

The relative incidence of different etiologic subgroups of FUO vary throughout the world. Locations in Asia had three to four times greater rate of infectious causes for FUO compared to Europe.[13] In comparison, centers in Europe found a significantly higher relative incidence of "no etiology ever found" in FUO cases. Presumably, the increased availability of rapid diagnostic testing resulted in the establishment of diagnosis in patient who would have previously been identified as FUO by 14 to 21 days.[13]

Historically, infectious etiologies have been the predominant cause of FUO in both children and adults throughout the world. When comparing studies by similar authors over time, the incidence of infectious causes has decreased over time.[11,13,14] This is presumably also related to faster diagnosis of many of these infectious etiology,[17] although decreasing rates of many previously common infectious agents can also be contributing to these results. FUO in children (including adolescents) have even higher relative rates of infectious etiology than adults. Relative rates of infectious triggers of pediatric FUO vary widely in studies (17%–50%)[6,8] while infectious causes of FUO in adults ranges closer to 15% to 35%.[5]

Within the US, a single site study of pediatric FUO reported viral etiology in almost 9% of cases caused by agents including Epstein Barr virus, cytomegalovirus, other herpes viruses, metapneumovirus, and enterovirus. Bacterial infections were often localized infections (septic arthritis, gluteal abscess, parapneumonic effusion, intraabdominal infection, endocarditis). Specific bacterial pathogens identified included

**Table 1**
**Causes of fever of unknown origin (FUO)**

Infectious

| | | |
|---|---|---|
| Abscesses | Bacterial diseases | Rickettsiae |
| Abdominal | Actinomycosis | African tick-bite fever |
| Brain | Bartonella henselae (cat- | Anaplasmosis |
| Dental | scratch) | Ehrlichia canis |
| Hepatic | Brucellosis | Ehrlichiosis (E chaffeensis, |
| Paraspinal | Campylobacter | E ewingii) |
| Pelvic | Chlamydia | Q fever (Coxiella burnetii) |
| Perinephric | Francisella tularensis | Rocky Mountain spotted |
| Rectal | (tularemia) | fever |
| Retroperitoneal | Listeria monocytogenes | Tick-borne typhus |
| Subphrenic | (listeriosis) | Spirochetes |
| Psoas | Meningococcemia | Borrelia burgdorferi (Lyme |
| Infected urachal cyst | (chronic) | disease) |
| Vertebral | Mycobacterium (non- | Relapsing fever (Borrelia |
| Viruses | tuberculosis) | recurrentis) |
| Adenovirus | Mycoplasma pneumoniae | Leptospirosis |
| Arborviruses | Neisseria meningitis | Rat-bite fever (Spirillum |
| Cytomegalovirus | (chronic) | minus) |
| Epstein-Barr virus | Rat-bite fever | Syphilis |
| Hanta Virus | (Streptobacillus | Parasitic diseases |
| Hepatitis viruses | moniliformis) | Amebiasis |
| HIV | Salmonella | Babesiosis |
| Human picornavirus | Tuberculosis | Giardiasis |
| Fungal diseases | Whipple disease | Leishmania |
| Blastomycosis | Yersiniosis | Malaria |
| (extrapulmonary) | Tuberculosis | Toxoplasmosis |
| Coccidioidomycosis | Localized infections | Trichinosis |
| (disseminated) | Cholangitis | Trypanosomiasis |
| Histoplasmosis | Infective endocarditis | Visceral larva migrans |
| (disseminated) | Lymphogranuloma | (Toxocara canis/cati) |
| | venereum | |
| | Mastoiditis | |
| | Osteomyelitis | |
| | Pneumonia | |
| | Pyelonephritis | |
| | Psittacosis | |
| | Sinusitis | |

Non-Infectious Immune-Mediated Diseases

| | | |
|---|---|---|
| Rheumatologic diseases | Miscellaneous inflammatory | Granulomatous diseases |
| Autoimmune cholangitis | Hemophagocytic | Granulomatosis with |
| Aortitis | syndromes | polyangiitis |
| Behçet disease | Kawasaki disease | Crohn disease |
| Juvenile dermatomyositis | Kikuchi-Fujimoto disease | Granulomatous colitis |
| Juvenile idiopathic arthritis | Immunoblastic | Granulomatous hepatitis |
| Rheumatic fever | lymphadenopathy | Granulomatous peritonitis |
| Sjögren syndrome | Löfgren syndrome | Sarcoidosis |
| Systemic lupus | Periodic fever syndromes | Ulcerative colitis |
| erythematosus | Schnitzler syndrome | Vasculitis syndrome |
| Polyarteritis nodosa | Subacute necrotizing | |
| | lymphadenitis | |

(continued on next page)

**Table 1**
*(continued)*

Malignancies

| | | |
|---|---|---|
| Hodgkin disease | Atrial myxoma | Cholesterol granuloma |
| Non-Hodgkin's Lymphoma | Hepatocellular carcinoma | Inflammatory pseudotumor |
| Leukemia | Neuroblastoma | Pheochromocytoma |
| Wilms tumor | Other solid tumor malignancies | Lymphomatoid granulomatosis |
| | | Myeloproliferative syndromes |

Other

| | | |
|---|---|---|
| Hypersensitivity diseases | Miscellaneous | Miscellaneous (continued) |
| Drug fever | Addison disease | Paroxysmal |
| Hype eosinophilic syndrome | Castleman disease | hemoglobinurias |
| Hypersensitivity pneumonitis | Chronic active hepatitis | Pericarditis |
| Serum sickness | Cyclic neutropenia | Poisoning |
| Weber-Christian disease | Diabetes insipidus (central and nephrogenic) | Postpericardiotomy syndrome |
| Familial & Hereditary | Drug fever | Pulmonary embolism |
| Anhidrotic ectodermal dysplasia | Factitious fever | Resorbing hematoma |
| Autonomic neuropathies | Hemoglobinopathies | Retroperitoneal fibrosis |
| Fabry disease | Hemolytic anemias | Rosai-Dorfman disease |
| Familial dysautonomia | Hypothalamic-central fever | Thrombophlebitis |
| Familial Hibernian fever | Infantile cortical hyperostosis | Thyrotoxicosis, thyroiditis |
| Familial Mediterranean fever | Metal fume fever | Thrombotic thrombocytopenic purpura |
| Hypertriglyceridemia | Pancreatitis | Venoocclusive disease |
| Ichthyosis | Parathyroid apoplexy | Vitamin B 12 deficiency |
| other autoinflammatory diseases | | |
| Sickle cell crisis | | |
| Spinal cord/brain injury | | |

Adapted from Steenhoff, A., *Fever of Unknown Origin*, in *Nelson textbook of pediatrics*, R. Kliegman, and colleagues, Editors. 2016, Elsevier: Philadelphia, Pennsylvania. p. 1397 to 1402.; with permission.

Bartonella, Clostridium difficile, Ehrlichiosis, and Staphylococcus. Although rare, fungal infections were also noted in his study.[10]

Non-infectious inflammatory disease (NIID) conditions including autoinflammatory, autoimmune, and collagen vascular diseases are common causes of FUO. The most common causes of NIID conditions in children included juvenile idiopathic arthritis (JIA), inflammatory bowel disorders, and systemic lupus erythematosus.[7,8] Increasing relative incidence of NIID conditions causing FUO is occurring over time. It is hypothesized that better diagnostic testing has allowed more diagnosis of immune-mediated disease to be made in patients with FUO who would have previously lacked any definitive diagnosis. The true relative incidence of non-infectious inflammatory conditions is difficult to compare between studies as some separate out collagen vascular disease as a category but classify other inflammatory conditions (including inflammatory bowel diseases) with rheumatological/collagen vascular diseases. There is also debate on whether some conditions such as Kawasaki disease, Kikuchi Fujimoto, periodic fever syndromes, or monogenic autoinflammatory disorders would be considered as non-infections inflammatory versus "other" causes of FUO. However, the overall entire non-infectious inflammatory/autoimmune conditions are thought to make up at between 10% and 30% of FUO[6,8,10]

There is mixed evidence of changes in the relative rates of malignancy-related FUO. Although infectious etiologies are decreasing compared to other etiologies, better imaging techniques may also result in earlier diagnosis of malignancy (thereby resulting in relatively proportion decrease in malignancy-related diagnosis as well). The overall relative incidence of malignancy in children and adolescents ranged from < 5% to almost 18%.[6,8,10] However, when broken down by age, older children and adolescents made up approximately 5% of cases.[6] The most common malignancies include lymphoma (Hodgkin's and non-Hodgkin lymphoma) and leukemia. Other malignancy reported in children and adolescents include Wilms tumor, neuroblastoma, myelodysplastic syndromes,[8] and hepatocellular carcinoma.[10]

Other causes of FUO are vast. As mentioned above, some studies include multiple inflammatory or immune-mediated diseases such as Kawasaki disease (and presumably similar disease states such as multisystem inflammatory syndrome in children (MIS-C)) and Kikuchi Fujimoto (necrotizing lymphadenitis) as part of the "other" category.[7,17] However, additional etiologies include blood clots (pulmonary embolism, deep vein thrombosis or hematomas in closed spaces, central etiology (dysautonomia, diabetes insipidus, central thermoregulation issues), and hyperthyroid. Important etiology within the "other" category that need to be excluded include factitious, drug related, "habitual" hyperthermia (condition in which exam, history and minimal work up is reassuring in patients with temperatures > 100 but <101 F persistently (low grade).[18]

Fevers of unknown origin for which no cause is ever determined can range from 20% to almost 45% of pediatric cases.[6,8] As diagnosis of infections, malignancy and immune dysregulation syndromes continue to be quicker, many predict this category of "unknown" etiology may continue to grow over time.

There are significant differences is the etiology of FUO based on geography. In a recent systemic review/meta-analysis of data, etiology of FUO varied significantly depending on geographic location. The highest prevalence of infectious etiology of FUO was found in southeast Asia at 49% of their cases. Inflammatory disorders were found in approximately 20% of all cases worldwide but the highest prevalence was in the western pacific region with 34% of their cases being from inflammation conditions. Cancer was found in 15% of all studies with the highest rate (at 24%) in the eastern Mediterranean region. Similarly, "other" etiology for FUO was found in 6% of cases but up to 9% in the western Pacific region.[19,20]

The combination of local geographic exposure affecting incidence of FUO as well as the changes in diagnostic tools over time makes it difficult to isolate out or compare information in adolescents alone. Most data in adolescents comes from pediatric case reports. However, understanding adult data is also important to understand the trends from pediatric through adulthood to better understand adolescent populations.

In comparison to children 5 and under, older children and adolescents are four times more likely to have connective tissue disorder at almost 20% of all FUO. The rates of immune disorder/connective tissue disorder was especially elevated in older children and adolescents in whom fever had persisted for > 28 days.[6]

### Considerations

Understanding the underlying health conditions and exposure history of patients is critical to appreciating the urgency and direction of work up for patients with FUO. As a result, patients who develop FUO can also be subdivided into categories. Traditionally, the vast majority of patients who developed FUO were otherwise fairly healthy. These patients are considered to have "classic" FUO. This is to separate them from three other distinct categories of "FUO." In the early 1990s, additional patient categories were proposed including health care associated fevers, neutropenic FUO, and human immunodeficiency virus (HIV)-related FUO.[2] Overtime, the categories including neutropenic and HIV related were combined with other immunocompromised state resulting in a new category of immunodeficiencies related FUO.[21] Additionally, a category of FUO in returned travelers has also been proposed.[3]

The initial criteria for neutropenic FUO included patients with an absolute neutrophil count (ANC) of less than 500 per mm3[5] or 1000 per mm3 who had fevers on multiple occasions of at least 101 F for with a negative work up for at least 3 days.[2] The overwhelming majority of FUOs in this category are thought to be from infectious etiology, even with a negative work up. Other special considerations within this category include drug-induced fevers (chemotherapy or other drug), underlying malignancy or other immune deregulatory disorder. Special emphasis of physical examination should focus on IV sites, lungs, perianal and skin folds.

As noted above, the subcategory of FUO in persons living with HIV/AIDS was proposed in 1991 (prior to the availability of retroviral therapy). However, as the risks of various etiology of FUO are likely related to underlying immune function rather than HIV itself, we recommend that patients with advanced HIV/AIDS who develop FUO be considered as one group of FUO in the immunocompromised host category.[21]

Individuals with immunocompromised states presenting with FUO can have a wide range of disease processes. This category includes patients with chemotherapy-induced neutropenia, immunosuppressant therapy for hematologic or solid organ transplantation, chronic corticosteroid use, use of biological modifying agents (eg, monoclonal antibody therapy or TNF alpha blockers), or individuals with advanced HIV with or without acquired immunodeficiency syndrome (HIV/AIDS).[21] Because of the vast degree of various risk factors, work up, and empiric treatment recommendations for people within this category, complete recommendations for this category is beyond the scope of this article. Unlike recommendations to withhold antibiotics in most "classic" FUO, patients within in category are recommend to start empiric antibiotics and antifungal therapy given the potential seriousness of infections in this population.

Criteria for health care associated FUO includes a hospitalized patient with multiple fevers of greater than 101 F (38.3 C) for at least 3 days which were not present or developing prior to admission. Work up must be negative with cultures negative for at least 48 hours.[2,5] Etiology of FUO in this cohort of patients includes health care-associated infections (eg, Clostridium difficile), post-operative complications (including deep vein thrombosis or pulmonary embolism), wound infections, line-associated infections, drug fevers and fevers from underlying disease process for which the patient is admitted.[2]

Given different exposure and potential evaluation, FUO in the returning traveler is proposed to be considered its own category. FUO in this population are felt to include more infectious processes. However, as traveling to a location will often result in the similar risks to a traveler as the local risk of endemic disease in that location, a focus on traveling should rather focus on endemic diseases in all the different locations for which a person has lived or stayed in. For providers in the US, this can include being familiar with local risk factors for various parts of the country, but also include many tropical diseases not commonly seen in the US as well as disease such as tuberculosis (TB) and other infections for which the incidence is higher in other countries. (See also Evaluation later in discussion).

## APPROACH

When patients initially present to medical attention for prolonged fevers, the initial steps should always be attempting to verify that fevers truly exist. Whenever possible, the documentation of fevers in the medical system is ideal. However, as many adolescents with FUO are otherwise healthy with outpatient evaluations, this can be more challenging. Families should be encouraged to document fevers at least twice daily using a fever diary. This can demonstrate not only the existence of fevers, but also identify frequency, severity, and any patterns of fevers.

Factitious features may be accidental (broken home thermometer, belief that reported temperatures must "add 1° to axillary temperatures"). However, history should also evaluate for the possibility of true factious fever.

A compete review of current and past history is essential in the evaluation of FUO. History should include any previous episodes of prolonged or unidentifiable fevers, preceding illnesses, and extensive exposure history (**Table 2**). Risk factors for tuberculosis exposure need to be evaluated including: exposure to individuals with TB,

---

**Table 2**
**Initial Evalution**

**History**

| Exposure | Family History | Other History |
|---|---|---|
| Sick Contacts | Recurrent Fever Syndromes | Local/National Travel |
| Animals | Unexplained or Frequent | International Travel |
| International Travers | Fevers in Childhood | Weight loss |
| Blood products (tattoos, | Autoimmune diseases | Anorexia |
| piercings, transfusions) | Medication | Sexual Activity/Prevention |
| Contaminated Water | Prescribed | of STD |
| (including wells) | Over the Counter | Immunization |
| Fresh water | Herbal Therapy | Medications |
| Tick & Mosquito | Illicit Drug Use | Recent Illnesses |
| Others with tuberculosis | | |
| Unpasteurized Foods | | |

**Key Exam Findings**

| Skin | Abdominal | Temperature |
|---|---|---|
| Rashes | Pain | Blood Pressure |
| Petechia | Organomegaly | Heart Rate |
| Focal abnormalities | Stool changes | Documented Weight |
| Lymphadenopathy | Musculoskeletal | changes |
| Mucosal Changes | Joint Swelling | Linear Growth Curve Pattern |
| Conjunctivitis | Bony Tenderness | |
| | Myalgia | |

**Minimum evaluation**

| Blood culture (x2) | Chest X ray | Consider: |
|---|---|---|
| Urinalysis ± Urine culture | | Abdominal Imaging |
| Complete blood count (CBC) | | HIV Testing |
| with differential | | QuantiFERON/PPD |
| Complete metabolic panel | | |
| Peripheral Smear | | |
| Erythrocyte Sedimentation | | |
| Rate (ESR) | | |
| C Reactive Protein (CRP) | | |

Adapted from Chusid, M.J., *Fever of Unknown Origin in Childhood.* Pediatr Clin North Am, 2017. 64(1): p. 205 to 230.; with permission

chronic cough, homelessness, incarceration or institutionalization, immigration or international travelers. Additionally a patient's HIV status and home environment including previous or current history of living on a reservation or history of international travel should also be examined.[9]

A thorough physical exam is also essential. If the patient is febrile at the time of examination, vitals should be evaluated for any compensatory changes to heart rate or blood pressure. Growth curves should be evaluated for height velocity and weight gain over time. Key exam findings are also described in **Table 2**. In addition to the examination performed in the office or hospital, any history of abnormal findings (abnormal joint findings, evanescent rash, and so forth) are also important to ask about.[9]

Concerning "red flags" in the history should include unexplained weight loss, anorexia, focal symptoms, or persistent high fever. Concerning physical exam findings include organomegaly, rash, clubbing, lymphadenopathy or any focal findings.[9]

Current definition for FUO includes a minimum investigative work up without finding an identifiable cause (see **Table 2**). This includes complete blood count, metabolic panel, erythrocyte sedimentation rate, C reactive protein, and urinalysis with culture and blood cultures in addition to a chest x-ray. Although some studies indicate abdominal imaging should be included in initial evaluation, this is not part of the standard work up for pediatric patients with FUO.[13]

## EVALUATION

Assuming this initial work up is negative, further work up is recommended based on clues provided by repeated examination of history and/or progression of any exam findings. Finding diagnostic clues on history, exam or labs can more than double (72% vs 30%) the chance of making a diagnosis in FUO.[14]

The fever curve itself is important for the evaluation of possible etiology. Fevers can be recurrent (fever which had resolved and then restarted), periodic (fever with a regular pattern of recurrence) or persistent.

In individuals who present with periodic or recurrent fevers ("chronic episodic fever of unknown origin"), it is important to consider periodic fever, aphthous stomatitis, pharyngitis, adenitis (PFAPA), cyclic neutropenia, or one of the several monogenetic recurrent fever syndromes. Monogenetic recurrent fever syndromes include tumor necrosis factor (TNF) receptor-associated periodic fever (TRAPS), Familiar Mediterranean Fever (FMF), cryopyrin-associated periodic fever (CAPS), mevalonate kinase deficiency (MKD, hyper IgD or HIDS).[18] Most recurrent fever syndromes present before the age of 5 and are therefore unlikely to present with new onset FUO in adolescents. However, if history suggests previous recurrent episodes for multiple years, these could be considered. Additionally, FMF and TRAPS can occasionally present later in life and should be considered in adolescents with periodic fevers of unknown etiology.[7] Fevers associated with TRAPS typically last 7 to 21 days with gaps between fever episodes lasting months to years. Associated physical exam findings include migratory myalgias with skin erythema, conjunctivitis, and periorbital edema. FMF can cause periodic fevers of 1 to 3 days duration with periods between fever episodes of weeks to years. Exam findings in FMF include rash, polyserositis, and scrotal pain (in males) or abdominal pain.[7]

Providers caring for adolescent presenting with recurrent fever must also consider a high probability of sequential limited self-resolving fevers (such as back-to-back illnesses). If history suggests exposures or symptoms of recurrent self-limiting illnesses, watchful waiting may be the most appropriate next step. If, however, the degree of recurrent illness seems out of proportion to local epidemiology or exposure history, providers could consider evaluation for acquired immunodeficiencies.

In adolescents with persistent FUO, a step-wise approach for the investigation of the FUO is recommended.[14] Other than chest x-ray (CXR) and blood cultures, most of the initial minimum work up is used to guide subsequent evaluation testing. Any abnormalities in initial lab work should have focused subsequent testing. Additional clues obtained by repeatedly collecting history and serial examination of patients should also guide subsequent testing.

Any patient with significant exposure history (travel, animal exposure, tick/mosquito exposure) or suggestive work up should have targeted special consideration testing (**Table 3**). Patients with abdominal findings should be evaluated for intraabdominal abscess, inflammatory bowel, cholangitis and infectious hepatitis viruses. On the other hand, patients with skin and joint manifestations may benefit from a focus on rheumatological or other inflammatory conditions (including genetic and recurrent fever syndromes). Skin manifestations such as splinter hemorrhages could suggest infective endocarditis.

Additional work up can include further immunologic evaluation, screening tests for various malignancies where available and targeting non-culture-based infectious work up (especially PCR/NAAT testing for difficult to culture infectious agents). More extensive imaging can also be considered based on focused concerns (see **Table 3**).

Care should also be taking to avoid false positives given the extensive and potentially continuing work up of fever in patients who otherwise appear well without any "red flags." As with any testing, frequent testing of low prevalent disease often result in more false positive than true positive. This can lead to unnecessary evaluation with financial and emotional implications for the patient and their family.

### Imaging

At minimum, a normal CXR is a requirement for investigation prior to establishing a diagnosis of FUO. Some studies also include normal abdominal and pelvis ultrasound and/or CT abdomen and pelvis to qualify as a FUO.[13,14] In the pediatric population, many question the standard use of abdominal imaging in patients without any abdominal symptoms (abdominal pain, organomegaly, bowel changes or abnormalities on complete metabolic panel).[10] However, abdominal imaging is commonly performed as part of a later step of the approach toward FUO in both adults and pediatrics (if not performed earlier).

Additional imaging modalities could be considered based on higher suspicion of possible etiology. For example, if there is any history concerning for inflammatory bowel disease, CT or MRI enterography could be considered. Alternatively, whole-body MRI could be considered for patients suspected to have occult osteomyelitis or chronic recurrent multifocal osteomyelitis.

Multiple adults study suggest that it is cost-effective to consider an early PET CT scan in patients with FUO. PET scan can detect inflammation due to infections, noninfectious inflammatory disease and malignancies, all of which are common etiology of FUO. PET-CT has been demonstrated to be cost-effective in adult studies primarily by decreasing the length of hospital admission.[22] Even in cases where a definitive diagnosis cannot be made, using previous testing and PET-CT can result in ability to obtain a targeted biopsy site sooner allowing for more rapid diagnosis (and therefore shorter hospitalization). Although there are some studies involving the use of PET-CT in children for inflammation with or without FUO,[23] the role of PET-CT is less clear in pediatrics. In addition to the concerns of cost, radiation exposure and utility,[6] the availability of PET CT in most pediatric centers is also significantly limited.

| Table 3 Advanced work up for FUO | | |
|---|---|---|
| **Initial Considerations** | | |
| QuantiFERON/TB Screen | Ferritin | Abdominal Imaging |
| CSF studies and culture | LDH | Echocardiogram |
| Stool O& P | Uric Acid | CT Abdomen/Pelvis |
| HIV testing | ANA | CT Chest |
| EBV Antibody/NAAT/PCR | Rheumatoid Factor | CT Sinus |
| CMV Antibody/NAAT/PCR | ds DNA | Whole Body MRI |
| Stool culture/NAAT/PCR | quantitative immunoglobulin levels | |
| Adenovirus NAAT/PCR | Thyroid-stimulating hormone (TSH) | |
| Mycoplasma NAAT/PCR | Complement - C3, C4, CH50 | |
| | Antibody response to vaccine (titers) | |
| | ANCA, ASMA, ASCA, LKM | |
| **Special Considerations** | | |
| Animal Exposures | "Travel" Related | Other Exposure |
| Brucella (Goats, cattle) | Malaria smear (endemic areas) | Naegleria (water) |
| Q fever (Sheep) | Dengue | Legionella (water) |
| Salmonella | Chikungunya | Toxocara (pica) |
| Bartonella antibodies (cats, fleas) | Hantavirus | Ticks/Mosquitos |
| Lymphocytic choriomeningitis (mice) | Coccidiomycosis | Lyme disease |
| Baylisascaris (raccoon) | Blastomycosis | Rickettsia (multiple) |
| Psittacosis (Birds) | Histoplasmosis | Borrelia (non-lyme) |
| Toxoplasmosis (Cat) | Paracoccidiomycosis | |
| Rat Bite Fever (rat) | Human T lymphocytic virus (HTLV) | |
| | Visceral Leishmaniasis | |
| | Cryptococcus | |
| **Advanced Considerations** | | |
| PET - CT | Biopsy | Next-generation sequencing for infectious agents |
| Whole body MRI | | Genome Testing panel vs whole genome vs whole exome |

*Abbreviaitons:* ANCA, antineutrophilic cytoplasmic antibody; ASCA, anti-saccharomyces cerevisiae antibody; ASMA, anti-smooth muscle antibody; CT, computerized tomography; MRI, magnetic resonance imaging; NAAT–nucleic acid amplification testing; PCR, polymerase chain reaction.
    Adapted from: Chusid, M.J., *Fever of Unknown Origin in Childhood.* Pediatr Clin North Am, 2017. 64(1): p. 205 to 230.; with permission.

## OUTCOMES

Outcomes related to FUO are typically correlated to the outcomes associated with the underlying etiology found. Older articles have reported 6% to 9% mortality rate in pediatric FUO. More recent publications in pediatrics suggest overall good prognosis in almost all patients with FUO.

Interestingly, one studying looking at long-term follow-up in adults with FUO did demonstrate a slightly higher incidence of malignancy for up to a year post-FUO (not diagnosed during the FUO evaluation). This was primarily due to increased rates of Hodgkin's lymphoma and non-Hodgkin's lymphoma as well as myelodysplastic/

myeloproliferative disorders.[24] Limited follow-up studies in pediatrics demonstrate that most recover without sequela, although there are a few cases later diagnosed with JIA or other causes of their previous FUO (such as recurrent intussusception) when followed for several years after FUO episode.[25] Another follow-up study in pediatrics demonstrates some patients will go on to develop a diagnosis of autoimmune or inflammatory disorders (such as uveitis, Crohn's).[26]

## FUTURE DIRECTIONS

Current technology has dramatically changed the dynamic of FUO over the past 100 years. As more, faster, cheaper, and better diagnostic technology continues to become available, more etiologies that would have otherwise been undiagnosable FUO will be recognized. On the other hand, more rapid diagnosis may further decrease the total incidence of FUO in the future, as fewer patients will have persistentent fevers for 2 or 3 weeks without an identifiable cause. However, to be able to follow changes over time, diagnostic criteria will need to be consistent, and studies will need to be conducted to determine the true incidence of FUO in the general population (or in the various FUO subset populations).

Already, tertiary centers and research studies are using advanced technology to diagnose infections and genetic autoimmune/inflammatory conditions which could present at FUO. Next generations sequencing of human plasma looking for infectious DNA is commercially available in the US and other parts of the world. This can potentially detect more infectious processes which would be responsible for FUO.[27]

Genomic sequencing is already being used to diagnosis monogenic autoimmune periodic fever syndromes. Additional genetic tests are likely to be discovered for more NIID processes in the future. Genome sequencing has been used to identify host factors related to fevers. FUO are often called uncommon presentations of common diseases. One study examined whole exome genome in 15 cases of FUO in China (seven later found to have infectious causes). Some were found to have genetic predisposition for infectious risk (GATA 2, CFTR mutation) with almost half the cases mentioning a genetic variant of uncertain significance in genes of interest related to fever pathway or risk factors for infectious disease.[28] This novel approach to identifying human host pathways may explain why common diseases are presenting in an uncommon fashion is intriguing, but care must be taken to minimize overinterpretation, especially in variants of uncertain significance.

Metabolomics refers to the study patterns of small molecule metabolites (lipids, sugars, amino acids, and so forth) to determine what causes those small molecule patterns. This can be analyzed using nuclear magnetic resonance (NMR) spectroscopy or mass spectroscopy. Commercially available products already exist to identify the name of microbial growth on plates in microbiology labs. However, metabolomics may be used increasing in patient-derived samples. Research studies have demonstrated the ability to detect infectious pathogen signs in hosts.[29] However, like other developing technologies, care in interpretation must be used as previously identified "signals" of infection were later identified to be non-specific inflammatory signals rather than unique targets to specific infectious disease processes.

Many of these developing technologies are currently expensive and of uncertain significance in FUO. However, it is possible that with further study and more cost-effective models, one or several of these may become of use in FUO in the future. More rigorous study would need to be conducted to ensure these more broad range "shot gun" approaches to FUO do not yield more incidental positive results which are not related to the patient's actual condition.

## DISCUSSION

Better culture and non-culture techniques (eg NAAT/PCR) for infectious etiology, improved imaging (CT, MRI, PET) and more, faster available testing for non-infectious immunologic disorders has dramatically changed the nature of FUO work up since it was first recognized over 100 years ago. Despite this, fever of unknown origin remains a diagnostic dilemma for many providers. With significant variation in the incidence of etiology of FUO throughout the world and limited data in the US, it can be challenging to fully appreciate the etiology of FUO in adolescents within the US.

Although rates of infectious etiology for FUO may be decreasing, this still appears to account for the largest percentage of FUOs for which an identifiable cause is found in both children and adults. Adolescents do have increasing connective tissue and other NIID etiology at higher rates than general pediatric populations. Despite advances in technology, a large percentage of FUO remain without identifiable etiology even after fevers resolve.

## SUMMARY

Fevers of unknown origin (FUO) remain a diagnostic dilemma. The differential remains broad with etiology most commonly including infectious, autoimmune, and malignant related. A significant portion of adolescents with FUO may never have an identifiable etiology found. However, the prognosis of FUO without determined etiology and in the absence of "red flag" symptoms is overall reassuring.

## CLINICS CARE POINTS

- To be considered a FUO, a fever should be present for > 14 to 21 days with negative/ reassuring exam and lab evaluation including CBC with differential, complete metabolic panel, urinalysis, urine and blood culture, ESR, CRP, CXR.
- In clinical practice, more rapid investigation for prolonged fevers is often started by 7 days into fever
- Fever history should differentiate between recurrent, periodic, and persistent fever
- Extensive exposure history and serial physical exams are important steps toward a targeted approach to work up classic FUO
- While over 200 possible etiology exist, patients with FUO often go undiagnosed.
- Prognosis is generally favorable in patients with FUO without "red flag" symptoms, especially in those without identifiable etiology after work up

## DISCLOSURE

The author has no disclosures.

## REFERENCES

1. Petersdorf RG, Beeson PB. Fever of unexplained origin: report on 100 cases. Medicine 1961;40(1):1–30.
2. Durack DT. Fever of unknown origin ? reexamined and redefined. Curr Clin Top Inf Dis 1991;11:35–51.
3. Haidar G, Singh N. Fever of Unknown Origin. N Engl J Med 2022;386(5):463–77.

4.  Bleeker-Rovers CP, Vos FJ, de Kleijn EMHA, et al. A prospective multicenter study on fever of unknown origin: the yield of a structured diagnostic protocol. Medicine (Baltimore) 2007;86(1):26–38.

5.  Knockaert DC, Vanderschueren S, Blockmans D. Fever of unknown origin in adults: 40 years on. J Intern Med 2003;253(3):263–75.

6.  Kim Y.S., Kim K.R., Kang J.M., et al., Etiology and clinical characteristics of fever of unknown origin in children: a 15-year experience in a single center, *Korean J Pediatr*, 60 (3), 2017, 77–85.

7.  Manthiram K, Edwards KM, Long SS. Prolonged, Recurrent and Periodic Fever Syndromes. In: Long SS, Prober CG, Fischer M, editors. Principles and practice of pediatric infectious diseases E-Book. Philadelphia, PA: Elsevier Health Sciences; 2022. p. 117–28.

8.  Chow A, Robinson JL. Fever of unknown origin in children: a systematic review. World Journal of Pediatrics 2011;7(1):5.

9.  Chusid MJ. Fever of Unknown Origin in Childhood. Pediatr Clin North Am 2017; 64(1):205–30.

10. Antoon J.W., Peritz D.C., Parsons M.R., et al., Etiology and Resource Use of Fever of Unknown Origin in Hospitalized Children, *Hosp Pediatr*, 8 (3), 2018, 135–140.

11. Iikuni Y., Okada J., Kondo H., et al., Current Fever of Unknown Origin 1982-1992, *Internal Medicine*, 33 (2), 1994, 67–73.

12. Chouchane S, Chouchane CH, Ben Meriem CH, et al. Les fièvres prolongées de l'enfant. Étude rétrospective de 67 cas Prolonged fever in children. Retrospective study of 67 cases. Archives de pédiatrie 2004;11:1319–25.

13. Fusco FM, Pisapia R, Nardiello S, et al. Fever of unknown origin (FUO): which are the factors influencing the final diagnosis? A 2005-2015 systematic review. BMC Infect Dis 2019;19(1):653.

14. Gaeta GB, Fusco FM, Nardiello S. Fever of unknown origin: a systematic review of the literature for 1995–2004. Nucl Med Commun 2006;27(3):205–11.

15. Cho CY, Lai CC, Lee ML, et al. Clinical analysis of fever of unknown origin in children: A 10-year experience in a northern Taiwan medical center. J Microbiol Immunol Infect 2017;50(1):40–5.

16. Arnow PM, Flaherty JP. Fever of unknown origin. Lancet 1997;350(9077):575–80.

17. Steenhoff A., Fever of Unknown Origin, In: Kliegman R., St Geme J.W., Blum N.J., et al., *Nelson textbook of pediatrics*, 2020, Elsevier; Philadelphia, Pennsylvania, 1397–1402.

18. Attard L., Tadolini M., De Rose D.U., et al., Overview of fever of unknown origin in adult and paediatric patients, *Clin Exp Rheumatol*, 36 (Suppl 110), 2018, 10–24.

19. Wright WF, Betz JF, Auwaerter PG. Prospective Studies Comparing Structured vs Nonstructured Diagnostic Protocol Evaluations Among Patients With Fever of Unknown Origin: A Systematic Review and Meta-analysis. JAMA Netw Open 2022; 5(6):e2215000.

20. Wright WF, Yenokyan G, Auwaerter PG. Geographic Influence Upon Noninfectious Diseases Accounting for Fever of Unknown Origin: A Systematic Review and Meta-Analysis. Open Forum Infect Dis 2022;9(8):ofac396.

21. Wright W.F., Mulders-Manders C.M., Auwaerter P.G., et al., Fever of unknown origin (FUO)– A call for new research standards and updated clinical management, *Am J Med*, 135 (2), 2022, 173–178.

22. Minamimoto R. Optimal use of the FDG-PET/CT in the diagnostic process of fever of unknown origin (FUO): a comprehensive review. Jpn J Radiol 2022;40(11): 1121–37.

23. Jasper N, Däbritz J, Frosch M, et al. Diagnostic value of [(18)F]-FDG PET/CT in children with fever of unknown origin or unexplained signs of inflammation. Eur J Nucl Med Mol Imaging 2010;37(1):136–45.
24. Søgaard K.K., Farkas D.K., Leisner M.Z., et al., Fever of Unknown Origin and Incidence of Cancer, *Clin Infect Dis*, 75 (6), 2022, 968–974.
25. Talano J-AM, Katz BZ. Long-term follow-up of children with fever of unknown origin. Clinical pediatrics 2000;39(12):715–7.
26. Miller LC, Sisson BA, Tucker LB, et al. Prolonged fevers of unknown origin in children: Patterns of presentation and outcome. J Pediatr 1996;129(3):419–23.
27. Dong Y, Gao Y, Chai Y, et al. Use of Quantitative Metagenomics Next-Generation Sequencing to Confirm Fever of Unknown Origin and Infectious Disease. Front Microbiol 2022;13:931058.
28. Guo W, Feng X, Hu M, et al. The Application of Whole-Exome Sequencing in Patients With FUO. Front Cell Infect Microbiol 2021;11:783568.
29. Tounta V., Liu Y., Cheyne A., et al., Metabolomics in infectious diseases and drug discovery, *Molecular Omics*, 17 (3), 2021, 376–393.

# Acquired Demyelinating Syndromes

Dominic O. Co, MD, PhD

## KEYWORDS

- Acquired demyelinating syndromes • Multiple sclerosis • Transverse myelitis
- Optic neuritis • Acute demyelinating encephalomyelitis

## KEY POINTS

- Acquired demyelinating syndromes (ADS) are a group of inflammatory demyelinating conditions comprising transverse myelitis, optic neuritis, acute demyelinating encephalomyelitis, or some combination of these.
- Different ADS have different tendencies to relapse and will respond to different types of anti-inflammatory and immune suppressive treatment.
- These differences in relapse tendencies and treatment make it important to be able to distinguish among the different types of ADS to institute the appropriate management plan.
- Clinical, laboratory, and MRI findings can be used to distinguish between the different types of ADS.

## INTRODUCTION

Acquired demyelinating syndrome (ADS) is an umbrella term for a diverse group of inflammatory/autoimmune demyelinating conditions. ADS can be thought of as including the "elemental" syndromes of acute transverse myelitis (ATM), optic neuritis (ON) and acute demyelinating encephalomyelitis (ADEM) that are often monophasic. However, recurrent attacks of the same demyelinating syndrome or combinations of these elemental syndromes can combine in various ways to form chronic disorders, such as multiple sclerosis, neuromyelitis optic spectrum disorders (NMOSD), and myelin oligodendrocyte glycoprotein antibody-associated disease (MOGAD). There are a few key differences between these various syndromes that make it important to differentiate them from each other. While all typically respond to steroids, they differ in their propensity to recur and accumulate long-term neurologic damage, and therefore the need to monitor for recurrence and to institute steroid-sparing therapy to prevent recurrence. In addition, there can be significant differences in their responsiveness to

Division of Allergy, Immunology, Rheumatology, Department of Pediatrics, University of Wisconsin School of Medicine and Public Health, Clinical Science Center (CSC), H6/572, 600 Highland Avenue, Madison, WI 53792, USA
E-mail address: doco@wisc.edu

Med Clin N Am 108 (2024) 93–105
https://doi.org/10.1016/j.mcna.2023.05.017
0025-7125/24/© 2023 Elsevier Inc. All rights reserved.

steroid-sparing therapies. Not only can the "wrong" therapy be ineffective for a particular ADS, it may even exacerbate that ADS.

In the past few decades, there has been significant and rapid progress in understanding and subclassifying the different types of ADS. In particular, the discovery of antibodies that associate with particular clinical phenotypes and predict prognosis and response to therapy has deepened our understanding. However, rapid accumulation of data has made the literature difficult to parse, since, for example, antibody data may not be available for older studies and patients are now classified with different, overlapping terminology (**Box 1**). This review will begin with descriptions of the elemental syndromes, then describe the more well-defined chronic syndromes of NMOSD, MOGAD, and multiple sclerosis.

## DISCUSSION
### Transverse Myelitis

Transverse myelitis (TM) is an immune-mediated demyelinating disease primarily affecting the spinal cord. It is an isolated monophasic illness in the majority of patients,[1] but could also represent the initial attack of a chronic relapsing demyelinating condition. It comprises approximately 20% of all pediatric-acquired demyelinating syndromes.[2] It has an annual incidence of one to two per 100,000 children.[1,3] The mean age of onset ranges from 8 to 11 years of age, but a bimodal distribution has also been reported with another group of patients presenting before the age of 5 years.[1,3,4]

A history of preceding infection is found in approximately 2/3 of patients.[1,3] The symptoms typically evolve over hours to days and often begin with back pain followed by the motor and sensory symptoms, which are typically bilateral. In the most severe cases, motor symptoms may present as hyporeflexive weakness (spinal shock), though eventually the more typical pattern of hyperreflexia evolves over days to weeks.[5] In the early stages, the hyporeflexic period can raise concern for Guillain-Barre syndrome. The sensory symptoms manifest either positively as neuropathic

---

**Box 1**
**Terms for different acute demyelinating syndromes**

ADS are referred to by many overlapping terms, some of which are listed later in discussion.
- Transverse myelitis (TM) – inflammatory demyelination of the spinal cord
- Optic neuritis (ON) – inflammatory demyelination of the optic nerve
- Acute demyelinating encephalomyelitis (ADEM) – multifocal inflammatory demyelination with associated encephalitis
- Chronic relapsing inflammatory optic neuritis (CRION) – a syndrome of recurrent episodes of optic neuritis
- Multiphasic demyelinating encephalomyelitis (MDEM) – a syndrome of recurrent episodes of ADEM
- Neuromyelitis optica (NMO) – classically, a chronic/relapsing syndrome characterized by the simultaneous occurrence of transverse myelitis and optic neuritis
- Neuromyelitis optica spectrum disorders (NMOSD) – a category of NMO-like disorders that recognizes the broader spectrum of demyelinating disease that is associated with AQP4-IgG (also known as NMO-IgG) which includes the classic presentation of simultaneous transverse myelitis and optic neuritis, but also either alone or in combination with other neurologic syndromes such as area postrema syndrome, and so forth (see **Box 2**)
- Myelin oligodendrocyte glycoprotein antibody-associated diseases (MOGAD) – Similar to NMOSD, a spectrum of demyelinating syndromes associated with MOG-IgG positivity.
- Multiple sclerosis (MS) – The classic inflammatory demyelinating disorder characterized by multiple characteristic demyelinating lesions distributed in space and time.

pain or as numbness with a sensory level. Bowel and bladder dysfunction are common as well.

Cerebrospinal fluid (CSF) studies typically demonstrate elevated protein and a lymphocytic pleocytosis. Because ATM can represent a first attack of either multiple sclerosis, NMO spectrum disorder, or MOGAD, testing should be sent for CSF oligoclonal bands, serum aquaporin-4 autoantibodies (AQP4-IgG), and serum myelin oligodendrocyte glycoprotein autoantibodies (MOG-IgG). CSF testing is available for AQP4-IgG, but it is not clear if it adds much diagnostically since most patients positive in the CSF are also positive in serum.[6] It should be noted that MOG-IgG testing in the CSF is not widely available, but recent studies have suggested that CSF testing may increase sensitivity and may identify a different subset of patients with a worse prognosis.[7]

MRI should demonstrate T2 hyperintense and FLAIR lesions predominantly in the white matter, though sometimes gray matter can also be involved. The lesions are often enhancing. Certain MRI patterns can be suggestive of other ADS. For example, longitudinally extensive transverse myelitis (LETM) is suggestive of NMOSD or MOGAD, whereas multiple lesions are associated with MOGAD or later progression to MS.[8] Brain MRI is typically normal in TM and lesions found in the brain should raise concern for later progression to MS.

### Optic Neuritis

Optic neuritis is an inflammatory attack on one or both optic nerves. As with TM, it can be an isolated episode or can be the initial attack in a chronic autoimmune disease. ON presents with eye pain and decreased visual acuity. Patients may have defects in color vision and visual fields as well. The symptoms present over hours to days with peak visual loss occurring within several days of onset.[9] In patients greater than 10 year old, it is more likely to present unilaterally, whereas younger patients are more likely to present with bilateral disease.[10] On examination, patients may demonstrate a relative afferent pupillary defect if only one eye is affected. MRI will show thickening, T2 hyperintensity, and contrast enhancement in the optic nerves.

Large case series have shown that optic neuritis occurs as an isolated episode in 48% to 69% of patients.[11] MS is less likely to occur in patients with bilateral presentation. Serum testing for AQP4-IgG and MOG-IgG is suggestive of NMOSD and MOGAD, respectively. CSF oligoclonal bands predict evolution to MS. The specific pattern of MRI lesions can be a clue to more specific etiologies. For example, longitudinally extensive optic nerve lesions (ie, > 50% the length of the optic nerve) are more likely to represent NMOSD or MOGAD. In addition, demyelinating lesions in the brain predict later evolution to MS.

### Acute Disseminated Encephalomyelitis

Acute disseminated encephalomyelitis (ADEM) is characterized by the sudden and first-time onset of multifocal immune-mediated inflammatory CNS demyelination in the setting of encephalopathy (not attributable to fever). The typical age of presentation is between 3 and 8 years.[12,13] It is often preceded by a viral infection or in some cases an immunization, but in many cases has no identifiable trigger.[14,15] Other clinical features include fever, gait disturbance, and speech impairment, whereas laboratory features include cerebrospinal fluid pleocytosis and increased CSF protein levels. Electroencephalogram (EEG) typically reveals diffuse slowing.[15] The time from onset to maximal symptoms is 4 to 7 days.[12] No controlled trials have been done in ADEM and treatment guidelines are based on observational studies and expert opinion. Initial treatment is typically with high-dose IV steroids (30 mg/kg/d, max

1000 mg per day) for 3 to 5 days followed by a 4 to 6 week taper of oral steroids. Initial improvement may take several days. Typically, patients will have complete resolution of neurologic symptoms over 4 to 6 weeks. In situations with severe manifestations (eg, severe vision loss, refractory seizures, and so forth) or failure to improve, second-line therapies such as plasma exchange or IVIG are added.[12]

Technically, ADEM is defined as having no new clinical or radiographic features 3 months after symptom onset.[16] However, a first bout of ADEM can be followed by recurrent episodes of ADEM (multiphasic disseminated encephalomyelitis, MDEM) or by attacks of other types of inflammatory demyelination such as TM or ON that result in later reclassification as a different ADS. The presence of CSF-restricted oligo-clonal bands, serum AQP4-IgG, are serum MOG-IgG during initial presentation are all predictive of later relapse.

### Neuromyelitis Optic Spectrum Disorders

NMO spectrum disorders are a group of autoimmune disorders affecting the CNS that were initially identified by the presentation of ON and TM that evolved in a fashion distinct from multiple sclerosis. The concept has undergone significant evolution since the diagnostic criteria were first proposed in 1999. A key turning point in the under-standing of NMO, as it was then known, was the discovery of IgG antibodies to aquaporin-4 (AQP4-IgG), which brought to light a range of different presentations that shared this underlying pathophysiology. As a result, the diagnostic criteria were revised in 2015 and the condition was renamed NMO spectrum disorder (NMOSD, **Box 2**).[17] NMOSD is rare in children comprising 0.6%-3.7% of all pediatric ADS.[18] However, the relapsing nature of NMOSD and therefore the need to monitor for relapses and/or institute preventive treatment makes it important to identify and distin-guish from monophasic forms of ADS. In addition, certain treatments for MS (eg, interferon-β, natalizumab, and fingolimod) have been shown to cause flares of NMOSD, making it particularly important to distinguish from MS.[18]

Patients with NMOSD present most commonly with optic neuritis and/or longitudi-nally extensive transverse myelitis (LETM), which are at the core of the original diag-nostic criteria.[18] Symptomatically, these present similarly to their elemental forms as described above, though may be more severe. One distinguishing feature of NMOSD-related ON or TM is that they occur together or in association with other neurologic syndromes (see later in discussion and **Box 2**). As alluded to above, the presence of AQP4-IgG in the serum is a key diagnostic feature as well. NMOSD-associated ON typically demonstrates longitudinally extensive inflammation of the optic nerve involving more than half its length with frequent bilateral involvement. Simi-larly, NMOSD-associated TM is typically longitudinally extensive, though LETM is often found in other pediatric neuroinflammatory disorders (such as MOGAD) and is less distinctive than it is in adult NMOSD.[19]

In addition to the classic presentation of ON and LETM, NMOSD can also present with a number of other neurologic syndromes.[19] Patients with NMOSD can present with area postrema syndrome (APS), a syndrome of intractable vomiting and hiccups associated with MRI lesions in the area postrema/dorsal medulla.[20] Other brainstem syndromes can also occur presenting with diplopia, facial palsy, dysarthria, vestibular ataxia, eye movement abnormalities, and trigeminal neuralgia.[19,21,22] Lesions of the diencephalon can lead to the syndrome of inappropriate diuretic hormone secretion (SIADH), hypotension, sleep abnormalities (hypersomnia, narcolepsy), amenorrhea-galactorrhea syndrome, or behavioral changes. Patients can also present with lesions involving the cerebral hemispheres resulting in hemiparesis, visual field defects, and encephalopathy similar to ADEM, though these are more often associated with

---

**Box 2**
**Diagnostic criteria for NMOSD**

Diagnostic criteria for NMOSD with AQP4-IgG
1. At least 1 core clinical characteristic
2. Positive test for AQP4-IgG using the best available detection method (cell-based assay strongly recommended)
3. Exclusion of alternative diagnoses

Diagnostic criteria for NMOSD without AQP4-IgG or NMOSD with unknown AQP4-IgG status
1. At least 2 core clinical characteristics occurring as a result of one or more clinical attacks and meeting all of the following requirements:
    a. At least 1 core clinical characteristic must be optic neuritis, acute myelitis with LETM, or area postrema syndrome
    b. Dissemination in space (2 or more different core clinical characteristics)
    c. Fulfillment of additional MRI requirements, as applicable
2. Negative tests for AQP4-IgG using the best available detection method, or testing unavailable
3. Exclusion of alternative diagnoses

Core clinical characteristics
1. Optic neuritis
2. Acute myelitis
3. Area postrema syndrome: episode of otherwise unexplained hiccups or nausea and vomiting
4. Acute brainstem syndrome
5. Symptomatic narcolepsy or acute diencephalic clinical syndrome with NMOSD-typical diencephalic MRI lesions
6. Symptomatic cerebral syndrome with NMOSD-typical brain lesions

Additional MRI requirements for NMOSD without AQP4-IgG and NMOSD with unknown AQP4-IgG status
1. Acute optic neuritis: requires brain MRI showing
    a. normal findings or only nonspecific white matter lesions, OR
    b. optic nerve MRI with T2-hyperintense lesion or T1-weighted gadolinium-enhancing lesion extending over 1/2 optic nerve length or involving optic chiasm.
2. Acute myelitis: requires associated intramedullary MRI lesion extending over 3 contiguous segments (LETM) OR 3 contiguous segments of focal spinal cord atrophy in patients with history compatible with acute myelitis
3. Area postrema syndrome: requires associated dorsal medulla/area postrema lesions
4. Acute brainstem syndrome: requires associated periependymal brainstem lesions

*Adapted from* Ref.[17]

---

positivity for MOG-IgG.[19] Interestingly, NMOSD has also been associated with both other organ-specific autoimmunity (celiac disease, autoimmune thyroid disease, type 1 diabetes) and systemic autoimmune disease (systemic lupus erythematosus, Sjogren syndrome) as well as other CNS autoantibodies.[18,22]

### Myelin Oligodendrocyte Glycoprotein Antibody Disease

MOG-IgG-associated disease (MOGAD) is a class of ADS with positive serologic testing for antibodies against myelin oligodendrocyte glycoprotein (MOG), a minor protein component of the myelin sheath. Patients with MOGAD were previously grouped with patients with NMOSD or ADEM depending on their clinical presentation, but as more data has accumulated about these patients, they have been reclassified as a distinct disease entity due to differences in their disease course and recommended management. The International MOGAD Panel has recently reviewed the distinctive features of MOGAD and proposed diagnostic criteria (**Box 3**)[23].

---

**Box 3**
**Proposed diagnostic criteria for MOGAD**

*1, 2, and 3 all required:*

1. At least one core clinical demyelinating event
   a. Optic neuritis
   b. Myelitis
   c. Acute demyelinating encephalomyelitis
   d. Cerebral monofocal or polyfocal deficits
   e. Brainstem or cerebellar deficits
   f. Cerebral cortical encephalitis often with seizures

2. Positive MOG-IgG test
   a. Clear positive serum testing OR
   b. Low positive, positive without titer, or negative serum but positive CSF requires
      i. Negative testing for AQP4-IgG AND
      ii. At least one supporting clinical or MRI features
         1. Optic neuritis
            a. Simultaneous bilateral involvement
            b. greater than 50% of optic nerve involved
            c. Optic sheath involvement
            d. Optic disc edema (on the fundoscopic examination)
         2. Myelitis
            a. Longitudinally extensive myelitis
            b. Central cord lesion or "H-sign" (involvement of the gray matter noted on axial slices)
            c. Conus lesion
         3. Brain, brainstem, or cerebral syndrome
            a. Multiple ill-defined T2 lesions in supratentorial and often infratentorial white matter
            b. Deep gray matter involvement
            c. Ill-defined T2 lesions of the pons, middle cerebral peduncle, or medulla
            d. Cortical lesion with or without lesional and overlying meningeal enhancement

3. Exclusion of other diagnoses including multiple sclerosis

*Reprinted with permission from* Elsevier. The Lancet Neurology, 2023;22(3):268-282. Doi:10.1016/S1474-4422(22)00431-8.

Patients with MOGAD most commonly present with ADEM (33%-65% of patients with MOGAD), but can also present with optic neuritis (10%-67%) or least commonly with transverse myelitis (0%–35%).[24] As a newer category of ADS, less is known about MOGAD, and it is the subject of increasing study. The differences between MOGAD and other ADS depend on the particular presenting syndrome, and will be discussed later. In general, patients with ADS positive for MOG tend to be younger, which may reflect the larger proportion of patients with MOGAD presenting with ADEM. A positive MOG-IgG at presentation is also associated with a higher risk of relapse that the idiopathic ADS syndromes, but patients with MOG-IgG-positive NMOSD are less likely to relapse than AQP4-IgG-positive NMOSD.[25] It may be helpful to follow MOG-IgG positivity over time, because persistent positivity confers a higher risk of relapse than in patients who become MOG-IgG negative.[24]

Patients with MOGAD who present with ADEM are clinically similar to other patients who present with ADEM. A small series of 33 patients with ADEM found that the sole clinical distinction at presentation between patients with MOG-IgG-positive and patients with MOG-IgG-negative was that patients with MOG-IgG-positive were more likely to have emotional or behavioral symptoms.[26] However, patients with MOG-

IgG-positive tended to have higher CSF cell counts and more likely to have abnormal spinal MRI. There was also a higher risk of long-term cognitive impairment and epilepsy in patients with MOGAD.

In contrast to patients with MOGAD presenting with ADEM, patients with MOGAD presenting with optic neuritis were older, typically between 13 and 18 years of age. Similar to patients with AQP4-IgG-positive, patients with MOGAD ON presented with severe deficits in visual acuity, had high rates of longitudinally extensive optic nerve lesions on MRI, and developed evidence of long-term axonal damage on OCT.[24] However, patients with MOGAD ON were more likely to have enhancement of perineural and orbital soft tissue on MRI than patients with NMOSD. In addition, they had better functional visual recovery similar to patients with MS-associated or double seronegative optic neuritis than patients with NMOSD.[24]

Patients with MOGAD presenting with TM were the least common, and therefore less is known about them. Similar to patients with MOGAD ON, their disability is often severe at onset with many being wheelchair bound and having bowel/bladder dysfunction. Similar to patients with AQP4-IgG-positive, patients with MOGAD TM present frequently with LETM and have central gray matter involvement leading to flaccid hyporeflexia. However, patients with MOGAD are more likely to have conus involvement and therefore bowel/bladder involvement.[24]

### Multiple Sclerosis

Multiple sclerosis (MS) is the prototypical inflammatory demyelinating condition that presents in a relapsing-remitting course in the majority of children. Compared to adults with MS, children with MS appear to have a more severe inflammatory disease characterized by a higher "annualized relapse rate" (ARR, a standard measure of the average number of MS attacks per year)[27] and a higher burden of lesions.[28] Despite more severe attacks, accumulation of disability is slower in children, thought to be due to a higher ability to recover from attacks and to the inherent plasticity of the developing brain.[29] Only 20% of ADS is ultimately diagnosed as MS and the treatment can differ significantly from the treatment of other demyelinating conditions such as NMOSD or MOGAD.[29]

Children with MS can present with long tract involvement (65% of patients), brainstem symptoms (37%) optic neuritis (34%), transverse myelitis (7%), and ADEM (15%). Of note, adolescents are less likely to present with ADEM and are more likely to present with a combination of the other syndromes. The diagnosis of MS is made by the McDonald criteria, (**Table 1**) with the most recent revision in 2017.[30] The criteria explicitly caution about their use in children under 11 years of age, though the criteria have been found to perform well in children with a sensitivity of 71% and specificity of 95%.[31]

Though spinal cord lesions are frequently seen in MS, they typically are not longitudinally extensive as seen in NMOSD or MOGAD.[3] Optic neuritis in patients eventually diagnosed with MS is typically unilateral and with less frequent and less severe optic nerve edema on fundoscopy.[32] In addition, optic nerve MRI usually shows short segment lesions without the involvement of the optic nerve sheath or optic chiasm.[32] AQP4-IgG and MOG-IgG are typically negative in MS. CSF pleocytosis and protein may be similarly abnormal in patients with MS and other demyelinating syndromes. However, CSF-restricted oligoclonal bands are helpful in distinguishing MS from other ADS, similar to adult disease.[29,33] There have been efforts to identify other markers of progression to MS. In one promising study, the T cell activation marker, soluble CD27 (sCD27) was found to be higher in children with clinically definite MS than patient with either monophasic ADS or non-MS relapsing ADS.[34]

**Table 1**
**McDonald criteria for multiple sclerosis**

| Number of Clinical Attacks | Lesions with Objective Evidence[a] | Additional Data Needed for MS Diagnosis |
|---|---|---|
| ≥ 2 | ≥ 2 | None |
| ≥ 2 | 1 with clear historical evidence of prior attack and a lesion in a distinct anatomic location | None |
| ≥ 2 | 1 | Dissemination in space as demonstrated by an additional clinical attack implicating a different CNS site or by MRI |
| 1 | ≥ 2 | Dissemination in time demonstrated by an additional clinical attack or by MRI§ OR demonstration of CSF-specific oligoclonal bands |
| 1 | 1 | Dissemination in space demonstrated by MRI or an additional clinical attack implicating a different CNS site AND One of the following: • CSF-specific oligoclonal bands • Dissemination in time demonstrated by ◦ an additional clinical attack ◦ MRI |

[a] An abnormality on neurologic examination, imaging (MRI or optical coherence tomography), or neurophysiological testing (visual evoked potentials) that corresponds to the anatomic location suggested by the symptoms.

*Reprinted with permission from* Elsevier. The Lancet Neurology, 2018;17(2):162-173. doi:10.1016/S1474-4422(17)30470-2.

### Approach

The key task in the approach to the first presentation of an ADS is to determine if the patient fits a well-described relapsing ADS such as MS, NMOSD or MOGAD, or if the patient has other features suggesting a tendency toward relapse. **Table 2** lists some of the distinctive features of the well-described relapsing ADS. Initial clues to the classification of ADS come from the history. The age at presentation is an important detail since MS is less likely to occur in patients younger than 11 years and NMOSD is overall less common in children, whereas MOGAD is more common as a proportion of recurrent ADS. A history of preceding infection is commonly found with presentations of typically monophasic transverse myelitis and also with MOGAD, likely because of its association with ADEM and the frequent association of ADEM with preceding infection.

The phenotype of the clinical presentation is a key variable. For example, patients presenting with ADEM are more likely to meet the criteria for MOGAD than NMOSD and least likely to have MS. Conversely, MS and NMOSD are more likely to present with optic neuritis and/or transverse myelitis. ON in patients with MS is more likely to be unilateral whereas ON that presents with NMOSD and MOGAD is often bilateral. The imaging findings can also provide clues to the specific ADS. Both NMOSD and MOGAD are likely to have longitudinally extensive lesions in the optic nerve with ON and in the spinal cord with TM. Finally, CSF biomarkers are helpful in distinguishing between these different syndromes with oligoclonal bands associated with MS, AQP4-IgG with NMOSD, and MOG-IgG with MOGAD. In the case of MOGAD, serial

**Table 2**
**Distinguishing features of acquired demyelinating syndromes**

| | NMOSD | MOGAD | MS |
|---|---|---|---|
| Onset < 11 y | Uncommon | Common | Uncommon |
| Prodromal Illness | Uncommon | Common | Uncommon |
| Likelihood of relapse | Common | Occasional | Common |
| Optic neuritis | Often bilateral<br>Often severely impaired at the onset<br>High risk for poor recovery<br>MRI: longitudinally extensive lesions, may involve chiasm and optic tract | Often bilateral<br>Often severely impaired at the onset<br>Typically good recovery<br>MRI: longitudinally extensive lesions, often involving optic nerve sheath | Typically unilateral<br>Typically mild to moderately impaired<br>Typically good recovery<br>MRI: Focal T2 optic nerve lesions not involving the optic nerve sheath |
| Transverse Myelitis | Poor clinical recovery<br>MRI: LETM pattern most common<br>Does not typically involve conus medullaris | Good clinical recovery<br>MRI: LETM pattern most common<br>Commonly involves conus medullaris | Good clinical recovery between attacks<br>MRI: Short focal T2 lesions |
| Acute disseminated encephalomyelitis | Occasional | Most frequent manifestation | Uncommon |
| Oligoclonal bands | Rare | Rare | Frequent |
| Serum AQP4-IgG | Frequent | 0% | Rare |
| Serum MOG-IgG | Rare | 100% | Rare |

*Adapted from Refs.*[23,40]

MOG-IgG titers can be additionally helpful since MOG-IgG can become negative over time, whereas persistently positive titers correlate with an increased risk of relapse.

## FUTURE DIRECTIONS - NOVEL BIOMARKERS

Significant progress has been made in the last few decades with the discovery of AQP4-IgG and MOG-IgG. There is promising work in progress to identify new bio-markers in ADS. AQP4-IgG and MOG-IgG are both typically measured in serum. While there has not been evidence that CSF levels of AQP4-IgG add much to management, there have been some promising studies that CSF MOG-IgG may increase sensitivity and perhaps identify a subset of patients with a worse prognosis.[7,35] Studies of general markers of neuronal or glial cell injury such as neurofilament, glial fibrillary acid protein (GFAP), myelin basic protein (MBP) and tau protein have demonstrated a correlation with disease activity but some have also suggested the ability to distinguish between different ADS.[36–38] Though these were initially assayed in CSF, for some antibodies, serum levels appear to also be useful. CSF cytokine profiles have been shown to differentiate MOGAD and NMOSD from MS in both pediatric and adult patients.[39] Measures of the T cell activation marker soluble CD27 (sCD27) in the CSF have been shown to predict evolution to MS in both adult and pediatric patients.[34]

## SUMMARY

The field has come to understand that ADS are a collection of different conditions that share the common pathophysiology of inflammatory demyelination. Despite this commonality, differences in clinical presentation, autoantibodies, and MRI findings now allow us to identify ADS subtypes that are likely to relapse. In addition, understanding these subtypes allows us to choose therapies that are more likely to be effective. Future research will help to identify other markers that might identify yet more subtypes and to develop more effective therapies to treat these conditions.

## CLINICS CARE POINTS

- NMO-IgG and MOG-IgG are key in distinguishing NMOSD and MOGAD, respectively, from other ADS.
- CSF oligoclonal bands are suggestive of eventual development of MS.
- Among other MRI findings, longitudinally extensive lesions of the spinal cord or optic nerve are more suggestive of NMOSD and MOGAD rather than MS or other ADS.

## DISCLOSURE

The author has nothing to disclose.

## ACKNOWLEDGMENTS

The author would like to acknowledge Jennifer Kwon, MD for critical review of the manuscript.

## REFERENCES

1. Theroux LM, Brenton JN. Acute Transverse and Flaccid Myelitis in Children. Curr Treat Options Neurol 2019;21(12):64.

2. Banwell B, Kennedy J, Sadovnick D, et al. Incidence of acquired demyelination of the CNS in Canadian children. Neurology 2009;72(3):232–9.

3. Absoud M, Greenberg BM, Lim M, et al. Pediatric transverse myelitis. Neurology 2016;87(9 Supplement 2):S46–52.

4. Kahn I. Acute Transverse Myelitis and Acute Disseminated Encephalomyelitis. Pediatr Rev 2020;41(7):313–20.

5. Wolf VL, Lupo PJ, Lotze TE. Pediatric Acute Transverse Myelitis Overview and Differential Diagnosis. J Child Neurol 2012;27(11):1426–36.

6. Jarius S, Wildemann B. Aquaporin-4 antibodies (NMO-IgG) as a serological marker of neuromyelitis optica: a critical review of the literature. Brain Pathol Zurich Switz 2013;23(6):661–83.

7. Carta S, Cobo CA, Armangué T, et al. Significance of Myelin Oligodendrocyte Glycoprotein Antibodies in CSF: A Retrospective Multicenter Study. Neurology 2023;100(11):e1095–108.

8. Dubey D, Pittock SJ, Krecke KN, et al. Clinical, Radiologic, and Prognostic Features of Myelitis Associated With Myelin Oligodendrocyte Glycoprotein Autoantibody. JAMA Neurol 2019;76(3):301–9.

9. Yeh EA, Graves JS, Benson LA, et al. Pediatric optic neuritis. Neurology 2016; 87(9 Supplement 2):S53–8.

10. Waldman AT, Stull LB, Galetta SL, et al. Pediatric optic neuritis and risk of multiple sclerosis: meta-analysis of observational studies. J AAPOS Off Publ Am Assoc Pediatr Ophthalmol Strabismus 2011;15(5):441–6.

11. Park KA, Yang HK, Han J, et al. Characteristics of Optic Neuritis in South Korean Children and Adolescents: A Retrospective Multicenter Study. J Ophthalmol 2022;2022:4281772.

12. Wang CX. Assessment and Management of Acute Disseminated Encephalomyelitis (ADEM) in the Pediatric Patient. Paediatr Drugs 2021;23(3):213–21.

13. Paolilo RB, Deiva K, Neuteboom R, et al. Acute Disseminated Encephalomyelitis: Current Perspectives. Child Basel Switz 2020;7(11):210.

14. Esposito S, Di Pietro GM, Madini B, et al. A spectrum of inflammation and demyelination in acute disseminated encephalomyelitis (ADEM) of children. Autoimmun Rev 2015;14(10):923–9.

15. Monllor AS, Saura MA, Fernández CM, et al. Acute Disseminated Encephalomyelitis. A Fourteen Years Review (P5.139). Neurology 2016;86(16 Supplement): P5139.

16. Krupp LB, Tardieu M, Amato MP, et al. International Pediatric Multiple Sclerosis Study Group criteria for pediatric multiple sclerosis and immune-mediated central nervous system demyelinating disorders: revisions to the 2007 definitions. Mult Scler J 2013;19(10):1261–7.

17. Wingerchuk DM, Banwell B, Bennett JL, et al. International consensus diagnostic criteria for neuromyelitis optica spectrum disorders. Neurology 2015;85(2):177–89.

18. Tenembaum S, Chitnis T, Nakashima I, et al. Neuromyelitis optica spectrum disorders in children and adolescents. Neurology 2016;87(9 Supplement 2):S59–66.

19. Tenembaum S, Yeh EA. Pediatric NMOSD: A Review and Position Statement on Approach to Work-Up and Diagnosis. Front Pediatr 2020;8:339.

20. Chitnis T, Ghezzi A, Bajer-Kornek B, et al. Pediatric multiple sclerosis: Escalation and emerging treatments. Neurology 2016;87(9 Supplement 2):S103–9.

21. Martins C, Moura J, Figueiroa S, et al. Pediatric neuromyelitis optica spectrum disorders in Portugal: A multicentre retrospective study. Mult Scler Relat Disord 2022;59:103531.

22. Baghbanian SM, Asgari N, Sahraian MA, et al. A comparison of pediatric and adult neuromyelitis optica spectrum disorders: A review of clinical manifestation, diagnosis, and treatment. J Neurol Sci 2018;388:222–31.

23. Banwell B, Bennett JL, Marignier R, et al. Diagnosis of myelin oligodendrocyte glycoprotein antibody-associated disease: International MOGAD Panel proposed criteria. Lancet Neurol 2023;22(3):268–82.

24. Bruijstens AL, Lechner C, Flet-Berliac L, et al. E.U. paediatric MOG consortium consensus: Part 1 - Classification of clinical phenotypes of paediatric myelin oligodendrocyte glycoprotein antibody-associated disorders. Eur J Paediatr Neurol EJPN Off J Eur Paediatr Neurol Soc 2020;29:2–13.

25. Lechner C, Baumann M, Hennes EM, et al. Antibodies to MOG and AQP4 in children with neuromyelitis optica and limited forms of the disease. J Neurol Neurosurg Psychiatry 2016;87(8):897–905.

26. Baumann M, Sahin K, Lechner C, et al. Clinical and neuroradiological differences of paediatric acute disseminating encephalomyelitis with and without antibodies to the myelin oligodendrocyte glycoprotein. J Neurol Neurosurg Psychiatry 2015;86(3):265–72.

27. Deiva K. Pediatric onset multiple sclerosis. Rev Neurol (Paris) 2020;176(1–2):30–6.

28. Waubant E, Chabas D, Okuda DT, et al. Difference in Disease Burden and Activity in Pediatric Patients on Brain Magnetic Resonance Imaging at Time of Multiple Sclerosis Onset vs Adults. Arch Neurol 2009;66(8):967–71.

29. Jakimovski D, Awan S, Eckert SP, et al. Multiple Sclerosis in Children: Differential Diagnosis, Prognosis, and Disease-Modifying Treatment. CNS Drugs 2022;36(1):45–59.

30. Thompson AJ, Banwell BL, Barkhof F, et al. Diagnosis of multiple sclerosis: 2017 revisions of the McDonald criteria. Lancet Neurol 2018;17(2):162–73.

31. Fadda G, Brown RA, Longoni G, et al. MRI and laboratory features and the performance of international criteria in the diagnosis of multiple sclerosis in children and adolescents: a prospective cohort study. Lancet Child Adolesc Health 2018;2(3):191–204.

32. Bennett JL, Costello F, Chen JJ, et al. Optic neuritis and autoimmune optic neuropathies: advances in diagnosis and treatment. Lancet Neurol 2023;22(1):89–100.

33. Mikaeloff Y, Caridade G, Assi S, et al. on behalf of the KIDSEP Study Group. Prognostic Factors for Early Severity in a Childhood Multiple Sclerosis Cohort. Pediatrics 2006;118(3):1133–9.

34. Wong YYM, van der Vuurst de Vries RM, van Pelt ED, et al. T-cell activation marker sCD27 is associated with clinically definite multiple sclerosis in childhood-acquired demyelinating syndromes. Mult Scler J 2018;24(13):1715–24.

35. Kim HJ, Palace J. Should We test for IgG Antibodies Against MOG in Both Serum and CSF in Patients With Suspected MOGAD? Neurology 2023;100(11):497–8.

36. Armangue T, Capobianco M, de Chalus A, et al. U. paediatric MOG consortium. E.U. paediatric MOG consortium consensus: Part 3 - Biomarkers of paediatric myelin oligodendrocyte glycoprotein antibody-associated disorders. Eur J Paediatr Neurol EJPN Off J Eur Paediatr Neurol Soc 2020;29:22–31.

37. Wong YYM, Bruijstens AL, Barro C, et al. Serum neurofilament light chain in pediatric MS and other acquired demyelinating syndromes. Neurology 2019;93(10):e968–74.

38. van der Vuurst de Vries RM, Wong YYM, Mescheriakova JY, et al. High neurofilament levels are associated with clinically definite multiple sclerosis in children and adults with clinically isolated syndrome. Mult Scler J 2019;25(7):958–67.

39. Kaneko K, Sato DK, Nakashima I, et al. CSF cytokine profile in MOG-IgG+ neurological disease is similar to AQP4-IgG+ NMOSD but distinct from MS: a cross-sectional study and potential therapeutic implications. J Neurol Neurosurg Psychiatry 2018;89(9):927–36.
40. Fadda G, Armangue T, Hacohen Y, et al. Paediatric multiple sclerosis and antibody-associated demyelination: clinical, imaging, and biological considerations for diagnosis and care. Lancet Neurol 2021;20(2):136–49.

# Common Variable Immunodeficiency

Allison Remiker, MD[a],*, Kristina Bolling, APNP[b],
James Verbsky, MD, PhD[b,c]

## KEYWORDS

- Common variable immunodeficiency • Primary immune deficiency • Autoimmunity
- Hypogammaglobulinemia

## KEY POINTS

- Common variable immunodeficiency (CVID) is the most common primary immune deficiency resulting from many different monogenic conditions.
- A key feature of CVID is hypogammaglobulinemia causing an increased risk of infections and majority of patients are treated with immunoglobulin.
- There is significant clinical heterogeneity in CVID with infectious and noninfectious complications including pulmonary and gastrointestinal symptoms, along with an increased risk of autoimmunity and cancer.

## INTRODUCTION

Common variable immunodeficiency (CVID), also known as acquired hypogammaglobulinemia, is the most common primary immune deficiency. It is characterized as a clinical syndrome representing a heterogenous group of disorders that exhibit a common phenotype of abnormal B cell differentiation with impaired production of specific immunoglobulin. Clinical manifestations are variable and include acquisition of recurrent bacterial infections after a period of wellness, polyclonal lymphoproliferation, autoimmunity (especially immune mediated cytopenias [IMCs]), pulmonary disease, liver disease, enteropathy, granulomas, and a propensity for development of malignancy.[1–4]

Although highly variable, the mean onset of symptoms in patients with CVID is in the third decade of life. There remains a considerable delay, up to 10 years, between the

---

[a] Division of Hematology/Oncology/Blood and Marrow Transplantation, Department of Pediatrics, Medical College of Wisconsin, and Children's Wisconsin, Milwaukee, WI, USA; [b] Division of Allergy and Clinical Immunology, Department of Pediatrics, Medical College of Wisconsin, and Children's Wisconsin, Milwaukee, WI, USA; [c] Division of Rheumatology, Department of Pediatrics, Medical College of Wisconsin, and Children's Wisconsin, Milwaukee, WI, USA
* Corresponding author. Medical College of Wisconsin, 8701 Watertown Plank Road, MRFC 3018, Milwaukee, WI 53226.
E-mail address: aremiker@mcw.edu

Med Clin N Am 108 (2024) 107–121
https://doi.org/10.1016/j.mcna.2023.06.012
0025-7125/24/© 2023 Elsevier Inc. All rights reserved.

onset of symptoms and the diagnosis of CVID.[5-8] Interestingly, often affected individuals may develop IMCs during early childhood and acquire symptoms of immunodeficiency during the second or third decade of life.

Clinical heterogeneity has led to diagnostic challenges and difficulties in the development of optimal treatment plans for patients with CVID. Individualized evaluations based on assessment of an immunologic profile are important, as defects in intrinsic B-cell function, intrinsic T-cell defects, as well as abnormalities in tumor necrosis factor (TNF) receptors have all been identified as potential sites of immune dysregulation in CVID, making the clinical syndrome "variable". Broad genetic screening (whole exome sequencing or extensive genetic panels) should be considered in patients with CVID with an early onset and/or severe phenotype as monogenic defects will be found in more than 25% of such patients.[9] Diagnostic evaluations are important in guiding targeted therapeutic options for patients. Early recognition, prompt management, and disease surveillance are the keys to improving the lives of patients affected by CVID.

## DEFINITIONS

With the underlying clinical and genetic heterogeneity in CVID, there is not a specific laboratory test or clinical finding that defines CVID. The identification of CVID relies on diagnostic criteria. There are 3 most commonly applied clinical criteria described by The European Society for Immunodeficiencies (ESID) Registry, Ameratunga and colleagues,[2,3,10] and the International Consensus Document (ICON), as outlined in **Boxes 1–3**.

---

**Box 1**
**The European Society for Immunodeficiencies registry: common variable immunodeficiency[1]**

At least one of the following:
- Increased susceptibility to infection
- Autoimmune manifestations
- Granulomatous disease
- Unexplained polyclonal lymphoproliferation
- Affected family member with antibody deficiency

AND marked decrease of IgG and marked decrease of IgA with or without low IgM levels (measured at least twice; <2 SD of the normal levels for their age)

AND at least one of the following:
- Poor antibody response to vaccines (and/or absent isohemagglutinins); that is, absence of protective levels despite vaccination where defined
- Low switched memory B cells (<70% of age-related normal value)

AND secondary causes of hypogammaglobulinemia have been excluded (eg, infection, protein loss, medication, malignancy)

AND diagnosis is established after the fourth year of life (but symptoms may be present before)

AND no deficiency of profound T-cell deficiency, defined as 2 out of the following (y = years of life):
- CD4 numbers/μL: 2 to 6 <300, 6 to 12 y < 250, >12 y < 200
- % naïve of CD4: 2 to 6 y <25%, 6 to 16 y <20%, >16 y <10%
- T-cell proliferation absent

Adapted from Odnoletkova I, Kindle G, Quinti I, Grimbacher B, Knerr V, Gathmann B, et al. The burden of common variable immunodeficiency disorders: a retrospective analysis of the European Society for Immunodeficiency (ESID) registry data. Orphanet journal of rare diseases. 2018;13(1):201.

---

**Box 2**
**New diagnostic criteria for common variable immune deficiency[10]**

A. Must meet all major criteria
   - Hypogammaglobulinemia: IgG below 5 g/L for adults
   - No other cause identified for immune defect
   - Age >4 years

B. Clinical sequelae directly attributable to in vivo failure of the immune system (1 or more criteria)
   - Recurrent, severe, or unusual infections
   - Poor response to antibiotics
   - Breakthrough bacterial infections despite prophylactic antibiotics
   - Infections despite immunization with the appropriate vaccine, for example, HPV disease
   - Bronchiectasis and/or chronic sinus disease
   - Inflammatory disorders or autoimmunity

C. Supportive laboratory evidence (3 or more criteria)
   - Concomitant deficiency or reduction of IgA (<0.8 g/L) and/or IgM (<0.4 g/L)
   - Presence of B cells but reduced memory B-cell subsets and/or increased CD21 low subsets by flow cytometry
   - IgG3 deficiency (<0.2 g/L)
   - Impaired vaccine responses compared with age-matched controls
   - Transient responses to vaccines compared with age-matched controls
   - Absent isohemagglutinins (if not blood group AB)
   - Serologic support for autoimmunity in Section B, for example, positive Coombs test
   - Sequence variations of genes predisposing to CVID, for example, TACI, BAFFR, MSH5, etc.

D. Presence of any one of relatively specific histologic markers of CVID (not required for diagnosis but presence increases diagnostic certainty)
   - Lymphoid interstitial pneumonitis
   - Granulomatous disorder
   - Nodular regenerative hyperplasia of the liver
   - Nodular lymphoid hyperplasia of the gut
   - Absence of plasma cells on gut biopsy

---

## BACKGROUND
### Epidemiology

CVID affects approximately 1:20,000 to 1:50,000 live births.[1] The prevalence is highly variable due to differences in the diagnostic criteria as outlined above (see "Definitions"). The development of recurring infections can occur at any time, but the peak incidence typically occurs between 16 and 20 years of age.[5–8] The United States (40.2%) has the highest documented prevalence rates of CVID, with the Middle East (2.6%) and Africa (1.3%) having the lowest.[11,12] However, this is thought to be influenced by limited availability of diagnostic methods and conglomerate data.

### Pathophysiology

The etiology of CVID is largely unknown, and there are no characteristic immunologic findings in these patients other than hypogammaglobulinemia and poor vaccine responses. However, with the advent of next generation sequencing, a considerable portion of patients with CVID demonstrate a genetic defect. Variants in *TACI* are found in approximately 5% to 10% of patients and increase the risk of developing CVID, whereas biallelic mutations always lead to the development of CVID.[13–18] Other monogenic disorders that have been described in patients with a diagnosis of CVID include ICOS, TNFRSF13 C (BAFF-R), TNFSF12 (TWEAK), CD19, CD81, CR2 (CD21), MS4A1 (CD20), TNFRSF7 (CD27), IL21, IL21 R, LPS-responsive beige -like anchor protein

---

**Box 3**
**International Consensus Document: common variable immunodeficiency disorders[2]**

1. Most patients will have at least 1 of the characteristic clinical manifestations (infection, autoimmunity, lymphoproliferation). However, a diagnosis of CVID may be conferred on asymptomatic individuals who fulfill criteria 2 to 5, especially in familial cases.

2. Hypogammaglobulinemia should be defined according to the age adjusted reference range for the laboratory in which the measurement is performed. The IgG level must be repeatedly low in at least 2 measurements more than 3 weeks apart in all patients. Repeated measurement may be omitted if the level is very low (<100–300 mg/dL depending on age), other characteristic features are present, and it is considered in the best interest of the patient to initiate therapy with IgG as quickly as possible.

3. IgA or IgM level must also be low.

4. It is strongly recommended that all patients with an IgG level of more than 100 mg/dL should be studied for responses to T-dependent (TD) and T-independent (TI) antigens, whenever possible. In all patients undergoing such testing, there must be a demonstrable impairment of response to at least 1 type of antigen (TD or TI). At the discretion of the practitioner, specific antibody measurement may be dispensed with if all other criteria are satisfied and if the delay incurred by prevaccination and postvaccination antibody measurement is thought to be deleterious to the patient's health.

5. Other causes of hypogammaglobulinemia must be excluded.

6. Genetic studies to investigate monogenic forms of CVID or for disease-modifying polymorphisms are not generally required for diagnosis and management in most of the patients, especially those who present with infections only without immune dysregulation, autoimmunity, malignancy, or other complications. In these latter groups of patients, however, single gene defects may be amenable to specific therapies (eg, stem cell therapy) and molecular genetic diagnosis should be considered when possible.

---

(LRBA), CTLA4, PRKCD, PLCG2, NFKB1, NFKB2, PIK3CD, PIK3R1, VAV1, RAC2, BLK, XIAP, SH2D1A, IKZF1 (IKAROS), IRF2BP2, and PTEN[19] (**Table 1**). There is some controversy as to whether patients with a monogenic defect should be diagnosed as CVID, but these disorders exhibit defective immunoglobulin levels and vaccine titers and meet diagnostic criteria for CVID.

Patients with CVID can be grouped into 2 categories: one group that exhibits hypogammaglobulinemia without other noninfectious complications, and a group with autoimmunity and inflammatory complications.[5] Since the common usage of immunoglobulin replacement, patients with only infectious complications have a milder course compared with those with noninfectious complications which exhibit increased morbidity and mortality.

One interesting aspect and hypothesis regarding the etiology of CVID addresses the clinical observation that patients with CVID have years of normal immune function before developing hypogammaglobulinemia, and that these patients often have autoimmune features (eg, autoimmune cytopenias) years before developing CVID. Some of these patients have gain-of-function variants in T- and B-cell signaling proteins (eg, CTLA4, LRBA, PIK3CD, PLCG2) supporting the hypothesis that CVID may be a gain-of-function defect leading to autoimmunity and eventual B-cell senescence and late onset hypogammaglobulinemia.[20] However, the genetic defects described vary greatly, and thus there are likely a number of different etiologies of CVID.

**Table 1**
**Genetic defects associated with common variable immunodeficiency**

| Gene | Genetic Disorder | Gene Function |
|---|---|---|
| BLK | BLK dysfunction | B-cell receptor signaling |
| CD19 | CD19 deficiency | B-cell signaling |
| CD81 | CD81 deficiency | Interacts with CD19 and mediates signal transduction events |
| CR2 (CD21) | CD21 deficiency | Inhibits activation, proliferation, and antibody production in B cells |
| CTLA4 | CTLA4 deficiency | Inhibits and regulates T-cell expression, function, and trafficking |
| ICOS | ICOS deficiency | T-cell activation |
| IKZF1 (IKAROS) | IKAROS haploinsufficiency | Regulates lymphoid differentiation |
| IL21 | IL-21 deficiency | Stimulates and activates cell cycle regulators and promotes cell proliferation |
| IL21 R | IL-21 receptor deficiency | Transduces the growth promotion of IL21, and proliferates and differentiates lymphocytes |
| IRF2BP2 | IRFBP2 loss of function | B-cell development and T-cell homeostasis |
| LRBA | LRBA deficiency | Interacts with CTLA4 in cytotoxic T-cell expression, function, and trafficking |
| MS4A1 (CD20) | CD20 deficiency | Development and differentiation of B cells |
| NFKB1 | NFKB1 deficiency | Regulates proinflammatory and immune system gene expression |
| NFKB2 | NFKB2 deficiency | Regulates proinflammatory and immune system gene expression |
| PIK3CD | PIK3CD gain of function | Regulates T cell, B cell, mast cell, neutrophil, and dendritic cell function |
| PIK3R1 | PIKR1 deficiency | Regulates T- and B-cell development and function |
| PLCG2 | PLCG2 deficiency | Signals cell growth, maturation, and migration |
| PRKCD | PRKCD deficiency | B-cell proliferation and apoptosis |
| PTEN | PTEN deficiency | Maintains immune system homeostasis through downstream effects of lymphocyte, cytokine, and growth factor receptors |
| VAV1 | Vav1 deficiency | Regulates T-cell function |
| RAC2 | RAC2 gain of function and RAC2 deficiency | Actin remodeling and activates neutrophil superoxide production |
| SH2D1A (SAP) | X-linked lymphoproliferative disease (XLP) | T-cell activation |
| TACI | TACI deficiency | B lymphocyte class switching |

(continued on next page)

**Table 1**
**(continued)**

| Gene | Genetic Disorder | Gene Function |
|---|---|---|
| TNFSF12 (TWEAK) | TWEAK deficiency | Induce apoptosis and regulate angiogenesis |
| TNFRSF7 (CD27) | CD27 deficiency | Regulates survival and activation of lymphocytes and development of cytotoxic T cells |
| TNFRSF13 C (BAFF-R) | BAFF receptor deficiency | Enhances B-cell survival and regulates the peripheral B-cell population |
| XIAP | XIAP deficiency | Apoptosis prevention through caspase inhibition |

**Table 2**
**Common infectious complications of common variable immunodeficiency**

| Site of Infection | Clinical Manifestations | Most Common Pathogens |
|---|---|---|
| Sinopulmonary | • Pneumonia<br>  ○ Bronchiectasis<br>  ○ Interstitial lung disease<br>• Sinusitis<br>• Bronchitis<br>• Otitis<br>  ○ Hearing loss<br>• Conjunctivitis | • Streptococcus pneumoniae<br>• Haemophilus influenzae<br>• Moraxella catarrhalis<br>• Mycoplasma pneumoniae<br>• Pneumocystis jirovecii<br>• Human herpesvirus 8 (HHV8) |
| Gastrointestinal | • Acute infectious diarrhea<br>• Refractory and/or chronic diarrhea ± weight loss and malabsorption<br>• Gastritis<br>• Bacterial overgrowth<br>• Hepatitis | • Giardia lamblia<br>• Campylobacter jejuni<br>• Salmonella species<br>• Norovirus<br>• Helicobacter pylori<br>• Cytomegalovirus<br>• Cryptosporidium<br>• Hepatitis B<br>• Hepatitis C |
| Urinary | • Cystitis<br>• Pyelonephritis | • Mycoplasma species<br>• Ureaplasma species |
| Central nervous system | • Meningitis | • Neisseria meningitidis |
| Joints | • Septic arthritis (monoarthritis or polyarthritis) | • Streptococcus species<br>• Mycoplasma species |
| Skin | • Verrucae vulgaris (warts)<br>• Molluscum<br>• Herpes labialis<br>• Herpes gingivostomatitis<br>• Shingles<br>• Impetigo<br>• Cellulitis<br>• Abscesses<br>• Oral candidiasis | • Human papilloma virus (HPV)<br>• Molluscum contagiosum virus (MCV)<br>• Herpes simplex virus (HSV)<br>• Herpes zoster<br>• Streptococcus species<br>• Staphylococcus aureus<br>• Candida albicans |
| Systemic | • Septicemia | • Streptococcus pneumoniae<br>• Neisseria meningitidis<br>• Haemophilus influenzae |

## DISCUSSION
### Clinical Manifestations

#### Infectious complications of common variable immunodeficiency

Acute and chronic infections are the most common clinical manifestation and a hallmark feature of CVID, and a major cause of morbidity and mortality affecting more than 90% of patients.[5] The most common pathogens infect the upper and lower respiratory and gastrointestinal tracts, although many organ systems can be affected (**Table 2**).[6,21–26]

*Sinopulmonary infections.* Symptoms may be acute, chronic, or recurrent. The most common pathogens to consider include *Streptococcus pneumoniae*, *Haemophilus influenzae*, and *Mycoplasma* species.

- Pneumonia
- Bronchitis
- Sinusitis
- Otitis
- Conjunctivitis

Respiratory tract involvement is very common in CVID and is a major cause of morbidity and mortality.[26–31] Respiratory tract involvement can be infectious or noninfections and can affect the upper or lower respiratory tract. Because of this it is essential to screen patients with CVID for respiratory involvement, and it is recommended to do this with a high-resolution chest CT (HRCT) to define pulmonary pathology. Chest radiographs and pulmonary function tests are not sensitive to diagnosis all the possible respiratory tract complications in CVID. As an example, HRCT of the chest detected bronchiectasis in 64% of individuals with CVID and interstitial lung disease (ILD) in 31% of patients with CVID, whereas pulmonary function tests (PFTs) and routine chest x-ray (CXR) detected these abnormalities in only 6% of patients.[32] It is also important to repeat the CT after 6 months of immunoglobulin replacement therapy to be determined if any pulmonary findings were the result of untreated infection.

Most patients with CVID present with recurrent upper or lower respiratory tract infections, including bronchitis, sinusitis, otitis media, and pneumonia. Encapsulated bacteria (eg, *H. influenzae, S. pneumoniae*) are the most common organisms involved, but atypical bacteria (eg, *Mycoplasma* and *Ureaplasma* spp.) are also an important pathogen.[5,21,33] Opportunistic infections (eg, *Pneumocystis* spp.) are uncommon and occur in less than 10% of patients.[23] Empiric treatment of pulmonary infections in CVID must include antibiotics against common encapsulated respiratory bacteria as well as well as atypical bacteria such as *Mycoplasma* spp. and *Ureaplasma* spp. Bronchiectasis is the most common pulmonary complication in CVID, occurs in over 30% of patients, and is the result of repeat respiratory infections. It is not clear whether immunoglobulin replacement therapy can prevent the development of bronchiectasis in patients with CVID, as often this finding is present before a diagnosis of CVID is made.[25] Bronchiectasis in patients with CVID is managed similar other causes of bronchiectasis (eg, hypertonic saline or $\beta_2$-agonists, chest physiotherapy, empiric treatment with macrolides).[34–36]

*Gastrointestinal infections.* Symptoms are often acute but can also be refractory or chronic. Causes include most commonly infections with *Giardia lamblia*, norovirus, *Salmonella* species, and *Campylobacter jejuni*.[12,37,38] Sources of clean water are essential for patients with CVID to prevent infections from water-borne pathogens.

- Acute infectious diarrhea
- Refractory and/or chronic diarrhea ± weight loss and malabsorption
- Bacterial overgrowth
- Gastritis

- Hepatitis

### Central Nervous System Infections

- Meningitis

### Joints

- Septic arthritis

### Skin

- Verrucae vulgaris (warts)[39]
- Molluscum contagiosum
- Herpes labialis
- Herpes gingivostomatitis
- Shingles
- Impetigo
- Cellulitis
- Abscesses
- Oral candidiasis

### Systemic

- Septicemia

## NONINFECTIOUS COMPLICATIONS OF COMMON VARIABLE IMMUNODEFICIENCY
### Pulmonary Disease

A diffuse interstitial lung disease known as granulomatous and lymphocytic interstitial lung disease (GLILD) occurs in 10% to 25% of patients with CVID. This entity has the following pathologic findings: peribronchiolar and interstitial lymphoid infiltration; granuloma; organizing pneumonia; and variable amounts of fibrosis. Untreated GLILD can cause progressive pulmonary fibrosis, and a pathology study of 16 patients with GLILD demonstrated significant fibrosis in over 40% of patients at the time of diagnosis.[40] The presence of granulomatous lung disease and adenopathy results in the diagnosis of sarcoidosis in many of these patients, although this disorder is distinct from sarcoidosis.[28,29,40–42] HRCT in GLILD often demonstrate mediastinal adenopathy, ground-glass abnormalities, areas of consolidation, and small and large nodules typically in the lower lung zones, which contrasts with sarcoidosis which is predominantly upper lung zone disease.[42,43] In comparison to sarcoidosis GLILD exhibits a poor response to corticosteroid therapy, panhypogammaglobulinemia, a high prevalence of autoimmune disease (eg, immune thrombocytopenia [ITP]), and a history of recurrent infections.[40,42] Patients with GLILD can also exhibit hepatosplenomegaly, diffuse adenopathy, widespread granulomas, and an increased risk of developing lymphoma.[28,29,42] Thus, GLILD appears to be a multisystemic lymphoproliferative and granulomatous disease. Splenomegaly and widespread lymphadenopathy are common findings. Granulomas in GLILD are not limited to the lung but may be found in virtually any organ including bone marrow, liver, spleen, and lymph nodes.

Importantly, this lung disease is refractory to IVIG therapy alone and other immunosuppressants are often needed.[26,28–31,44] Corticosteroids are the most commonly used immunosuppressive agent for this disorder although relapse is common and it is unclear if they alter disease progression.[45] In one of the largest treatment series to date, 39 patients with GLILD were treated with a combination of rituximab and an anti-metabolite (eg, azathioprine or mycophenolate) with improvement of radiographic abnormalities and pulmonary function without an increased incidence of infection.[46]

Other treatments have included monotherapy with rituximab, low-dose cyclosporin, tacrolimus, infliximab, and CTLA4-Ig (immunoglobulin) in patients with CTLA4 haploin-sufficiency or LRBA deficiency.[47–51]

As mentioned above all patients with CVID should have an HRCT of the chest and pulmonary function testing at baseline, after initiation of Ig replacement and periodi-cally thereafter. In addition, any patient with HRCT findings consistent with GLILD should undergo open lung biopsy, as needle biopsies may not obtain enough tissue to exclude other parenchymal diseases of the lung as well as lymphoma. Video assis-ted thoracoscopic surgery is the most common technique to obtain sufficient tissue for diagnosis, although other techniques (eg, cryobiopsy) have shown some promise.

### Autoimmunity

Autoimmune conditions are a common presentation in CVID, present in 25% to 30% of patients.[52–54] Autoimmunity can be the initial indication of CVID, most often in chil-dren than in adults. Autoimmune hematologic conditions (also known as IMCs), including ITP, autoimmune hemolytic anemia (AIHA), autoimmune neutropenia (AIN), or a combination of 2 or more (Evans syndrome [ES]), are the most frequently identified autoimmune conditions thought to be secondary to underlying immune dysregulation associated with CVID. AIHA and ES in particular are recognized as prominent features in inborn errors of immunity and immune dysregulation disorders, with AIHA having at least an 830-fold higher risk than the general population.[53,55,56] Sixty-five percent of patients with ES were found to have an underlying immune-related monogenic disor-der when evaluated in a recent study, warranting assessment for immune dysregula-tion and immunodeficiency in such patients.[57] Other autoimmune manifestations include gastrointestinal conditions (eg, inflammatory bowel disease, autoimmune hep-atitis), skin conditions (eg, alopecia totalis, vitiligo, psoriasis), endocrine conditions (eg, autoimmune hyperthyroidism or hypothyroidism), and rheumatologic conditions (eg, cutaneous vasculitis, systemic lupus erythematosus, sicca syndrome).[52–54]

### Lymphoproliferative Disease/Malignancy

Lymphoproliferative disease and increased susceptibility toward development of ma-lignancy occurs in patients with defective immune function. The etiology of the increased risk of lymphoproliferation in CVID is likely multifactorial including gain-of-function genetic diseases, genetic polymorphisms in DNA repair, radiosensitivity, cytokine stimulation, viral infections, and T- and B-cell dysregulation. The most frequently diagnosed cancers include lymphoid and gastric malignancies. Patients with polyclonal lymphadenopathy have the most increased risk of lymphoid malig-nancy, in particular non-Hodgkin B-cell lymphoma. However, impaired immunity against Epstein-Barr virus and *Helicobacter pylori* coupled with chronic atrophic gastritis and stomach metaplasia have been attributed to an increased risk in devel-opment of gastric cancer.[58,59]

### Enteropathy

Chronic enteropathy is a complication associated with CVID, which is complex with variable presentations including villous atrophy, chronic bacterial overgrowth, chronic exudative enteropathy, and chronic enteritis. Clinical features include chronic diar-rhea, malnutrition, abdominal pain, and anasarca, which in some cases leads to parental nutrition requirements. Histology may show a variety of abnormalities including increased intraepithelial lymphocytes, villous blunting, nodular lymphoid hy-perplasia, crypt distortion, apoptosis, and paucity of plasma cells. Treatment for this disorder can be difficult and there are no standard therapies, and trials of medications used to treat inflammatory bowel disease are trialed empirically.[38]

### Liver Disease (Nodular Regenerative Hyperplasia)

Nodular regenerative hyperplasia (NRH) is a rare but serious complication found in a subset of patients with CVID affecting approximately 5% of individuals. NRH is illustrated by intra-hepatic vasculopathy leading to hepatocyte injury and hepatocyte regeneration, which forms characteristic nodules. The presence of nodules in turn compresses the hepatic parenchyma, as well as central and portal veins causing downstream effects including portal hypertension, esophageal varices, and splenomegaly with associated neutropenia and thrombocytopenia due to splenic congestion. A severe stage of NRH is described as an autoimmune hepatitis (AIH)-like disease with inflammatory features superimposed by an NRH background. Patients with AIH-like liver disease have significant morbidity and mortality requiring aggressive treatment making early recognition important.[60]

### Evaluations

If a patient's clinical presentation is suspicious for CVID, a comprehensive evaluation of the immune system should be performed.[1,2,10,61]

### Initial evaluation

- Complete blood count with differential
- Reticulocyte count (if anemia present)
- Lymphocyte subset analysis by flow cytometry for T-, B-, and NK-cell enumeration
- Serum immunoglobulins (IgG, IgA, IgM, IgE)

Typical findings of CVID include low serum immunoglobulin levels by age of hypogammaglobulinemia. Other causes of hypogammaglobulinemia should be considered including protein loss through the renal or gastrointestinal systems and medications (eg, steroids, antiepileptics). This initial assessment will differentiate if a patient has findings that may be compatible with CVID and if abnormal, should be referred to a subspecialist (typically an Immunologist) for further evaluations and management.

### Secondary evaluation

- Protein and polysaccharide vaccine responses
- B-cell maturation testing by flow cytometry
- T-cell functional testing by mitogen stimulation
- PFTs and lung CT scan after a trial of immunoglobulin replacement
- Evaluation for gastrointestinal or hepatic dysfunction
- Genetic testing

### Therapeutic options

The antibody deficiency in CVID is treated with Ig replacement either in intravenous form (IVIG) or subcutaneous administration (SCIG). Regular dosing of Ig can prevent the majority of infections. Patients with CVID will have lifelong Ig therapy.

IVIG for CVID or other primary immune deficiencies is initiated in the range of 400 to 600 mg/kg/mo. With IV administration, Ig levels follow a peak and trough pattern, and the trough level is monitored periodically. Although troughs are monitored to assure a basic minimum level, dosing is adjusted according to the patients' symptoms and frequency of infections. Many patients, particularly those without significant noninfectious complications, will do well at lower doses. Other patients will require higher dosing, which tends to be more common in patients with enteropathy, bronchiectasis, or significant ongoing sinus disease. IVIG is initially administered monthly. Common side effects during or after infusion include headache and nausea. Side effects from infusions can be minimized by good pre-hydration, infusion rate control and premedication with analgesics, antihistamines, and steroids if needed.

SCIG is initiated similarly at 400 to 600 mg/kg/mo with increases based on symptoms. The total monthly Ig dose is divided over the number of infusions planned per month. It is designed for self-administration by the patient, or by a caregiver. Patients generally infuse once a week, every other week dosing is possible. Serum IgG levels remain more consistent with SCIG therapy compared with IVIG therapy and trough levels do not need to be monitored. SCIG is generally better tolerated than IVIG. Side effects are restricted to local reactions such as erythema, itching, or swelling which improve with continued use. Systemic side effects do not usually occur.

However on Ig therapy patients receive passive immunity for all vaccines and thus these patients do not need routine vaccinations and boosters. Any serologic testing, such as vaccine titers or antibody levels to infectious organisms, is no longer valid while on Ig therapy. Certain vaccines that promote T-cell responses, such as human papilloma virus (HPV), Varicella-Zoster virus (VZV), influenza, and COVID can be given.

## SUMMARY

CVID is characterized as a heterogenous group of disorders exhibiting a common phenotype of abnormal B-cell differentiation with impaired production of specific immunoglobulin. The clinical manifestations are variable and include acquisition of recurrent bacterial infections, lymphoproliferation, autoimmunity, pulmonary disease, gastrointestinal disease, granulomas, and an increased risk of cancer. Although many different types of infections can occur, sinopulmonary infections are the most common. The onset of the disease can be at any age, but the peak incidence occurs in ages 16 to 20 years. The diagnosis of CVID is complex, as there is not one specific laboratory finding associated with the disease. There are several clinical criteria models used in practice, all of which indicate patients should have hypogammaglobulinemia, defective vaccine responses, age greater than 4 years, and exclusion of other causes of immunoglobulin deficiency. The management of CVID consists of regular immunoglobulin replacement therapy, prevention of infections, and vigilant surveillance for complications.

## CLINICS CARE POINTS

- CVID is a primary immune deficiency characterized by hypogammaglobulinemia and frequent or recurrent infections.
- Patients with CVID should have comprehensive immune system evaluations including enumeration of immunoglobulins and vaccine responses.
- Clinicians caring for patients with CVID should consider co-morbidities including pulmonary and gastrointestinal disease, as well as a risk for autoimmunity and cancer.
- Regular immunoglobulin replacement is a key factor in the management of patients with CVID.
- Infection prevention in patients with CVID is important including routine vaccinations and use of a clean water source for prevention of parasitic infections.

## DISCLOSURE

The authors declare that the research was conducted in the absence of any commercial or financial relationships that could be construed as a potential conflict of interest.

## REFERENCES

1. Odnoletkova I, Kindle G, Quinti I, et al. The burden of common variable immunodeficiency disorders: a retrospective analysis of the European Society for Immunodeficiency (ESID) registry data. Orphanet J Rare Dis 2018;13(1):201.
2. Bonilla FA, Barlan I, Chapel H, et al. International Consensus Document (ICON): Common Variable Immunodeficiency Disorders. J Allergy Clin Immunol Pract 2016;4(1):38–59.
3. Seidel MG, Kindle G, Gathmann B, et al. The European Society for Immunodeficiencies (ESID) Registry Working Definitions for the Clinical Diagnosis of Inborn Errors of Immunity. J Allergy Clin Immunol Pract 2019;7(6):1763.
4. Tagye SG, Al-Herz W, Bousfiha A, et al. Human Inborn Errors of Immunity: 2022 Update on the Classification from the International Union of Immunological Societies Expert Committee. J Clin Immunol 2022;42(7):1473.
5. Cunningham-Rundles C, Bodian C. Common variable immunodeficiency: clinical and immunological features of 248 patients. Clin Immunol 1999;92(1):34–48.
6. Resnick ES, Moshier EL, Godbold JH, et al. Morbidity and mortality in common variable immune deficiency over 4 decades. Blood 2012;119(7):1650–7.
7. Chapel H, Lucas M, Lee M, et al. Common variable immunodeficiency disorders: division into distinct clinical phenotypes. Blood 2008;112(2):277–86.
8. Quinti I, Soresina A, Spadaro G, et al. Long-term follow-up and outcome of a large cohort of patients with common variable immunodeficiency. J Clin Immunol 2007;27(3):308–16.
9. Ameratunga R, Lehnert K, Woon S-T. All patients with common variable immunodeficiency disorders (CVID) should be routinely offered diagnostic testing. Front Immunol 2019;10:2678.
10. Ameratunga R, Woon S-T, Gillis D, et al. New diagnostic criteria for common variable immune deficiency (CVID), which may assist with decisions to treat with intravenous or subcutaneous immunoglobulin. Clin Exp Immunol 2013;174(2): 203–11.
11. Hammarström L, Vorechovsky I, Webster D. Selective IgA deficiency (SIgAD) and common variable immunodeficiency (CVID). Clin Exp Immunol 2000;120(2):225.
12. Gathmann B, Mahlaoui N, CEREDIH, Gérard L, et al. Clinical picture and treatment of 2212 patients with common variable immunodeficiency. J Allergy Clin Immunol 2014;134(1):116.
13. Zhang L, Radigan L, Salzer U, et al. Transmembrane activator and calcium-modulating cyclophilin ligand interactor mutations in common variable immunodeficiency: clinical and immunologic outcomes in heterozygotes. J Allergy Clin Immunol 2007;120(5):1178–85.
14. Pan-Hammarstrom Q, Salzer U, Du L, et al. Reexamining the role of TACI coding variants in common variable immunodeficiency and selective IgA deficiency. Nat Genet 2007;39(4):429–30.
15. Salzer U, Chapel HM, Webster AD, et al. Mutations in TNFRSF13B encoding TACI are associated with common variable immunodeficiency in humans. Nat Genet 2005;37(8):820–8.
16. Castigli E, Wilson SA, Garibyan L, et al. TACI is mutant in common variable immunodeficiency and IgA deficiency. Nat Genet 2005;37(8):829–34.

17. Poodt AE, Driessen GJ, de Klein A, et al. TACI mutations and disease suscepti-
    bility in patients with common variable immunodeficiency. Clin Exp Immunol
    2009;156(1):35–9.

18. Mohammadi J, Liu C, Aghamohammadi A, et al. Novel mutations in TACI
    (TNFRSF13B) causing common variable immunodeficiency. J Clin Immunol
    2009;29(6):777–85.

19. Bogaert DJ, Dullaers M, Lambrecht BN, et al. Genes associated with common
    variable immunodeficiency: one diagnosis to rule them all? J Med Genet 2016;
    53(9):575–90.

20. Abolhassani H, Hammarström L, Cunningham-Rundles C. Current genetic land-
    scape in common variable immune deficiency. Blood 2020;135(9):656–67.

21. Oksenhendler E, Gérard L, Fieschi C, et al. Infections in 252 patients with com-
    mon variable immunodeficiency. Clin Infect Dis 2008;46(10):1547.

22. Gathmann B, Goldacker S, Klima M, et al. The German national registry for pri-
    mary immunodeficiencies (PID). Clin Exp Immunol 2013;173(2):372.

23. Lucas M, Lee M, Lortan J, et al. Infection outcomes in patients with common var-
    iable immunodeficiency disorders: relationship to immunoglobulin therapy over
    22 years. J Allergy Clin Immunol 2010;125(6):1354.

24. Roifman CM, Rao CP, Lederman HM, et al. Increased suspectibility to Myco-
    plasma infection in patients with hypogammaglobulinemia. Am J Med 1986;
    80(4):590.

25. Quinti I, Soresina A, Spadaro G, et al. Long-term follow-up and outcomes of a
    large cohort of patients with common variable immunodeficiency. J Clin Immunol
    2007;27(3):308.

26. Busse PJ, Farzan S, Cunningham-Rundles C. Pulmonary complications of com-
    mon variable immunodeficiency. Ann Allergy Asthma Immunol 2007;98(1):1.

27. Baumann U, Routes JM, Soler-Palacin P, et al. The Lung in Primary Immunodefi-
    ciencies: New Concepts in Infection and Inflammation. Front Immunol 2018;9:
    1837.

28. Wehr C, Kivioja T, Schmitt C, et al. The EUROclass trial: defining subgroups in
    common variable immunodeficiency. Blood 2008;111(1):77–85.

29. Bates CA, Ellison MC, Lynch DA, et al. Granulomatous-lymphocytic lung disease
    shortens survival in common variable immunodeficiency. J Allergy Clin Immunol
    2004;114(2):415–21.

30. Arnold DF, Wiggins J, Cunningham-Rundles C, et al. Granulomatous disease:
    distinguishing primary antibody disease from sarcoidosis. Clin Immunol 2008;
    128(1):18–22.

31. Buckley RH. Pulmonary complications of primary immunodeficiencies. Paediatr
    Respir Rev 2004;5(Suppl A):S225–33.

32. Maarschalk-Ellerbroek LJ, de Jong PA, van Montfrans JM, et al. CT screening for
    pulmonary pathology in common variable immunodeficiency disorders and the
    correlation with clinical and immunological parameters. J Clin Immunol 2014;
    34(6):642–54.

33. Gelfand EW. Unique susceptibility of patients with antibody deficiency to myco-
    plasma infection. Clin Infect Dis 1993;17(Suppl 1):S250–3.

34. Nair GB, Ilowite JS. Pharmacologic agents for mucus clearance in bronchiec-
    tasis. Clin Chest Med 2012;33(2):363–70.

35. Wong C, Jayaram L, Karalus N, et al. Azithromycin for prevention of exacerba-
    tions in non-cystic fibrosis bronchiectasis (EMBRACE): a randomised, double-
    blind, placebo-controlled trial. Lancet 2012;380(9842):660–7.

36. Altenburg J, de Graaff CS, Stienstra Y, et al. Effect of azithromycin maintenance treatment on infectious exacerbations among patients with non-cystic fibrosis bronchiectasis: the BAT randomized controlled trial. JAMA 2013;309(12):1251–9.

37. Agarwal S, Mayer L. Pathogenesis and treatment of gastrointestinal disease in antibody deficiency syndromes. J Allergy Clin Immunol 2009;124(4):658.

38. Uzzan M, Ko HM, Mehandru S, et al. Gastrointestinal Disorders Associated with Common Variable Immune Deficiency (CVID) and Chronic Granulomatous Disease (CGD). Curr Gastroenterol Rep 2016;18(4):17.

39. Zarezadeh Mehrabadi A, Aghamohamadi N, Abolhassani H, et al. Comprehensive assessment of skin disorders in patients with common variable immunodeficiency (CVID). J Clin Immunol 2022;42(3):653–64.

40. Rao N, Mackinnon AC, Routes JM. Granulomatous and lymphocytic interstitial lung disease: a spectrum of pulmonary histopathologic lesions in common variable immunodeficiency–histologic and immunohistochemical analyses of 16 cases. Hum Pathol 2015;46(9):1306–14.

41. Fasano MB, Sullivan KE, Sarpong SB, et al. Sarcoidosis and common variable immunodeficiency. Report of 8 cases and review of the literature. Medicine 1996; 75(5):251–61.

42. Verbsky JW, Routes JM. Sarcoidosis and Common Variable Immunodeficiency: Similarities and Differences. Semin Respir Crit Care Med 2014;35(3):330–5.

43. Torigian DA, LaRosa DF, Levinson AI, et al. Granulomatous-lymphocytic interstitial lung disease associated with common variable immunodeficiency: CT findings. J Thorac Imag 2008;23(3):162–9.

44. Mechanic LJ, Dikman S, Cunningham-Rundles C. Granulomatous disease in common variable immunodeficiency. Ann Intern Med 1997;127(8 Pt 1):613–7.

45. Hurst JR, Verma N, Lowe D, et al. British Lung Foundation/United Kingdom Primary Immunodeficiency Network Consensus Statement on the Definition, Diagnosis, and Management of Granulomatous-Lymphocytic Interstitial Lung Disease in Common Variable Immunodeficiency Disorders. J Allergy Clin Immunol Pract 2017;5(4):938–45.

46. Chase NM, Verbsky JW, Hintermeyer MK, et al. Use of combination chemotherapy for treatment of granulomatous and lymphocytic interstitial lung disease (GLILD) in patients with common variable immunodeficiency (CVID). J Clin Immunol 2013;33(1):30–9.

47. Ng J, Wright K, Alvarez M, et al. Rituximab Monotherapy for Common Variable Immune Deficiency-Associated Granulomatous-Lymphocytic Interstitial Lung Disease. Chest 2019;155(5):e117–21.

48. Deya-Martinez A, Esteve-Sole A, Velez-Tirado N, et al. Sirolimus as an alternative treatment in patients with granulomatous-lymphocytic lung disease and humoral immunodeficiency with impaired regulatory T cells. Pediatr Allergy Immunol 2018; 29(4):425–32.

49. Franxman TJ, Howe LE, Baker JR Jr. Infliximab for treatment of granulomatous disease in patients with common variable immunodeficiency. J Clin Immunol 2014;34(7):820–7.

50. Lo B, Zhang K, Lu W, et al. Patients with LRBA deficiency show CTLA4 loss and immune dysregulation responsive to abatacept therapy. Science 2015; 349(6246):436–40.

51. Kiykim A, Ogulur I, Dursun E, et al. Abatacept as a long-term targeted therapy for LRBA deficiency. J Allergy Clin Immunol Pract 2019;7(8):2790–800.

52. Boileau J, Mouillot G, Gérard L, et al. Autoimmunity in common variable immunodeficiency: correlation with lymphocyte phenotype in the French DEFI study. J Autoimmun 2011;36(1):25.
53. Agarwal S, Cunningham Rundles C. Autoimmunity in common variable immunodeficiency. Ann Allergy Asthma Immunol 2019;123(5):454.
54. Mormile I, Punziano A, Riolo CA, et al. Common variable immunodeficiency and autoimmune disease: a retrospective study of 95 adult patients in a single tertiary care center. Front Immunol 2021;12:652487.
55. Wang J, Cunningham Rundles C. Treatment and outcome of autoimmune hematologic disease in common variable immunodeficiency (CVID). J Autoimmun 2005;25(1):57.
56. Sève P, Bourdillon L, Sarrot-Reynauld F, et al. Autoimmune hemolytic anemia and common variable immunodeficiency: a case-control study of 18 patients. Medicine (Baltim) 2008;87(3):177.
57. Hadjadi J, Aladjidi N, Fernandes H, et al. Pediatric Evans syndrome is associated with a high frequency of potentially damaging variants in immune genes. Blood 2019;134(1):9–21.
58. Yakaboski E, Fuleihan RL, Sullivan KE, et al. Lymphoproliferative disease in CVID: a report of types and frequencies form a US patient registry. J Clin Immunol 2020; 40(3):524–30.
59. Gangemi S, Allegra A, Musolino C. Lymphoproliferative disease and cancer among patients with common variable immunodeficiency. Leuk Res 2015;39(4): 389–96.
60. Fuss IJ, Friend J, Yang Z, et al. Nodular regenerative hyperplasia in common variable immunodeficiency. J Clin Immunol 2013;33(4):748–58.
61. Von Spee-Mayer C, Koemm V, Wehr C, et al. Evaluating laboratory criteria for combined immunodeficiency in adult patients diagnosed with common variable immunodeficiency. Clin Immunol 2019;203:59.

# Approach to Idiopathic Anaphylaxis in Adolescents

Jeanne E. Conner, MSN, RN, APNP[a], Joshua A. Steinberg, MD[a,b,*]

## KEYWORDS

- Anaphylaxis • Mast cell activation • Mastocytosis • Hereditary alpha tryptasemia
- Adolescent

## KEY POINTS

- Anaphylaxis is a potentially-life threatening syndrome of varied severity, presentation, and pathophysiology.
- Adolescents have increased risks for adverse outcomes from anaphylaxis and require unique support.
- Mast cell disorders, rare allergens, and cofactors may be etiologic factors in otherwise obscure cases of anaphylaxis.
- Mimic disorders may simulate anaphylaxis and require exclusion.
- A diagnosis of idiopathic anaphylaxis should only be considered only after an extensive review of rare causes and mimic disorders.

## INTRODUCTION

Anaphylaxis is a potentially fatal acute syndrome resulting from the acute activation of cells including mast cells, basophils, and other effector cells. Symptoms often present with sudden onset, and often involve cutaneous (urticaria/angioedema, itching, and flushing), gastrointestinal (nausea, vomiting, diarrhea, and cramps), hypotensive (pre-syncope, syncope, confusion, and reflex tachycardia), or respiratory (laryngeal stridor, bronchospasm, coughing, dyspnea, and wheezing) features. Often, 2 or more of these systems are involved concurrently; however, anaphylaxis can present with sudden onset of just 1 of the noncutaneous systems as well (**Fig. 1**).[1]

Common triggers for anaphylaxis in adolescents include food, drugs, and venom. Food allergy to either tree nuts or shellfish is the most common cause of anaphylaxis in this age group.[2] Venom and drug-induced anaphylaxis is more common in adolescents than in younger children.[2]

[a] Division of Allergy and Clinical Immunology, Department of Pediatrics, Medical College of Wisconsin, 9000 West Wisconsin Avenue. B440, Milwaukee, WI 53226, USA; [b] Section of Allergy, Department of Medicine, Clement J. Zablocki Veterans' Affairs Medical Center, 5000 West National Avenue, 1AN, Milwaukee, WI 53295, USA
* Corresponding author.
*E-mail address:* jsteinberg@mcw.edu

Med Clin N Am 108 (2024) 123–155
https://doi.org/10.1016/j.mcna.2023.05.018
0025-7125/24/Published by Elsevier Inc.

medical.theclinics.com

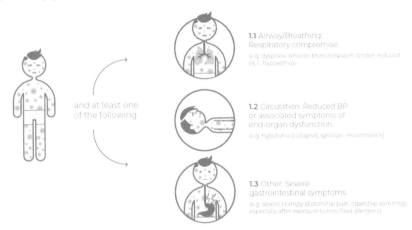

Anaphylaxis is highly likely when any one of the following **two criteria is fulfilled**

1. Acute onset of an illness (minutes to several hours) with involvement of the skin, mucosal tissue, or both (e.g. generalized hives, pruritus or flushing, swollen lips-tongue-uvula)

and at least one of the following

**1.1** Airway/Breathing: Respiratory compromise. (e.g. dyspnea, wheeze-bronchospasm, stridor, reduced PEF, hypoxemia)

**1.2** Circulation: Reduced BP or associated symptoms of end-organ dysfunction. (e.g. hypotonia [collapse], syncope, incontinence)

**1.3** Other: Severe gastrointestinal symptoms. (e.g. severe crampy abdominal pain, repetitive vomiting); especially after exposure to non-food allergens)

2. Acute onset of **hypotension**[a] or **bronchospasm** or **laryngeal involvement**[b] after exposure to a known or highly probable allergen for that patient (minutes to several hours), **even in the absence of typical skin involvement**.

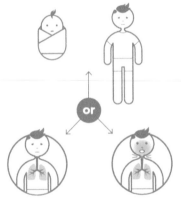

or

**Fig. 1.** WAO clinical criteria for diagnosis of anaphylaxis. BP, blood pressure; PEF, peak expiratory flow. [a]Hypotension defined as a decrease in systolic BP greater than 30% from that person's baseline, OR (i). Infants and children under 10 years: systolic BP less than (70 mm Hg + [2 × age in years]). (ii). Adults: systolic BP less than < 90 mm Hg. [b]Laryngeal symptoms include: stridor, vocal changes, odynophagia. Reproduced with permission from Cardona and colleagues 2020.[1]

The frequency of anaphylaxis is difficult to estimate; however, generally is thought to be increasing in developed and developing countries along with increases in the frequency of food allergy.[3] Adolescents have a disproportionate risk of fatal anaphylaxis.[3–5] Concerning adolescent behaviors such as rare utilization of epinephrine in emergencies,[6] insufficient perception of risk, and poor adoption of disease self-management strategies are commonplace.[7] Riskier exposures to food triggers are observed in adolescents; however, accidental food allergen exposures, misinformation, and inexperience seemed to be most prevalent.[8]

Generally, the cause for anaphylaxis is readily recognizable by a clinician because the cause often precedes symptom onset by only minutes. However, up to 17.5%

of pediatric cases can present with no clearly identifiable cause.[9] In these situations, a wide clinical differential and diagnostic evaluation is necessary before labeling the condition as idiopathic anaphylaxis.[10]

## Pathophysiology

The most common cause of anaphylaxis is via immunoglobulin E (IgE)-mediated mast cell and basophil degranulation. Following immunologic sensitization to a foreign protein, IgE antibodies specific to the protein are produced by B-cells and plasma cells. These allergen-specific IgE antibodies bind to IgE receptors on the cell surface of mast cells and basophils.[11]

With subsequent exposure to the allergen, the protein cross-links adjacent allergen-specific IgE on the mast cell or basophil membrane. This leads to downstream intracellular cascades and ultimate degranulation of preformed signaling mediators such as histamine and proteases to the extracellular space. These mediators then result in cascades of rapid physiologic change, including sudden vascular permeability, smooth muscle contraction, and additional immunologic system activation. These events culminate with the clinical syndrome of anaphylaxis.[11]

Besides signaling through IgE, binding of other mast cell and basophil cell-surface receptors can induce degranulation. Complement, cytokine, prostaglandin, leukotriene, drug, toxin, and other IgG receptors have been demonstrated to independently result in degranulation and cause clinical anaphylaxis. Additionally, neutrophils and macrophages can be activated, in an IgE and mast cell/basophil independent manner, and result in anaphylaxis.[12]

## Diagnostic Approach

When an adolescent presents with apparently unexplained anaphylaxis, a first necessary step is to obtain a detailed history[13] (**Box 1**). As anaphylaxis often begins outside of medical environments,[2] a clinician often depends on history from the patient or family members. Histories are subject to recall bias, second-hand information, and other omissions.

---

**Box 1**
**Essential features of the history in the evaluation of a patient who has experienced an episode of anaphylaxis. Reprinted with permission from Lieberman P. 2013[13]**

A. Detailed history of ingestants (foods/drugs) taken within 6 hours before the event.

B. Activity in which the patient was engaged at the time of the event.

C. Location of the event (home, school, work, indoors, or outdoors)

D. Exposure to heat or cold

E. Any related sting or bite

F. Time of day or night

G. Duration of the event

H. Recurrence of symptoms after initial resolution

I. The exact nature of the symptoms (eg, if cutaneous, determine whether flush, pruritus, urticaria, angioedema)

J. Assessing for physical factors or triggers

K. In a female, the relationship between the event and menstrual cycle

L. Was medical care given, and if so, what treatments were administered

Review of prehospital and emergency medical records for objective findings, in particular vital signs and evaluation of the airway and skin, is desirable for validation. Establishing a clear timeline of symptom onset and offset, especially in relationship to suspected triggers and treatments, is beneficial. Many suspected triggers can be deductively excluded from consideration if the exposure preceded symptoms by more than 2 hours; however, there are pertinent exceptions (galactose-alpha-1,3-galactose oligosaccharide motif [alpha-gal][14] and non-steroidal anti-inflammatory drugs [NSAIDs]).

Determining if the history and objective features meet anaphylaxis criteria should be the following step. To standardize diagnostic and treatment, the World Allergy Organization (WAO) established international criteria, most recently updated in 2020 (**Fig. 1**).[1] Multiple other guidelines and standards exist, however, many promulgated by national allergy organizations[15–18]; thus, there are some minor variances. Validation of the original 2005 National Institute of Allergy and Infectious Diseases/Food Allergy and Anaphylaxis Network (NIAID/FAAN) criteria within emergency departments had shown a high diagnostic negative predictive value (96.4%) and high sensitivity (95%), although the specificity was less ideal (82%).[16]

Despite these efforts at standardization, it is widely apparent that clinical utilization of diagnostic guidelines remains poor in prehospital and emergency settings, and anaphylaxis remains heavily underdiagnosed, underreported, and undertreated.[19]

### Immunoglobulin E-Mediated Allergy

#### Obscure food allergens
More than 90% of food allergies are triggered by egg, peanut, tree nut, fish, shellfish, sesame, wheat, milk, and soy; however, prevalence can vary extensively regionally (**Table 1**). As a result, other food triggers may be more obscure. Unusual allergens have been described, largely in case reports and case series, and the overall incidence is generally rare.

#### Ollen food syndrome
Pollen food syndrome is a very common disorder in atopic adolescents,[20] found in 5% to 48% of allergic children internationally. Symptoms often include rapid onset itchy mouth, throat discomfort, and occasional nausea following ingestion of fresh fruits, vegetables, legumes, or tree nuts. Cross-reactivity of food proteins with specific pollen proteins mediates this phenomenon. Cross-reactivities with profilin and pathogenesis-related class 10 (PR-10) proteins are generally mild and rarely induce anaphylaxis. However, other protein cross-reactivities to other proteins, such as to non-specific lipid transfer protein (nsLTP), are more commonly associated with anaphylaxis. The incidence of pollen food syndrome triggering anaphylaxis may range from 1.7% to 19% in varied studies.[21] Specific allergen component IgE serum testing, which can identify IgE binding specific cross-reactive protein components, are commercially available and may help identify higher risk pollen-food cross-reactivities.[22]

#### Food-exercise-induced anaphylaxis
Anaphylaxis symptoms occurring during or within an hour of exercise should prompt consideration of exercise itself being a trigger or a cofactor. The most common type of summation anaphylaxis, or anaphylaxis, which requires a trigger and a cofactor, is food-exercise-induced anaphylaxis (FEIA).[23,24] Trigger foods commonly associated with FEIA seem highly regionally variable, yet wheat proteins account for more than half of the cases in many studies.[23] Other common foods include tomato, celery, and shrimp. For some, no food cofactor is suggested, and the diagnosis is termed exercise-induced anaphylaxis (EIA).[25]

**Table 1**
Atypical or obscure triggers of anaphylaxis

| | Prevalence in Teens | Unique/Distinct Features | Diagnostic Tools |
|---|---|---|---|
| **IgE mediated** | | | |
| FEIA | Common | • Onset during exertion, up to 6 h following ingestion of specific food(s) (such as profilin, PR-10, nsLTP, others) <br> • Often aggravated by other cofactors (summation anaphylaxis) | Specific spices or herbs to common triggers: <br> • Wheat Tri a 19 (ω5-Gliadin), also Tri a 20/21/26/36 <br> • Celery <br> • Shellfish <br> • Peanut |
| Delayed mammalian meat allergy (alpha-gal polysaccharide) | Common | • Onset 4–6 h postprandially <br> • Prevalence related to endemicity specific ticks <br> • Reactions to mammalian but not avian meats <br> • Cross-reactivity with biologic drugs derived from mammalian cell lines 14 | • sIgE to alpha-gal, meats <br> • Skin testing |
| Spice allergens | Rare | • May be associated with pollen-food syndrome patterns | • sIgE to specific spices or herbs |
| Rare drug/vaccine allergens <br> • Gelatin[172] <br> • Neomycin[173] | Rare | | • Skin testing <br> • sIgE testing |
| Pollen-food syndrome (oral allergy syndrome) | Common | • Patterned sudden onset of multiple fruit/vegetable/nut/legume intolerances <br> • Often resolves if foods are cooked or heat treated <br> • Usually coexists with seasonal allergic rhinitis | • sIgE <br> • Component-resolved sIgE |
| Latex | Rare | • History of multiple surgical operations (including spina bifida) <br> • Cross-reactivity with banana, avocado, chestnut, and kiwifruit | • sIgE (note: low sensitivity) |

(continued on next page)

**Table 1**
*(continued)*

| | Prevalence in Teens | Unique/Distinct Features | Diagnostic Tools |
|---|---|---|---|
| Aeroallergen | Rare | • Marijuana<br>• Bee pollen | • sIgE testing<br>• Skin testing |
| **Non-IgE mediated** | | | |
| MRGPRX ligand | Common | • Can induce anaphylaxis on first exposure, without prior exposure to the drug | • Often associated with narcotics, vancomycin, quinolones, venoms, neuromuscular paralytics |
| NSAID/aspirin (aspirin exacerbated respiratory disease) | Common | • Triad of severe asthma, nasal polyposis and COX1 inhibitor reactions may not develop simultaneously<br>• Celecoxib (strict COX2 inhibitor) and acetaminophen generally tolerated | • Urine LTE4<br>• Aspirin challenge |
| Exercise induced (EIA) | Common | • Preceding history of exercise | • Develops with or without preceding food |
| Summation[24] | Rare | • two or more triggers (co-factors) required together or sequentially<br>• overlap with FEIA (above) | • history of 2 or more co-factors such as exercise, NSAID, menses, illness, alcohol, poor sleep |
| **Venom mediated** | | | |
| Mosquito | Rare | • Limited to endemic areas/seasons<br>• Follows bites | • Serum IgE |
| Fire ants | Common | • Limited to endemic areas<br>• Follows bites<br>• Benefits from venom immunotherapy | • Skin testing<br>• Serum IgE |
| Tick bites | Rare | • Limited to endemic areas in Europe and Australia<br>• Follows bites | • Serum IgE |

*Alpha-gal oligosaccharide motif anaphylaxis (delayed mammalian meat syndrome)*
Food proteins induce most food allergies; however, delayed mammalian meat syndrome is a clinically relevant oligosaccharide-mediated food allergy. Alpha-gal is foreign to humans and other higher order primates due to the loss of the alpha-gal glycosylase during evolution.[14] Most other mammals have retained the glycosylase, thus mammalian-sourced meats have the alpha-gal motif on many glycosylated proteins.

Patients sensitized to alpha-gal present with anaphylaxis following ingestion of mammalian meats such as beef and pork. Unlike protein-based food allergens that induce symptoms often within minutes after ingestion, alpha-gal-induced anaphylaxis is typically induced 4 to 6 hours after ingestion of mammalian meat. This can cause diagnostic delay because the association with meat may be difficult to deduce.[14]

Fascinatingly, the primary elicitor of sensitization to alpha-gal oligosaccharides is a tick bite. Patients at most risk tend to be hunters or hikers who live in endemic regions for specific ticks such as the Lone Star tick in North America, the Castor bean tick in Europe, and the Longhorn tick in Asia and Australia.[26] Patients with this syndrome may also develop anaphylaxis to certain biological drugs derived from mammalian cell lines.[14]

*Food dyes and additives*
In contrast to prevailing beliefs, synthetic food and drug dyes are rarely allergenic.[27] In contrast, naturally sourced dyes rarely trigger anaphylaxis. Dyes used from used in cosmetics and foods such as cochineal (carmine) extract derived from female *Dactylopius coccus* scale insects has been implicated.[28] Naturally sourced annatto seed coloring has also been associated with anaphylaxis.[29]

Generally, food additives and preservatives are very uncommon triggers of unexplained anaphylaxis.[30] Sulfite antioxidants, such as those in dried fruits generally trigger asthma rather than anaphylaxis.[31] Specific food additives implicated in anaphylaxis include mycoprotein used in vegan meat substitutes,[32] psyllium in fiber supplements,[33] erythritol in sugar-free products,[34–36] guar gum,[37] and inulin.[38,39]

*Spice and rare food allergies*
Herbal and spice allergies are generally rare.[40] Mustard is perhaps the most common, most extensively described in France with prevalence in children up to 6%.[41] Multiple case reports of anaphylaxis, most due to pollen cross-reactivities, have been described to chamomile,[42] fennel,[43] fenugreek,[44] oregano,[45] thyme,[45] coriander,[46,47] and others.

Dust mite-contaminated flour has been often implicated causing anaphylaxis. This syndrome, curiously often triggered following pancake ingestion, is most common in warm tropical environments where the mites can thrive.[48,49] Lupine flour, a legume powder added as a flour supplement popular in Europe, can trigger flour-associated anaphylaxis as well.[50]

There have been multiple case reports of bee pollen dietary supplements inducing anaphylaxis. Although sensitization is rare to insect-pollinated flower pollens, wind-pollinated flower pollens have been identified within bee pollen supplements.[51]

### Nonfood Immunoglobulin E-Mediated Allergies

Anaphylaxis to marijuana has been rarely reported.[52] Nearly 3 of 4 patients with marijuana allergy are sensitized to Can s 3, a protein cross-reactive with other foods and pollens.[53] Because adolescents often initiate marijuana use surreptitiously, a careful history elicitation may be helpful.

Natural rubber latex exposures in adolescents are likely primarily via surgical exposures, yet children can become sensitized to natural rubber latex at home and other environments.[54] Particular efforts to avoid natural rubber latex exposure in surgical suites, and most specifically to eliminate exposure for children with spina bifida, have resulted in markedly reduced incidence of latex anaphylaxis.[55] Although largely minimized, medical exposure to latex continues within developing nations and still exists in developed countries.[56] Anaphylaxis presenting during the maintenance phase of anesthesia should raise concerns for latex allergy.

### Obscure Venom Allergens

Envenomation from hymenoptera insects is a very common source of IgE-mediated anaphylaxis and given the pain from a sting often easily identifiable as a trigger. In contrast, other insect bites have been rarely associated with anaphylaxis.

Despite expanding global distribution of mosquitos, systemic immediate type hypersensitivities and anaphylaxis to mosquito venom seem very rare.[57,58] In one case, systemic mosquito allergy without evidence of specific immunoglobulin E (sIgE) sensitization was revealed to be due to systemic mastocytosis (SM).[59] Treatment with immunotherapy to whole mosquito body extracts may be beneficial.[60]

Imported fire ant (*Solenopsis invicta*) stings are nearly universal in endemic areas, with sting rates of ~51% within first weeks of arrival in endemic areas.[61] Children aged younger than 10 years in endemic areas have an attack rate of 55%, and 40% are stung monthly in peak seasonal exposure.[62] As such, the potential for allergic sensitization is significant, up to 17% within in endemic areas. The clinical phenotype of patients with fire ant-induced anaphylaxis seems clinically similar to those with hymenoptera stings.[63] Fire ant immunotherapy is highly efficacious.

Anaphylaxis to proteins (independent of alpha-gal hypersensitivity) in certain ticks has been described but poorly understood.[26] This is best described in Europe from pigeon tick (*Argas reflexus*) bites, and in Australia from the common bush tick (*Ixodes holocyclus*) bites.[64–66]

### Non–Immunoglobulin E-Mediated Allergy

#### Mastocyte-related G-protein coupled receptor X2

Mast cell degranulation via ligands binding the mastocyte-related G-protein coupled receptor X2 receptor has been identified as the etiologic factor for multiple non–IgE-mediated drug allergies and some venom reactions.[67] The receptor seems to be a polyvenom receptor, and interestingly many endogenous ligands (substance P, vasoactive intestinal peptide [VIP], cortistatin, and somatostatin) and exogenous medications (narcotics, neuromuscular paralytics, vancomycin, fluoroquinolones, and leuprolide) may induce anaphylaxis through this receptor. At the present time, loss-of-function polymorphisms have been described but gain of function or activating autoantibodies to this receptor has not yet been described.[67]

#### NSAID induced

AERD/NERD (aspirin-NSAID exacerbated respiratory disease), a COX1-inhibitor drug hypersensitivity, typically presents in young adults. The incidence in adolescence is uncertain; however, it was found to be 6% in a recent study with retrospective recall of age of onset.[68] Severe asthma and nasal polyposis may precede anaphylactic reactions to NSAIDs with this diagnosis, thus the diagnosis can be elusive in adolescence. Normal urine leukotriene E4 ($LTE_4$) levels may help exclude an AERD diagnosis.[69]

### Clonal Mast Cell Disorders

#### Mastocytosis

Mastocytosis is a neoplastic disorder leading to proliferation of mast cells and a common cause of obscure anaphylaxis (**Table 2**). Criteria and subtypes are promulgated by the WHO[70] and have been recently refined within a 2022 consensus.[71]

**Table 2**
**Mast cell disorders**

| | Prevalence in Adolescents | Unique Features | Diagnostic Tools |
|---|---|---|---|
| **Clonal mast cell disorders** | | | |
| MCAS (monoclonal subtype, MMAS) | Rare | • Episodic anaphylaxis-like symptoms *and* response to antimediators *and* biomarker evidence of mast cell activation<br>• Evidence of clonal surface markers or KIT mutation<br>• Not meeting WHO SM criteria | N-methylhistamine urine<br>Prostaglandin F2a<br>Prostaglandin D2<br>Leukotriene E4<br>Tryptase<br>Evidence of clonal surface markers or KIT mutation |
| CM | Common | • Pigmented macules/papules that urticate with pressure (Darier sign) or heat<br>• Often involutes during puberty<br>• Anaphylaxis risk associated with skin involvement, serum tryptase | Whole skin examination<br>Darier sign<br>Skin biopsy<br>SCORMA score[171] |
| SM (indolent) | Rare | • Risk of osteoporosis<br>• Venom-induced hypotension without venom allergy<br>• Frequent intolerance to alcohol and NSAIDs | Bone marrow biopsy<br>WHO diagnostic criteria<br>D816 V high-sensitivity PCR (ddPCR or allele specific) |
| SM (smoldering, aggressive) Mast cell leukemia | Extraordinarily rare | • Organ infiltration (B-symptoms):<br>• Hepatomegaly/splenomegaly, marrow infiltration<br>• Organ dysfunction (C-symptoms):<br>• Liver, splenic dysfunction<br>• Cytopenias<br>• Weight loss<br>• Malabsorption<br>• Osteoporosis | Evaluation for end-organ injury, hepatosplenomegaly<br>Blood count with differential, flow cytometry, hematopathology/genetics<br>DEXA (dual x-ray absorptiometry) bone density assessment scan<br>Oncology consultation |

(continued on next page)

**Table 2**
*(continued)*

| | Prevalence in Adolescents | Unique Features | Diagnostic Tools |
|---|---|---|---|
| **Nonclonal mast cell activation** | | | |
| HAT [85] | Common (Up to 1 in 20) | • Common in Caucasians<br>• Autosomal dominant inheritance<br>• Highly variable penetrance<br>• Severity associated with copy number<br>• Retained primary dentition common | • Baseline serum tryptase >6.5<br>• Tryptase gene copy number variation ddPCR test |
| Chronic urticaria/angioedema | Very common | • Autoimmune in ~40%, idiopathic in remainder<br>• Not due to drug allergy, but often aggravated by NSAIDs<br>• Only cold-induced urticaria associated with anaphylaxis risk | • Basophil activation test<br>• Anti-IgE autoantibodies<br>• Anti-CD24 autoantibodies<br>• Ice cube skin test |
| MCAS (nonclonal) | Rare | • Episodic anaphylaxis-like symptoms AND response to antimediators AND biomarker evidence of mast cell activation<br>• No evidence of clonal surface markers or KIT mutation<br>• Not meeting SM criteria | • N-methylhistamine urine<br>• Prostaglandin F2a<br>• Prostaglandin D2<br>• Leukotriene E4<br>• Tryptase<br>• No evidence of clonal surface markers or KIT mutation |
| Complement activation (CARPA) | Unknown | • Preceding exposure to nanomedicines or biological drugs | • C4, sC5a, sC3a<br>• Serum sC5-9<br>• Rheumatologic serologic and clinical evaluation |

**Cutaneous mastocytosis.** Cutaneous mastocytosis (CM) is a relatively common disease of childhood and adolescence. Maculopapular CM (MCPM)/urticaria pigmentosa (UP) is the most common subtype of CM of childhood, usually presenting within the first year of life.[72] Multiple polymorphic pigmented skin lesions are the primary symptom, which urticate with applied pressure (Darier's sign).

Anaphylaxis from CM in children and adolescents is unusual (up to 9%) but the risk is largely associated with extensive body surface area involvement or elevated basal serum tryptase.[73,74] Roughly 70% of children with CM carry a mutation within the *cKIT* gene, a mast cell growth-promoting tyrosine kinase. Only 30% are due to D816V associated mutations, whereas this is more than 90% in adult populations.[75]

More than 80% of children with MCPM/UP experience involution or resolution of CM lesions during adolescence.[76] Certain features of CM may suggest systemic disease, particularly a positive D816V peripheral blood mutation,[77] persistent tryptase elevation, and lack of involution after puberty.[78]

**Systemic mastocytosis.** SM is a rare hematologic neoplastic disorder of mast cells, which is definitively associated with a higher risk of spontaneous or minimally triggered anaphylaxis. The most prevalent type is indolent systemic mastocytosis (ISM). Not all adolescents who present with CM also have SM, unlike in adult populations. Advanced SM is extraordinarily rare in adolescent populations.[76] Nearly all pediatric SM presents with concomitant CM, unlike in adult populations.[79]

**Mast cell activation syndrome.** Consensus criteria for mast cell activation syndrome (MCAS) were developed in 2011 and reinforced by expert consensus in 2019.[80,81] There are 3 necessary conditions to be met for diagnosis (simplified).

1. spontaneous anaphylaxis, without other known cause,
2. acute elevation of a relevant biomarker with symptoms, and
3. clinical response to antimediator medications.

For patients meeting MCAS criteria, abnormalities on bone marrow and intestinal pathologic condition often but do not always demonstrate abnormal clustering, spindled cell morphology, and/or clonal markers.[82,83] Acute elevation with symptoms of biomarkers serum tryptase is found in roughly one-third, and elevations of urinary n-methylhistamine in over half, and of prostaglandin D2 in less than half with prostaglandin D2.[84] Prognosis seems excellent as two-thirds of MCAS patients experience complete or major response to antimediators such as antihistamines or mast cell inhibitors.[84]

### Nonclonal Mast Cell Disorders

### Hereditary alpha tryptasemia
Described first in 2016 as a genetically defined clinical disorder,[85] hereditary alpha tryptasemia (HAT) is a gene copy number variation with a clinical syndrome including in some series an increased risk of anaphylaxis.[85] Tryptase is a protease released exclusively by mast cells, encoded by sets of alpha and beta tryptase genes. The total gene copies of both alpha and beta tryptase (between alpha and beta) should equal 4; however, additional alpha gene copies can be observed in approximately 6% of Caucasian Americans. These additional copies of alpha-tryptase correlate with baseline serum tryptase levels as well as with HAT symptom severity.[85] Overexpression of $\alpha$-tryptase protein due to coinheritance of a linked overactive promoter seems to explain the observed serum tryptase concentrations.[86]

Genetic copy number variation testing via a droplet digital polymerase chain reaction (PCR) assays available to screen for HAT and has very high sensitivity and specificity for the disorder.[87] The wide variation of symptoms and penetrance with a set genotype is still poorly understood and debated.[85,88,89] Surprisingly, coexisting clonal mast cell disease may be present in 10% to 17% of HAT patients, so screening for both disorders may be necessary.[86,90,91]

### Cold-induced urticaria

Unlike other forms of chronic urticaria, patients with cold triggers have a high prevalence of anaphylaxis (up to 21%).[92] Most anaphylaxis cases follow exposure to cold water, which has a high heat of vaporization and enthalpy and can cool the core body temperature readily. Ice cube skin testing can help diagnose; however, it has low sensitivity for the diagnosis and risk for anaphylaxis in children and adolescents.[93]

## Mimic Disorders

Validation studies of clinical anaphylaxis criteria pose the hazard of false positives, leading to diagnostic misclassification.[16] Common mimic disorders (**Table 3**), which can present in adolescence include hereditary angioedema (HAE), panic and somatoform disorders, and inducible laryngeal obstruction. Additionally, extremely rare disorders such as neuroendocrine tumors could also present similarly to anaphylaxis.

### Neuroendocrine tumors

Neuroendocrine neoplasms such as carcinoid or VIPomas may episodically release hormones, causing mediator symptoms that can overlap with anaphylaxis.[94] Most carcinoids do not cause carcinoid syndrome due to first-pass hepatic metabolism; however, carcinoid tumors presenting in the lung or liver can produce anaphylaxis-mimicking episodic diarrhea, flushing (80%), and/or bronchospasm (25%).[95] Carcinoid symptoms can be triggered by cofactors such as anaphylaxis, including alcohol, exercise, or stress. Diagnostic screening via 5-hydroxyindoleacetic acid (5-HIAA), a serotonin metabolite, via a 24-hour urine collection is recommended. VIPomas similarly can produce profound secretory diarrhea and flushing and are often associated with elevated VIP serum levels and osmolality defects. Higher specificity studies including gallium-tracer based positron emission tomography/computed tomography (PET/CT) or PET/MRI have high diagnostic sensitivity for disease.[96]

### Bradykinin-mediated angioedema

Bradykinin-induced angioedema can seem indistinguishable from angioedema from histaminergic causes. However, angioedema from bradykinin induces neither hypotension nor urticaria, and it is not responsive to corticosteroids, epinephrine, or antihistamines. Generally, angioedema from bradykinin pathophysiology has a slower onset and much slower offset than with anaphylaxis.

**Hereditary angioedema.** HAE often initially presents in adolescence, with episodic recurrent vomiting and abdominal pain attacks and/or orofacial angioedema.[97] Attacks can be spontaneous or associated with menses but in contrast to anaphylaxis can be triggered by trauma such as dental procedures. Screening for HAE types I and II can be performed with convalescent complement 1 esterase inhibitor (C1INH; functional and quantitative) and C4 serum levels. HAE with normal C1INH remains diagnostically challenging; however, genetic sequencing for known mutations is commercially available.[98]

**ACE-I-induced angioedema.** Angioedema due to angiotensin-converting enzyme inhibitors (ACE-I) drugs is thought to be bradykinin mediated, and clinically the swelling

**Table 3**
**Anaphylaxis mimic disorders**

| | Prevalence | Distinct Features from Anaphylaxis | Shared Features with Anaphylaxis | Diagnostic Tools |
|---|---|---|---|---|
| **Neuroendocrine Disorders** | | | | |
| Carcinoid | Rare[94] | • Bowel obstruction<br>• Mesenteric ischemia<br>• Right heart failure<br>• Tricuspid regurgitation<br>• Pulmonary valve stenosis<br>• Prolonged hypotension (crisis)97 | Flushing<br>Hypotension | • Elevated 5-HIAA, urinary (24 h collection)<br>• Elevated chromogranin A<br>• $^{68}$Ga-DOTATATE or DOTATOC PET/CT response to somatostatin analogs |
| VIPoma | Rare | • Copious secretory diarrhea<br>• Hypokalemia<br>• Hypochlorhydria<br>• Weight loss<br>• Hypercalcemia<br>• Hyperglycemia | Diarrhea<br>Flushing | • Stool osmolarity gap<br>• Serum electrolytes<br>• Elevated serum VIP<br>• $^{68}$Ga-DOTATATE or DOTATOC PET/CT response to somatostatin analogs |
| Familial medullary thyroid carcinoma | Rare | • Telangiectasias<br>• Thyroid nodules | Flushing | • Elevated calcitonin<br>• Elevated carcinoembryonic antigen<br>• Family history (spontaneous disease rarely presents before the age of 20 years) |
| Pheochromocytoma | Rare | • Hypertension<br>• Diaphoresis<br>• Headaches<br>• Insulin resistance | Flushing<br>Tachycardia | • Elevated metanephrines/catecholamines<br>• Family history of MEN2, NF1, VHL or PHEO (spontaneous disease rare in adolescents)<br>• CT for adrenal mass |

(continued on next page)

**Table 3**
*(continued)*

| | Prevalence | Distinct Features from Anaphylaxis | Shared Features with Anaphylaxis | Diagnostic Tools |
|---|---|---|---|---|
| **Bradykinin Disorders** | | | | |
| HAE[97,168] | Rare | • Erythema marginatum<br>• Absent hypotension<br>• Absent urticaria<br>• Abdominal pain<br>• No response to corticosteroids, antihistamines, epinephrine | Angioedema<br>Vomiting | • Low basal/acute serum C1INH (functional or quantitative)<br>• Low C4<br>• Positive genetic screen for mutations: SERPIN1, Factor 12, PLG, ANGPT1, KNG1, MYOF |
| ACE-I induced angioedema | rare | • Absence of hypotension, urticaria, bronchospasm | Angioedema | • Preceding ACE-I exposure<br>• No biomarker |
| **Unexplained Disorders** | | | | |
| Systemic capillary leak syndrome (Clarkson's)[169,170] | Rare | • Hemoconcentration and hypoalbuminemia<br>• Prolonged episodic hypotension<br>• Common associations with monoclonal gammopathy, infection (COVID-19, dengue), drug triggers including IL2, autoimmunity (psoriasis) | Hypotension<br>Angioedema<br>Gastrointestinal symptoms | • Response to immunoglobulin |
| Inducible laryngeal obstruction (paradoxic vocal cord dysfunction) | Common | • Absent wheezing, hypotension, urticaria/flushing<br>• Inspiratory stridor<br>• On-off symptoms | Acute dyspnea<br>presyncope | • Pittsburgh VCD Index 115<br>• Laryngoscopy demonstrating abnormal inspiratory adduction of the vocal cords<br>• Spirometry demonstrating flattening of inspiratory flow volume loop |

**Exogenous Source**

| | | | | |
|---|---|---|---|---|
| COX1 inhibitors Aspirin/NSAIDs | Common | • Delayed onset symptoms after exposure (common) • Nasal polyps/severe asthma often precedes NSAID intolerance | Flushing Wheezing Bronchospasm Hypotension Diarrhea | • Urine LTE4 (high negative predictive value)[69] |
| Niacin (nicotinic acid) | Unknown | • Improvement with NSAIDs | Flushing Nausea Vomiting Pruritis | • Vitamin supplements/energy drinks transaminitis |
| Histidine (scombroid poisoning) | Rare | • Spoiled scromboid fish ingestion, without fish allergy • More than one person with simultaneous symptoms | No clinical distinguishing symptoms | Tryptase (acute level should be normal because there is no degranulation) |

**Psychiatric**

| | | | | |
|---|---|---|---|---|
| Somatoform | Common | • Absence of hypotension, wheezing, urticaria, and vomiting | Throat tightness common | Formal anaphylaxis criteria utilization |
| Panic attacks | Common | • Paresthesias • Absent urticaria/angioedema • Diaphoresis • Hyperventilation | Intense fear Shortness of breath | Formal anaphylaxis criteria utilization |
| Factitious (Munchausen's) | Unknown | • Secondary gain | Intentional access and exposure to known anaphylaxis trigger | Formal anaphylaxis criteria utilization |

can be poorly distinguished from HAE.[99] Although ACE-I are rarely used in adolescents; similar to adults, adolescents seem at risk for angioedema.[100] Continued angioedema despite cessation of an ACE-I drug has been described; however, whether this occurs in adolescents is unknown.[101] ACE-I-induced angioedema regrettably is a diagnosis of exclusion without a diagnostic biomarker to date.

### Exogenous
**Niacin (vitamin B3).** Adolescents are known to take multivitamins and nutritional supplements for purported benefits. Energy drinks are marketed to adolescents, and many contain milligram quantities of niacin per serving.[102] Niacin can induce anaphylaxis-mimicking flushing and hypotension via release of prostaglandin D2 ($PGD_2$) from mast cells and serotonin from platelets.[103] Diagnosis can be made rapidly via resolution after discontinuation of niacin. Although nondiagnostic, NSAIDs may help resolve symptoms by blocking prostaglandin.

**Histidine (scombroid) poisoning.** Consumption of spoiled pelagic fish, often in the scombroid family including tuna and grouper, can lead to postprandial anaphylaxis-like symptoms. These symptoms are caused by direct ingestion of histidine produced by spoilage bacteria, and the tyramine can be converted to histamine. Clues suggesting the poisoning include others with similar acute symptoms eating the same meal, and subsequent tolerance to fish.[104]

**Food additives.** Although commonly perceived by the public as allergens, food additives such as synthetic food dyes, glutamates, and benzoates are rarely triggers of pseudo-allergic symptoms in double-blinded challenges.[105] Similarly, naturally occurring food salicylates, vasoactive amines have minimal-quality or poor-quality data supporting risk of anaphylactic symptoms.[105] Low-histamine, dye or preservative-free diets are not presently endorsed by any organizational practice parameter for the management of idiopathic anaphylaxis or food allergies.

### Infectious
Evaluating patients for a history of potential exposure to helminths, in endemic areas, is recommended. Anaphylaxis from rupture of echinococcus cysts has been well described, often during surgery but it may be spontaneous.[106] Ingestion of raw or undercooked fish and cephalopods can lead to *Anisakis simplex* nematode infections, which have been associated with anaphylaxis. Disease is most common in Japan and Spain.[107] *Taenia solium* tapeworm-induced anaphylaxis and other allergic manifestations have been reported in rare cases.[108] Roundworm *Ascaris lumbricoides* infections have been associated with intense allergic reactions.[109]

### Upper airway
**Inducible laryngeal obstruction.** Stridulous, often inspiratory, dyspnea caused by paradoxic closure of the vocal cords may mimic airway angioedema and bronchospasm present with anaphylaxis. This syndrome has had a multitude of other names including vocal cord dysfunction and paradoxic vocal cord movement.[110] The overall prevalence in adolescents may be around 5% to 7%.[111]

A clinical index of suspicion can be bolstered via screening tools and intermittent flattening of inspiratory flow volume loops on spirometry.[110] The Pittsburgh Index, which uses variables of throat tightness, dysphonia, absence of wheezing, and triggering odors, has favorable screening sensitivity and specificity.[112] Direct laryngeal evaluation of abnormal movement via flexible rhinolaryngoscopy, using provocative maneuvers, is the gold standard diagnostic evaluation. Unfortunately, the sensitivity of these tests and provocative maneuvers is likely poor.[110]

Although multiple treatments have been studied, laryngeal/speech therapy or botulinum toxin therapy for refractory cases are commonly considered for long-term management. Pathophysiology, diagnosis, and treatment remain with significant knowledge gaps at the present time.[110]

### Psychiatric

**Somatoform disorder.** Proposed criteria for nonorganic symptoms mimicking anaphylaxis were developed in 1995, termed undifferentiated somatoform-idiopathic anaphylaxis.[113] In the original description, cutaneous and laryngeal symptoms were found in most patients, and these patients reported no response to medication. All the patients were ultimately diagnosed with undifferentiated somatoform disorder (DSM3). Over half of the patients had defensive responses to the consideration of a somatoform disorder.

A follow-up modern study found patients with somatoform anaphylaxis were more likely to complain of subjective throat tightness or swelling. Past psychiatric histories were not unique compared with confirmed anaphylaxis patients in this study.[114]

Somatic symptom disorder per the present international reference DSM 5[115] is defined as one or more somatic symptoms that cause distress or psychosocial impairment, and excessive thoughts about the seriousness, feelings including persistent or severe anxiety, or behaviors such as excessive time and energy devoted to the concern. There is no present subset defined in DSM 5 for somatic anaphylaxis.

**Fictitious (Munchausen's) anaphylaxis.** Fictitious (feigned or intentionally induced) anaphylaxis has been reported in multiple case reports.[116–119] In contrast to somatoform disorders, there is an intentional intent to deceive for secondary gain. Suspected cases should be referred to specialists in behavioral medicine.

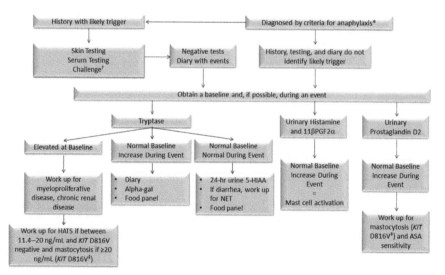

**Fig. 2.** Proposed diagnostic evaluation for occult anaphylaxis (excluding evaluation for non-neuroendocrine tumor mimic disorders). *Diagnosis according to accepted criteria. †Because challenges can have safety risks, a challenge should not be conducted if history is conclusive or serum-specific IgE is >15 kU/L and should be conducted with caution in patients with serum-specific IgE from 0.35 to 15 kU/L, in consideration with concurrent atopic diagnoses. ‡Peripheral blood. Reprinted with permission from the Idiopathic Anaphylaxis Yardstick, Carter M. et al. 2020.[10]

### Diagnostic Evaluation Workflow

A staged diagnostic approach is recommended to address both mimic disorder concerns, as well as anaphylaxis causes (**Fig. 2**). Routine screening with allergen skin prick testing, sIgE testing, and/or observed challenge to the allergen is recommended if there is a likely trigger.[10]

### Routine allergy evaluations

Established screening tools for allergen sensitization may assist if rare allergens are suspected. Commercial ELISA-like sIgE tests are widely available, and skin prick/intradermal testing is a standard diagnostic offered by allergists.

Whereas testing for aeroallergen and foods have reasonable test characteristics, drug allergy skin and sIgE testing generally has very poor sensitivity/specificity characteristics and is often unhelpful.[120] Graded supervised allergen challenges remain the gold standard for clinical exclusion of an allergy to a substance and should be considered if there is a low prechallenge concern for reactivity.[120] Basophil activation tests are an emerging diagnostic with some commercial availability but suffer from uncertain test characteristics and uncertain role in diagnostic evaluation.[121]

If no cause is evident but a trigger is still suspected, a patient diary may help recall of preceding triggers. Laboratory evaluation for mast cell biomarkers is often the next step (**Fig. 2**).

### Tryptase

Tryptase is a protease selectively produced by mast cells and is the most useful initial laboratory marker. Mature tryptase is produced following mast cell degranulation. It has a short half-life, peaking between 30-minute and 90-minute postanaphylaxis, and declining 2 hours after degranulation. Obtaining tryptase draws rapidly during suspected reactions can be helpful diagnostically. Significant tryptase elevation suggesting degranulation have been defined as levels greater than 120% of the baseline serum tryptase plus 2ng/dL.[122] A fractionated serum tryptase laboratory test can quantify mature from immature tryptase. Mature tryptase levels greater than 1 ng/dL may suggest recent degranulation, whereas low levels with high total tryptase suggest a high mast cell burden.[123]

### Other biomarkers

Mild anaphylaxis symptoms, and food-induced anaphylaxis, often do not present with elevated acute tryptase levels. Other biomarkers may be diagnostic for evidence of mast cell/basophil activation. Urinary N-methyl histamine, prostaglandin F2a or D2, and leukotriene E4 levels above normal may be noted following anaphylaxis. Serum histamine is a difficult biomarker is generally not recommended for the assessment of anaphylaxis.[124,125]

Complement-mediated anaphylaxis might be suggested if consumable components such as C4 are low acutely, and/or if soluble sC5-9 levels are elevated.[126] Complement activation-induced anaphylaxis (CARPA) has been proposed as the underpinning of anaphylaxis induced from nanoparticle and some biologic medicines, including coronavirus disease 2019 (COVID-19) mRNA vaccines.

### Convalescence

**Tryptase.** A baseline serum tryptase is a recommended initial screen for SM and HAT.[10] Basal serum tryptase less than 6.5 ng/mL are not observed with HAT but generally one supernumerary copy leads to tryptase levels 13.6 ng/mL (95% CI 12.6–14.4).[127] Baseline serum tryptase levels less than 11.4 ng/mL are uncommon with SM, whereas levels above 20 ng/mL suggest disease and are a minor criterion.

**KIT proto-oncogene receptor tyrosine kinase mutation.** High sensitivity allele-specific or digital droplet KIT proto-oncogene receptor tyrosine kinase (KIT) D816 V mutation serologic tests are available.[128] False negatives can occur due to low precursor frequency because mastocytosis and monoclonal mast cell disorders have somatic rather than germ-line mutations, and thus restricted to a mast cell hematopoetic lineage.[129] Sequencing for other KIT mutations in select exons is commercially available; however, the sensitivity may be poor.[75] In children/adolescents, the specific KIT mutation does not predict the evolution of disease.[130]

**Bone marrow evaluation.** Bone marrow biopsy remains the gold standard site for biopsy to consider clonal mast cell disorders and consider abnormal nonclonal disorders.[71] Special immunohistochemistry stains to identify mast cells with clonal markers,[131] and special genetic evaluations are required for diagnostic purposes.[75] Flow cytometry inclusive of CD117/CD25/CD2/CD35 can help identify rare clonal mast cell populations. Very rarely, mastocytosis can be missed on a bone marrow biopsy, and repeat biopsies, screening for extramedullary disease,[132] or expert pathologic review using special approaches might be necessary.[133]

*Acute treatment*
**Anaphylaxis self-recognition and self-management.** Often, anaphylaxis occurs outside of medical environments, which requires patient or parent self-recognition and initial management of anaphylaxis. The recognition (**Fig. 1**) and initial emergency management (**Fig. 3**) of anaphylaxis have been standardized.[1,17] These standards are generally uniform, without regard to the pathophysiology or etiologic cause.

Self-recognition and self-management are critical and can be taught to adolescents. Obstacles to anaphylaxis self-management in adolescents include recognition, self-efficacy to request assistance with peer pressures, needle phobia, and epinephrine not readily available.[134]

Rapid administration of intramuscular epinephrine, lying down with legs elevated, and emergency medical systems activation are initial management steps.

**Medical management.** Prehospital and hospital emergency medical management also includes IV fluid resuscitation, provision of bronchodilator and oxygen, and assessment and management of the airway as indicated by symptoms.[1] Adjunctive systemic corticosteroids and antihistamines are not required given the lack of evidence for benefit and a high number to treat. Provider discretion is still permitted for consideration of these medications for management.[18]

Prolonged observation periods are recommended if there is a high risk for second phase reaction. Major factors for prolonged observation include requiring 2 or more doses of epinephrine, severe initial symptoms, and an unknown trigger.[18] Escalation to intensive care unit level care is indicated if airway protection or need for central pressor support, and/or if there was cardiopulmonary arrest or end-organ injury. At discharge, provision and education about indications for epinephrine autoinjectors, written action plans, and follow-up care is required.[18]

*Prevention*
**Avoidance of known triggers.** For known triggers, avoidance represents first-line prevention.

- *Cold urticaria*: Avoidance of cold exposures with appropriate protective clothing, and avoidance of situations of risky exposure.[135]
- *(Food)/Exercise-induced anaphylaxis*: Patients with FEIA/EIA should exercise before breakfast on empty stomach, and exercising with epinephrine autoinjectors

## INITIAL TREATMENT

1. Have a written emergency protocol for recognition and treatment of anaphylaxis and rehearse it regularly.

2. Remove exposure to the trigger if possible, e.g. discontinue an intravenous diagnostic or therapeutic agent that seems to be triggering symptoms.

3. Assess the patient: Airway / Breathing / Circulation, mental status, skin and body weight (mass)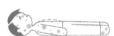

*Promptly and simultaneously, perform steps 4, 5 and 6*

4. Call for help: resuscitation team (hospital) or emergency medical services (community) if available.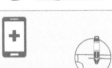

5. Inject epinephrine (adrenaline) intramuscularly in the mid-anterolateral aspect of the thigh, 0.01 mg/kg of a 1:1,000 (1 mg/ml) solution, maximum of 0.5 mg (adult) or 0.3 mg (child); record the time of the dose and repeat every 5-15 minutes, if needed. Most patients respond to 1 or 2 doses.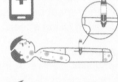

6. Place patient on the back or in a position of comfort if there is respiratory distress and/or vomiting; elevate the lower extremities; fatality can occur within seconds if patient stands or sits suddenly.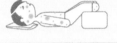

7. When indicated, give high-flow supplemental oxygen (6-8 L/minute), by face mask or oropharyngeal airway.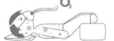

8. Establish intravenous access using needles or catheters with wide-bore cannula (14-16 gauge). Consider giving 1-2 liters of 0.9% (isotonic) saline rapidly (e.g. 5-10 ml/kg in the first 5-10 minutes to an adult; 10 ml/kg to a child).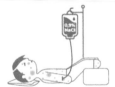

*In addition*

9. If indicated at any time, perform cardiopulmonary resuscitation with continuous chest compressions.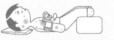

10. At frequent, regular intervals, monitor patient's blood pressure, cardiac rate and function, respiratory status, and oxygenation (monitor continuously, if possible).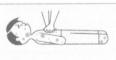

**Fig. 3.** WAO criteria for the initial treatment of anaphylaxis. Disclaimer: In no event shall WAO be liable for any damages arising out of any use of or reliance on this material (see www.worldallergy.org for full disclaimer). Not for commercial use. (*Source*: Cardona V, Ansotegui IJ, Fbisawa M et al. World Allergy Organization Anaphylaxis Guidance 2020. World Allergy Organization Journal 2020; 13(10):100472. Doi:https://doi.org/10.1016/j.waojou.2020.100472. Reproduced with permission from Cardona and colleagues 2020.[1])

and with a partner able to recognize, treat reactions, and call for emergency assistance.[25]

- *Drug allergy*: Strict avoidance of triggering or cross-reactive medications is the mainstay of present management.[120] Inpatient desensitization can permit safer exposure to the drug if a drug is medically necessary.
- *Food allergy*: Strict avoidance of triggering foods and cross-reactive foods is the mainstay of present management of anaphylaxis. Desensitization via oral immunotherapy has been intensely studied especially for peanut. There is strong evidence that oral immunotherapy (OIT) increases food tolerance; however, the benefit is often transient or marginal and with an increased risk of anaphylaxis compared with avoidance.[136]
- *Pollen-food syndrome*: Theoretically, subcutaneous and sublingual allergen immunotherapy could have benefit for pollen-food syndrome (PFS); however, there have been few studies to date with varied responses.[137,138] Strictly avoiding PFS foods that trigger anaphylaxis is recommended.

**Medications.** Treatment to suppress both the severity and frequency of spontaneous anaphylaxis has been poorly studied, and often medication trials are necessary to find a suitable controller. A threshold for when to initiate suppressive therapy has been defined as frequent idiopathic anaphylaxis, defined least 2 episodes during 2 months or at least 6 episodes during 12 months; however, this commonly used threshold was arbitrarily defined.[139]

Prolonged courses of systemic corticosteroids with oral antihistamines were initially recommended for unexplained anaphylaxis, often achieving disease stabilization and resolution.[139,140] The health risks for adolescents of prolonged systemic steroids are significant however, and a risk/benefit ratio consideration may be needed. Other approaches may need to be considered in adolescents.

- *H1:* Prophylactic use of newer (3rd generation) antihistamines following chronic urticaria guidelines is recommended for frequent idiopathic anaphylaxis[10]; however, there is minimal data supporting benefit to date. Urticaria guidelines recommend up to 4 times standard dosing over a day of newer H1 antagonists such as cetirizine/levocetirizine, fexofenadine, or loratadine/desloratadine.[141] These antihistamines, in contrast to earlier generations, have longer half-lives and less anticholinergic side effects.
- *H2:* The prophylactic benefit of H2 specific antagonists, such as famotidine, is uncertain. Famotidine can be considered in trial, however, especially if gastritis symptoms while taking systemic steroids concurrently.[10] In chronic urticaria, only 1 in 3 have clinical response to H2-specific antagonists.[141]
- *Leukotriene targeting drugs*: Leukotriene receptor antagonists, such as montelukast or zafirlukast, and 5-lipoxygenase inhibitors, such as zaluteon, have not been well studied in idiopathic anaphylaxis (IA).[10]
- *Mast cell inhibitors (MCI)*: Cromolyn has not been well studied in IA. Given poor absorption from the gastrointestinal (GI) tract, benefit is largely expected for GI symptoms only.
- *Combination medicines*:
  - Doxepin (H1/H2): Doxepin is an oral tricyclic drug with superpotent H1/h2 antagonism. Unfortunately, sedation, prolonged QTc intervals, and interaction with selective serotonin reuptake inhibitor (SSRI) antidepressants make use for anaphylaxis prophylaxis challenging in adolescents.[10]
  - Ketotifen (H1/MCI): Ketotifen, a first-generation oral antihistamine, has both mast cell stabilization and antihistamine properties. Benefit of ketotifen for

steroid-dependent IA has been reported[142,143]; however, evidence for superiority over other H1 antihistamines for pediatric mastocytosis is lacking.[144]
- o Rupatadine (H1/PAF): Rupatadine, a loratadine analog, has unique antiplatelet activating factor function.[145] PAF has been associated with hypotension and fatal anaphylaxis.[146] Benefit for prophylaxis or treatment of anaphylaxis is presently unknown.
- Immunosuppression/Immunomodulators:
  - o Calcineurin inhibitors: Data supporting immunosuppression in unexplained anaphylaxis is minimal; however, off-label use for chronic urticaria is more robust. Supportive data for the use of cyclosporine in chronic urticaria exist, and it is a second-line recommendation for management per international chronic urticaria guidelines.[141]
  - o Bruton's tyrosine kinase inhibitors (BTKi): Recent studies have found BTKi drugs abrogate mast cell degranulation via signaling via sIgE. Low doses of BTKi drugs are well tolerated and immunosuppression seems to be minimal.[147] Although not yet studied in idiopathic anaphylaxis, phase 2B chronic urticaria studies of remibrutinib were highly suppressive of symptoms at even the lowest dose studied.[148]
- Biologics
  - o *Anti-IgE*
    - Off-label benefit of omalizumab has been extensively reported in case series for IA and mast cell disorders; however, there have been few controlled studies. A major review of 55 CM, ISM, and MCAS patients demonstrated a complete response in more than 1%, a major response in 54% and a 21% a partial response. Response was sustained in three-fourths and seemed most beneficial for vasomotor and gastrointestinal symptoms.[149]
    - In contrast, a prospective RCT in frequent idiopathic anaphylaxis cohort however failed to find a significant benefit at 6 months with idiopathic anaphylaxis yet trended toward benefit and drug tolerance was good.[150]
    - Although not yet studied for unexplained or idiopathic anaphylaxis, there are several anti-IgE biologics under active evaluation for chronic urticaria. Ligelizumab has demonstrated benefit in chronic urticaria over omalizumab.[151,152] Candidate drugs TEV-45779 and UB-221 are also under study.[153,154]
  - o *Dupilumab (anti-Th2)*: Dupilumab, a marketed anti-interleukin 4 and 13 receptor (anti-IL4R/IL13R) biologic, has been under study for chronic urticaria with mixed positive and negative phase 3 trials.[155,156] Benefit for IA is limited to case reports to date.[157]
  - o *Anti-KIT*: KIT both a surface marker on mature mast cells and progenitor stem cells, thus is a challenging drug target. Phase I human studies of CDX-0159 seem to result in both a profound and durable mast cell compartment suppression.[158] There are no studies to date of use for idiopathic anaphylaxis.
  - o *Anti-SIGLEC8*: SIGLEC-8 is a surface receptor on mast cells, basophils, and eosinophils, and ligation induces apoptosis and suppression of mediator production.[159,160] AK002 (lirentelimab) is under study for chronic urticaria[161]; however, there are no studies to date of use for idiopathic anaphylaxis.

### Patient/family support and resources

The psychosocial impact of unexplained or IA in adolescents has been minimally studied. Adolescent and parent anxiety regarding food allergy have been extensively studied; a balanced level of anxiety promoting appropriate anaphylaxis preparedness without debilitating fears is often difficult to achieve.[162] A challenging consequence of severe or frequent anaphylaxis in adolescents is the development of post-traumatic stress disorder (PTSD).[163] Adolescents with medically unexplained syndromes are known to very commonly suffer from emotional distress, often not well addressed in the search for a suitable diagnosis and treatment plan.[164] Interventions focused on parental responses to illness and family communication seemed to be most beneficial in a systematic review.[164]

Provision of a written anaphylaxis emergency plan is recommended for all with food allergies.[165] Emergency anaphylaxis action plan form templates are widely available and free from many organizations, in many languages. Formal written and posted emergency action plans, as well as chronic illness accommodation plans, can provide the link between family, medical provider, and schools to ensure safety, preparedness and minimized impairment to the adolescent. Formally assessing and supporting the needs of adolescents in their transition to independent self-management of anaphylaxis is recommended by the age of 11 to 13 years.[166]

Adolescents and parents with medically unexplained or idiopathic disorders symptoms may be susceptible to pseudoscientific or alternative medicine treatments, presently a particularly common problem with mast cell disorders.[81] Multiple national nonprofit patient support organizations may offer community of support and guidance for patients with idiopathic or yet unexplained anaphylaxis. Often IA resources are housed within mastocytosis organizations such as the Canadian Mastocytosis society (Canada), the Mast Cell Society (US), UK Masto (UK), Assomast (FR), or the Selbsthilfeverein Mastozytose (GER).

### Provider support

Development of guidelines for the evaluation and management of idiopathic and occult anaphylaxis and screening for mimic disorders are in their infancy. The development of an idiopathic anaphylaxis yardstick: a set of practical recommendations published in 2020[10] is one of the first efforts to guide diagnostic efforts. Superspecialist referral networks are in development, particularly via the European Competence Network on Mastocytosis (ECNM) group, for obscure cases needing support.

There are emerging research networks to support unexplained anaphylaxis and to support researchers studying rare disorders. The ECNM provides expert referrals and scientific registry (ECNM Registry). Additionally, there is a long-standing etiologic study (NCT00719719) at the National Institutes of Health (US).[167]

### SUMMARY

1. Diagnosis
   a. In summary, clinical features suggestive of anaphylaxis, without a readily evident trigger, should prompt expanded diagnostic considerations.
   b. A comprehensive history and timeline of exposures and subsequent symptoms is the most useful diagnostic tool. Objective findings as available, such as vital signs and observations of the airway and skin, can help validate anaphylaxis or suggest an alternative disorder.
   c. Using anaphylactic diagnostic criteria is recommended given strong positive and negative predictive values.
   d. For obscure causes of anaphylaxis, a broad differential of rare food, drug, venom triggers should be considered, with additional consideration of summative anaphylaxis, which may involve 2 or more cofactors.
   e. Patients with unexplained anaphylaxis require evaluation for an underlying mast cell disorder. Multiple laboratory diagnostics can help confirm or refute certain etiologies and aid to narrow the differential diagnoses.

f. Referral to an allergy specialist is strongly recommended to guide evaluation when confronted with anaphylaxis of uncertain cause. Hematologist support is necessary to assist with the diagnosis of clonal mast cell disorders.

2. Management
   a. Medical management of anaphylaxis should follow guideline-based practices. This includes preparedness with epinephrine autoinjectors and extensive training with the adolescent and their family. Provision of written action plans is recommended.
   b. As adolescents mature, they should have guided support for symptom self-recognition and management responsibilities.
   c. Preparation with written emergency action plans and emergency simulations can reduce feared poor outcomes and provide confidence.
   d. As unexplained recurrent and unpredictable anaphylaxis can cause significant anxiety, addressing mental health concerns early and often with this invisible disability is important.
   e. Although medical options to prevent anaphylaxis without cause are presently few, there is significant hope that what is presently idiopathic will be later diagnosable.
   f. Existing pharmacologic drugs, many used off-label, may minimize the frequency and/or severity of reactions in the interim. Future medications in research and development offer significant hope for future control of anaphylaxis.

## DISCLOSURE

Neither author declares relevant financial conflicts of interest.

## REFERENCES

1. Cardona V, Ansotegui IJ, Ebisawa M, et al. World allergy organization anaphylaxis guidance 2020. World Allergy Organ J 2020;13(10):100472.
2. Grabenhenrich LB, Dölle S, Moneret-Vautrin A, et al. Anaphylaxis in children and adolescents: The European Anaphylaxis Registry. J Allergy Clin Immun 2016; 137(4):1128–37.e1.
3. Comberiati P, Spahn J, Peroni DG. Anaphylaxis in adolescents. Curr Opin Allergy Clin Immunol 2019;19(5):425–31.
4. Turner PJ, Campbell DE. Epidemiology of severe anaphylaxis: can we use population-based data to understand anaphylaxis? Curr Opin Allergy Clin Immunol 2016;16(5):441–50.
5. Pouessel G, Turner PJ, Worm M, et al. Food-induced fatal anaphylaxis: From epidemiological data to general prevention strategies. Clin Exp Allergy 2018; 48(12):1584–93.
6. Gallagher M, Worth A, Cunningham-Burley S, et al. Epinephrine auto-injector use in adolescents at risk of anaphylaxis: a qualitative study in Scotland, UK. Clin Exp Allergy 2011;41(6):869–77.
7. Nwaru BI, Sheikh A. Anaphylaxis in adolescents: a potential tripartite management framework. Curr Opin Allergy Clin Immunol 2015;15(4):344–9.
8. Gallagher M, Worth A, Cunningham-Burley S, et al. Strategies for living with the risk of anaphylaxis in adolescence: qualitative study of young people and their parents. Prim Care Respir J 2012;21(4):392–7.
9. Wright CD, Longjohn M, Lieberman PL, et al. An analysis of anaphylaxis cases at a single pediatric emergency department during a 1-year period. Ann Allergy Asthma Immunol 2017;118(4):461–4.

10. Carter MC, Akin C, Castells MC, et al. Idiopathic anaphylaxis yardstick: Practical recommendations for clinical practice. Ann Allergy Asthma Immunol 2020; 124(1):16–27.
11. Peavy RD, Metcalfe DD. Understanding the mechanisms of anaphylaxis. Curr Opin Allergy Clin Immunol 2008;8(4):310.
12. Finkelman FD, Khodoun MV, Strait R. Human IgE-independent systemic anaphylaxis. J Allergy Clin Immunol 2016;137(6):1674–80.
13. Lieberman P. Treatment of patients who present after an episode of anaphylaxis. Ann Allergy Asthma Immunol 2013;111(3):170–5.
14. Steinke JW, Platts-Mills TA, Commins SP. The alpha-gal story: lessons learned from connecting the dots. J Allergy Clin Immunol 2015;135(3):589–96.
15. Campbell RL, Hagan JB, Manivannan V, et al. Evaluation of national institute of allergy and infectious diseases/food allergy and anaphylaxis network criteria for the diagnosis of anaphylaxis in emergency department patients. J Allergy Clin Immunol 2012;129(3):748–52.
16. Loprinzi Brauer CE, Motosue MS, Li JT, et al. Prospective Validation of the NIAID/FAAN Criteria for Emergency Department Diagnosis of Anaphylaxis. J Allergy Clin Immunol Pract 2016;4(6):1220–6.
17. Muraro A, Worm M, Alviani C, et al. EAACI guidelines: Anaphylaxis (2021 update). Allergy 2022;77(2):357–77.
18. Shaker MS, Wallace DV, Golden DB, et al. Anaphylaxis—a 2020 practice parameter update, systematic review, and Grading of Recommendations, Assessment, Development and Evaluation (GRADE) analysis. J Allergy Clin Immun 2020;145(4):1082–123.
19. Sclar DA, Lieberman PL. Anaphylaxis: Underdiagnosed, Underreported, and Undertreated. Am J Med 2014;127(1 Supplement):S1–5.
20. Mastrorilli C, Cardinale F, Giannetti A, et al. Pollen-Food Allergy Syndrome: A not so Rare Disease in Childhood. Medicina 2019;55(10):641.
21. Skypala IJ. Can patients with oral allergy syndrome be at risk of anaphylaxis? Curr Opin Allergy Clin Immunol 2020;20(5):459–64.
22. Carlson G, Coop C. Pollen food allergy syndrome (PFAS): a review of current available literature. Ann Allergy Asthma Immunol 2019;123(4):359–65.
23. Kulthanan K, Ungprasert P, Jirapongsananuruk O, et al. Food-Dependent Exercise-Induced Wheals, Angioedema, and Anaphylaxis: A Systematic Review. J Allergy Clin Immunol Pract 2022;10(9):2280–96.
24. Calvani M, Anania C, Cuomo B, et al. Summation anaphylaxis: A challenging diagnosis. Pediatr Allergy Immunol 2020;31(Suppl 26):33–5.
25. Geller M. Clinical Management of Exercise-Induced Anaphylaxis and Cholinergic Urticaria. J Allergy Clin Immunol Pract 2020;8(7):2209–14.
26. Mateos-Hernández L, Villar M, Moral A, et al. Tick-host conflict: immunoglobulin E antibodies to tick proteins in patients with anaphylaxis to tick bite. Oncotarget 2017;8(13):20630–44.
27. Feketea G, Tsabouri S. Common food colorants and allergic reactions in children: Myth or reality? Food Chem 2017;230:578–88.
28. Takeo N, Nakamura M, Nakayama S, et al. Cochineal dye-induced immediate allergy: Review of Japanese cases and proposed new diagnostic chart. Allergol Int 2018;67(4):496–505.
29. Ramsey NB, Tuano KT, Davis CM, et al. Annatto seed hypersensitivity in a pediatric patient. Ann Allergy Asthma Immunol 2016;117(3):331–3.
30. Wilson BG, Bahna SL. Adverse reactions to food additives. Ann Allergy Asthma Immunol 2005;95(6):499–507.

31. Yang WH, Purchase EC. Adverse reactions to sulfites. CMAJ 1985;133(9): 865–7.
32. Jacobson MF, DePorter J. Self-reported adverse reactions associated with my-coprotein (Quorn-brand) containing foods. Ann Allergy Asthma Immunol 2018; 120(6):626–30.
33. Khalili B, Bardana EJ Jr, Yunginger JW. Psyllium-associated anaphylaxis and death: a case report and review of the literature. Ann Allergy Asthma Immunol 2003;91(6):579–84.
34. Sugiura S, Kondo Y, Tsuge I, et al. IgE-dependent mechanism and successful desensitization of erythritol allergy. Ann Allergy Asthma Immunol 2016;117(3): 320–1.e1.
35. Sugiura S, Kondo Y, Ito K, et al. A case of anaphylaxis to erythritol diagnosed by CD203c expression–based basophil activation test. Ann Allergy Asthma Immunol 2013;111(3):222–3.
36. Yunginger JW, Jones RT, Kita H, et al. Allergic reactions after ingestion of erythritol-containing foods and beverages. J Allergy Clin Immun 2001; 108(4):650.
37. Papanikolaou I, Stenger R, Bessot JC, et al. Anaphylactic shock to guar gum (food additive E412) contained in a meal substitute. Allergy 2007;62(7):822.
38. Gay-Crosier F, Schreiber G, Hauser C. Anaphylaxis from inulin in vegetables and processed food. N Engl J Med 2000;342(18):1372.
39. Franck P, Moneret-Vautrin D, Morisset M, et al. Anaphylactic reaction to inulin: first identification of specific IgEs to an inulin protein compound. Int Arch Allergy Immunol 2005;136(2):155–8.
40. Chen JL, Bahna SL. Spice allergy. Ann Allergy Asthma Immunol 2011;107(3): 191–9.
41. Sharma A, Verma AK, Gupta RK, et al. A Comprehensive Review on Mustard-Induced Allergy and Implications for Human Health. Clin Rev Allergy Immunol 2019;57(1):39–54.
42. Bravo E, Moreno E, Sola JP, et al. Anaphylatic reaction after chamomile tea consumption. Allergo Journal International 2022;31(2):56–7.
43. Borghesan F, Mistrello G, Amato S, et al. Mugwort-fennel-allergy-syndrome associated with sensitization to an allergen homologous to Api g 5. Eur Ann Allergy Clin Immunol 2013;45(4):130–7.
44. Aurich S, Spiric J, Engin A, et al. Report of a Case of IgE-Mediated Anaphylaxis to Fenugreek. J Investig Allergol Clin Immunol 2019;29(1):56–8.
45. Benito M, Jorro G, Morales C, et al. Labiatae allergy: systemic reactions due to ingestion of oregano and thyme. Ann Allergy Asthma Immunol 1996;76(5): 416–8.
46. Unkle DW, Ricketti AJ, Ricketti PA, et al. Anaphylaxis following cilantro ingestion. Ann Allergy Asthma Immunol 2012;109(6):471–2.
47. Brussino L, Nicola S, Giorgis V, et al. Beer anaphylaxis due to coriander as hidden allergen. BMJ Case Rep 2018;2018:bcr2018.
48. Sanchez-Borges M, Capriles-Hulett A, Fernandez-Caldas E. Oral mite anaphylaxis: who, when, and how? Curr Opin Allergy Clin Immunol 2020;20(3):242–7.
49. Sanchez-Borges M, Suarez Chacon R, Capriles-Hulett A, et al. Anaphylaxis from ingestion of mites: pancake anaphylaxis. J Allergy Clin Immunol 2013; 131(1):31–5.
50. de Jong NW, van Maaren MS, Vlieg-Boersta BJ, et al. Sensitization to lupine flour: is it clinically relevant? Clin Exp Allergy 2010;40(10):1571–7.

51. Choi J-H, Jang Y-S, Oh J-W, et al. Bee Pollen-Induced Anaphylaxis: A Case Report and Literature Review. Allergy, Asthma & Immunology Research 2015; 7(5):513.
52. Chatkin JM, Zani-Silva L, Ferreira I, et al. Cannabis-Associated Asthma and Allergies. Clin Rev Allergy Immunol 2019;56(2):196–206.
53. Decuyper II, Van Gasse AL, Faber MA, et al. Exploring the Diagnosis and Profile of Cannabis Allergy. J Allergy Clin Immunol Pract 2019;7(3):983–9.e5.
54. Ylitalo L, Alenius H, Turjanmaa K, et al. Natural rubber latex allergy in children: a follow-up study. Clin Exp Allergy 2000;30(11):1612–7.
55. Meneses V, Parenti S, Burns H, et al. Latex allergy guidelines for people with spina bifida. J Pediatr Rehabil Med 2020;13:601–9.
56. Parisi CAS, Kelly KJ, Ansotegui IJ, et al. Update on latex allergy: New insights into an old problem. World Allergy Organization Journal 2021;14(8):100569.
57. Galindo PAP. Mosquito bite hypersensitivity. Allergol Immunopathol 1998;26(5): 251–4.
58. Hassoun S, Drouet M, Sabbah A. [Anaphylaxis caused by a mosquito: 2 case reports]. Allerg Immunol (Paris) 1999;31(8):285–7. Anaphylaxie au moustique: à propos de 2 cas cliniques.
59. Reiter N, Reiter M, Altrichter S, et al. Anaphylaxis caused by mosquito allergy in systemic mastocytosis. Lancet 2013;382(9901):1380.
60. McCormack DR, Salata KF, Hershey JN, et al. Mosquito bite anaphylaxis: immunotherapy with whole body extracts. Ann Allergy Asthma Immunol 1995;74(1): 39–44.
61. Tracy JM, Demain JG, Quinn JM, et al. The natural history of exposure to the imported fire ant (Solenopsis invicta). J Allergy Clin Immun 1995;95(4):824–8.
62. Partridge ME, Blackwood W, Hamilton RG, et al. Prevalence of allergic sensitization to imported fire ants in children living in an endemic region of the southeastern United States. Ann Allergy Asthma Immunol 2008;100(1):54–8.
63. Szari SM, Adams KE, Quinn JM, et al. Characteristics of venom allergy at initial evaluation: Is fire ant hypersensitivity similar to flying Hymenoptera? Ann Allergy Asthma Immunol 2019;123(6):590–4.
64. Rolla G, Heffler E, Boita M, et al. Pigeon tick bite: A neglected cause of idiopathic nocturnal anaphylaxis. Allergy 2018;73(4):958–61.
65. Hilger C, Bessot J-C, Hutt N, et al. IgE-mediated anaphylaxis caused by bites of the pigeon tick Argas reflexus: Cloning and expression of the major allergen Arg r 1. J Allergy Clin Immun 2005;115(3):617–22.
66. Brown AF, Hamilton DL. Tick bite anaphylaxis in Australia. J Accid Emerg Med 1998;15(2):111–3.
67. Porebski G, Kwiecien K, Pawica M, et al. Mas-Related G Protein-Coupled Receptor-X2 (MRGPRX2) in Drug Hypersensitivity Reactions. Perspective. Front Immunol 2018;2018:9.
68. Bensko JC, McGill A, Palumbo M, et al. Pediatric-onset aspirin-exacerbated respiratory disease: Clinical characteristics, prevalence, and response to dupilumab. J Allergy Clin Immunol Pract 2022;10(9):2466–8.
69. Bochenek G, Stachura T, Szafraniec K, et al. Diagnostic Accuracy of Urinary LTE4 Measurement to Predict Aspirin-Exacerbated Respiratory Disease in Patients with Asthma. J Allergy Clin Immunol Pract 2018;6(2):528–35.
70. Arber DA, Orazi A, Hasserjian R, et al. The 2016 revision to the World Health Organization classification of myeloid neoplasms and acute leukemia. Blood 2016; 127(20):2391–405.

71. Leguit RJ, Wang SA, George TI, et al. The international consensus classification of mastocytosis and related entities. Virchows Arch 2023;482(1):99–112.

72. Akin C. How to evaluate the patient with a suspected mast cell disorder and how/when to manage symptoms. Hematology 2022;2022(1):55–63.

73. Brockow K, Jofer C, Behrendt H, et al. Anaphylaxis in patients with mastocytosis: a study on history, clinical features and risk factors in 120 patients. Allergy 2008;63(2):226–32.

74. Alvarez-Twose I, Vano-Galvan S, Sanchez-Munoz L, et al. Increased serum baseline tryptase levels and extensive skin involvement are predictors for the severity of mast cell activation episodes in children with mastocytosis. Allergy 2012;67(6):813–21.

75. Hoermann G, Sotlar K, Jawhar M, et al. Standards of Genetic Testing in the Diagnosis and Prognostication of Systemic Mastocytosis in 2022: Recommendations of the EU-US Cooperative Group. J Allergy Clin Immunol 2022;10(8):1953–63.

76. Lange M, Hartmann K, Carter MC, et al. Molecular Background, Clinical Features and Management of Pediatric Mastocytosis: Status 2021. Int J Mol Sci 2021;22(5). https://doi.org/10.3390/ijms22052586.

77. Carter MC, Bai Y, Ruiz-Esteves KN, et al. Detection of KIT D816V in peripheral blood of children with manifestations of cutaneous mastocytosis suggests systemic disease. Br J Haematol 2018;183(5):775–82.

78. Castells M, Metcalfe DD, Escribano L. Diagnosis and treatment of cutaneous mastocytosis in children: practical recommendations. Am J Clin Dermatol 2011;12(4):259–70.

79. Méni C, Bruneau J, Georgin-Lavialle S, et al. Paediatric mastocytosis: a systematic review of 1747 cases. Br J Dermatol 2015;172(3):642–51.

80. Valent P, Akin C, Arock M, et al. Definitions, criteria and global classification of mast cell disorders with special reference to mast cell activation syndromes: a consensus proposal. Int Arch Allergy Immunol 2012;157(3):215–25.

81. Weiler CR, Austen KF, Akin C, et al. AAAAI Mast Cell Disorders Committee Work Group Report: Mast cell activation syndrome (MCAS) diagnosis and management. J Allergy Clin Immun 2019;144(4):883–96.

82. Giannetti MP, Akin C, Hufdhi R, et al. Patients with mast cell activation symptoms and elevated baseline serum tryptase level have unique bone marrow morphology. J Allergy Clin Immunol 2021;147(4):1497–501.e1.

83. Hamilton MJ, Zhao M, Giannetti MP, et al. Distinct Small Intestine Mast Cell Histologic Changes in Patients With Hereditary Alpha-tryptasemia and Mast Cell Activation Syndrome. Am J Surg Pathol 2021;45(7):997–1004.

84. Hamilton MJ, Hornick JL, Akin C, et al. Mast cell activation syndrome: a newly recognized disorder with systemic clinical manifestations. J Allergy Clin Immunol 2011;128(1):147–152 e2.

85. Lyons JJ, Yu X, Hughes JD, et al. Elevated basal serum tryptase identifies a multisystem disorder associated with increased TPSAB1 copy number. Nat Genet 2016;48(12):1564–9.

86. Chovanec J, Tunc I, Hughes J, et al. Genetically determining individualized clinical reference ranges for the biomarker tryptase can limit unnecessary procedures and unmask myeloid neoplasms. Blood Adv 2022. https://doi.org/10.1182/bloodadvances.2022007936.

87. Lyons JJ. Hereditary Alpha Tryptasemia: Genotyping and Associated Clinical Features. Immunol Allergy Clin 2018;38(3):483–95.

88. Chollet MB, Akin C. Hereditary alpha tryptasemia is not associated with specific clinical phenotypes. J Allergy Clin Immun 2022;149(2):728–735e2.

89. Glover SC, Carter MC, Korošec P, et al. Clinical relevance of inherited genetic differences in human tryptases: Hereditary alpha-tryptasemia and beyond. Ann Allergy Asthma Immunol 2021;127(6):638–47.

90. Vanderwert FI, Sordi B, Mannelli F, et al. Screening for Hereditary Alpha-Tryptasemia in Subjects with Systemic Mastocytosis (SM) and Non-SM Mast Cell Activation Symptoms. Blood 2021;138:1500.

91. Greiner G, Sprinzl B, Górska A, et al. Hereditary α tryptasemia is a valid genetic biomarker for severe mediator-related symptoms in mastocytosis. Blood 2021; 137(2):238–47.

92. Prosty C, Gabrielli S, Le M, et al. Prevalence, Management, and Anaphylaxis Risk of Cold Urticaria: A Systematic Review and Meta-Analysis. J Allergy Clin Immunol Pract 2022;10(2):586–96.

93. Alangari AA, Twarog FJ, Shih MC, et al. Clinical features and anaphylaxis in children with cold urticaria. Pediatrics 2004;113(4):e313–7.

94. Farooqui ZA, Chauhan A. Neuroendocrine Tumors in Pediatrics. Glob Pediatr Health 2019;6. https://doi.org/10.1177/2333794X19862712. 2333794X19862712.

95. Cheung VT, Khan MS. A guide to midgut neuroendocrine tumours (NETs) and carcinoid syndrome. Frontline Gastroenterol 2015;6(4):264–9.

96. Mesquita CT, Palazzo IC, Rezende MF. Ga-DOTA PET/CT: the first-line functional imaging modality in the management of patients with neuroendocrine tumors. Radiol Bras 2022;55(2):VII–VIII.

97. Tachdjian R, Kaplan AP. A Comprehensive Management Approach in Pediatric and Adolescent Patients With Hereditary Angioedema. Clin Pediatr 2023;0(0). https://doi.org/10.1177/00099228231155703. 00099228231155703.

98. Maurer M, Magerl M, Betschel S, et al. The international WAO/EAACI guideline for the management of hereditary angioedema-The 2021 revision and update. Allergy 2022;77(7):1961–90.

99. Bezalel S, Mahlab-Guri K, Asher I, et al. Angiotensin-converting Enzyme Inhibitor-induced Angioedema. Am J Med 2015/02/01/2015;128(2):120–5.

100. Hom KA, Hirsch R, Elluru RG. Antihypertensive drug-induced angioedema causing upper airway obstruction in children. Int J Pediatr Otorhinolaryngol 2012;76(1):14–9.

101. Beltrami L, Zanichelli A, Zingale L, et al. Long-term follow-up of 111 patients with angiotensin-converting enzyme inhibitor-related angioedema. J Hypertens 2011;29(11):2273–7.

102. Robin S, Buchanan R, Poole R. Energy drinks and adolescents - A hepatic health hazard? J Hepatol 2018;68(4):856–7.

103. Papaliodis D, Boucher W, Kempuraj D, et al. Niacin-induced "flush" involves release of prostaglandin D2 from mast cells and serotonin from platelets: evidence from human cells in vitro and an animal model. J Pharmacol Exp Ther 2008;327(3):665–72.

104. Feng C, Teuber S, Gershwin ME. Histamine (Scombroid) Fish Poisoning: a Comprehensive Review. Clin Rev Allergy Immunol 2016;50(1):64–9.

105. Skypala IJ, Williams M, Reeves L, et al. Sensitivity to food additives, vaso-active amines and salicylates: a review of the evidence. Clin Transl Allergy 2015;5(1):34.

106. Minciullo P, Cascio A, David A, et al. Anaphylaxis caused by helminths: review of the literature. Eur Rev Med Pharmacol Sci 2012;16(11):1513–8.

107. Pravettoni V, Primavesi L, Piantanida M. Anisakis simplex: current knowledge. Eur Ann Allergy Clin Immunol. Aug 2012;44(4):150–6.
108. Minciullo PL, Cascio A, Isola S, et al. Different clinical allergological features of Taenia solium infestation. Clin Mol Allergy 2016;14(1):18.
109. Cooper PJ. Interactions between helminth parasites and allergy. Curr Opin Allergy Clin Immunol. Feb 2009;9(1):29–37.
110. Halvorsen T, Walsted ES, Bucca C, et al. Inducible laryngeal obstruction: an official joint European Respiratory Society and European Laryngological Society statement. Eur Respir J 2017;50(3). https://doi.org/10.1183/13993003.02221-2016.
111. Johansson H, Norlander K, Berglund L, et al. Prevalence of exercise-induced bronchoconstriction and exercise-induced laryngeal obstruction in a general adolescent population. Thorax 2015;70(1):57–63.
112. Traister RS, Fajt ML, Landsittel D, et al. A novel scoring system to distinguish vocal cord dysfunction from asthma. J Allergy Clin Immunol Pract 2014;2(1):65–9.
113. Choy AC, Patterson R, Patterson DR, et al. Undifferentiated somatoform idiopathic anaphylaxis: nonorganic symptoms mimicking idiopathic anaphylaxis. J Allergy Clin Immunol 1995;96(6 Pt 1):893–900.
114. Rosloff DA, Patel K, Feustel PJ, et al. Criteria positive and criteria negative anaphylaxis, with a focus on undifferentiated somatoform idiopathic anaphylaxis: A review and case series. Allergy Asthma Proc 2020;41(6):436–41.
115. Diagnostic A. Statistical manual of mental disorders fifth edition text revision (DSM-5-TR). Washington, DC, USA: American Psychiatric Association Publishing; 2022.
116. Bahna SL, Oldham JL. Munchausen stridor-a strong false alarm of anaphylaxis. Allergy Asthma Immunol Res 2014;6(6):577–9.
117. Khanal R, Sendil S, Oli S, et al. Factitious Disorder Masquerading as a Life-Threatening Anaphylaxis. Journal of Investigative Medicine High Impact Case Reports 2021;9. 23247096211006248.
118. Hendrix S, Sale S, Zeiss CR, et al. Factitious Hymenoptera allergic emergency: a report of a new variant of Munchausen's syndrome. J Allergy Clin Immunol 1981;67(1):8–13.
119. Wong H. Munchausen's syndrome presenting as prevarication anaphylaxis. Can J Allergy Clin Immunol 1999;4:299–300.
120. Khan DA, Banerji A, Blumenthal KG, et al. Drug allergy: A 2022 practice parameter update. J Allergy Clin Immunol 2022;150(6):1333–93.
121. Bogas G, Salas M, et al. The role of basophil activation test in drug allergy. Current Treatment Options in Allergy 2021;8(4):298–313.
122. Valent P, Bonadonna P, Hartmann K, et al. Why the 20% + 2 Tryptase Formula Is a Diagnostic Gold Standard for Severe Systemic Mast Cell Activation and Mast Cell Activation Syndrome. Int Arch Allergy Immunol 2019;180(1):44–51.
123. Lyons JJ. Inherited and acquired determinants of serum tryptase levels in humans. Ann Allergy Asthma Immunol 2021;127(4):420–6.
124. Laroche D, Vergnaud MC, Dubois F, et al. Plasma histamine and tryptase during anaphylactoid reactions. Agents Actions 1992/06/01 1992;36(2):C201–2.
125. Valent P, Akin C, Bonadonna P, et al. Proposed Diagnostic Algorithm for Patients with Suspected Mast Cell Activation Syndrome. J Allergy Clin Immunol Pract 2019;7(4):1125–1133 e1.
126. Szebeni J. Complement activation-related pseudoallergy: a stress reaction in blood triggered by nanomedicines and biologicals. Mol Immunol 2014;61(2):163–73.

127. Lyons JJ, Greiner G, Hoermann G, et al. Incorporating Tryptase Genotyping Into the Workup and Diagnosis of Mast Cell Diseases and Reactions. J Allergy Clin Immunol Pract 2022;10(8):1964–73.
128. Kristensen T, Vestergaard H, Bindslev-Jensen C, et al. Sensitive KIT D816V mutation analysis of blood as a diagnostic test in mastocytosis. Am J Hematol 2014;89(5):493–8.
129. Jara-Acevedo M, Teodosio C, Sanchez-Muñoz L, et al. Detection of the KIT D816V mutation in peripheral blood of systemic mastocytosis: diagnostic implications. Mod Pathol 2015;28(8):1138–49.
130. Meni C, Georgin-Lavialle S, Le Saché de Peufeilhoux L, et al. Paediatric mastocytosis: long-term follow-up of 53 patients with whole sequencing of KIT. A prospective study. Br J Dermatol 2018;179(4):925–32.
131. Sotlar K, George TI, Kluin P, et al. Standards of Pathology in the Diagnosis of Systemic Mastocytosis: Recommendations of the EU-US Cooperative Group. J Allergy Clin Immunol Pract 2022;10(8):1986–1998 e2.
132. Doyle LA, Hornick JL. Pathology of Extramedullary Mastocytosis. Immunology and Allergy Clinics 2014;34(2):323–39.
133. Reichard KK, Chen D, Pardanani A, et al. Morphologically Occult Systemic Mastocytosis in Bone Marrow: Clinicopathologic Features and an Algorithmic Approach to Diagnosis. Am J Clin Pathol 2015;144(3):493–502.
134. Knibb RC, Alviani C, Garriga-Baraut T, et al. The effectiveness of interventions to improve self-management for adolescents and young adults with allergic conditions: A systematic review. Allergy 2020;75(8):1881–98.
135. Maltseva N, Borzova E, Fomina D, et al. Cold urticaria – What we know and what we do not know. Allergy 2021;76(4):1077–94.
136. Braun C, Caubet J-C. Food oral immunotherapy is superior to food avoidance-CON. Ann Allergy Asthma Immunol 2019;122(6):569–71.
137. Cox L, Nelson H, Lockey R, et al. Allergen immunotherapy: A practice parameter third update. J Allergy Clin Immun 2011;127(1):S1–55.
138. Greenhawt M, Oppenheimer J, Nelson M, et al. Sublingual immunotherapy: A focused allergen immunotherapy practice parameter update. Ann Allergy Asthma Immunol 2017;118(3):276–282 e2.
139. Patterson R. Idiopathic anaphylaxis. Clin Rev Allergy Immunol 1999;17(4):425–8.
140. Ditto AM, Krasnick J, Greenberger PA, et al. Pediatric idiopathic anaphylaxis: experience with 22 patients. J Allergy Clin Immunol 1997;100(3):320–6.
141. Zuberbier T, Abdul Latiff AH, Abuzakouk M, et al. The international EAACI/GA2-LEN/EuroGuiDerm/APAAACI guideline for the definition, classification, diagnosis, and management of urticaria. Allergy 2022;77(3):734–66.
142. Patterson R, Fitzsimons EJ, Choy AC, et al. Malignant and corticosteroid-dependent idiopathic anaphylaxis: successful responses to ketotifen. Ann Allergy Asthma Immunol 1997;79(2):138–44.
143. Dykewicz MS, Wong SS, Patterson R, et al. Evaluation of ketotifen in corticosteroid-dependent idiopathic anaphylaxis. Ann Allergy 1990;65(5):406–10.
144. Kettelhut BV, Berkebile C, Bradley D, et al. A double-blind, placebo-controlled, crossover trial of ketotifen versus hydroxyzine in the treatment of pediatric mastocytosis. J Allergy Clin Immunol 1989;83(5):866–70.
145. Munoz-Cano R, Ainsua-Enrich E, Torres-Atencio I, et al. Effects of Rupatadine on Platelet- Activating Factor-Induced Human Mast Cell Degranulation Compared With Desloratadine and Levocetirizine (The MASPAF Study). J Investig Allergol Clin Immunol 2017;27(3):161–8.

146. Vadas P, Gold M, Perelman B, et al. Platelet-Activating Factor, PAF Acetylhydrolase, and Severe Anaphylaxis. N Engl J Med 2008;358(1):28–35.

147. Kaul M, End P, Cabanski M, et al. Remibrutinib (LOU064): A selective potent oral BTK inhibitor with promising clinical safety and pharmacodynamics in a randomized phase I trial. Clin Transl Sci 2021;14(5):1756–68.

148. Maurer M, Berger W, Gimenez-Arnau A, et al. Remibrutinib, a novel BTK inhibitor, demonstrates promising efficacy and safety in chronic spontaneous urticaria. J Allergy Clin Immunol 2022;150(6):1498–1506 e2.

149. Lemal R, Fouquet G, Terriou L, et al. Omalizumab Therapy for Mast Cell-Mediator Symptoms in Patients with ISM, CM, MMAS, and MCAS. J Allergy Clin Immunol Pract 2019;7(7):2387–95.

150. Carter MC, Maric I, Brittain EH, et al. A randomized double-blind, placebo-controlled study of omalizumab for idiopathic anaphylaxis. J Allergy Clin Immunol 2021;147(3):1004–1010 e2.

151. Maurer M, Gimenez-Arnau AM, Sussman G, et al. Ligelizumab for Chronic Spontaneous Urticaria. N Engl J Med 2019;381(14):1321–32.

152. Maurer M, Gimenez-Arnau A, Bernstein JA, et al. Sustained safety and efficacy of ligelizumab in patients with chronic spontaneous urticaria: A one-year extension study. Allergy 2022;77(7):2175–84.

153. Teva Pharmaceuticals. Study to Compare Efficacy and Safety of TEV-45779 With XOLAIR (Omalizumab) in Adults With Chronic Idiopathic Urticaria. ClinicalTrials.gov identifier: NCT04976192. 2023. Available at: https://www.clinicaltrials.gov/study/NCT04976192. Accessed June 27, 2023.

154. Kuo BS, Li CH, Chen JB, et al. IgE-neutralizing UB-221 mAb, distinct from omalizumab and ligelizumab, exhibits CD23-mediated IgE downregulation and relieves urticaria symptoms. J Clin Invest 2022;132(15). https://doi.org/10.1172/JCI157765.

155. Maurer M, Casale T, Saini S, et al. Dupilumab Significantly Reduces Itch and Hives in Patients With Chronic Spontaneous Urticaria: Results From a Phase 3 Trial (LIBERTY-CSU CUPID Study A). J Allergy Clin Immun 2022;149(2):AB312.

156. Update on ongoing Dupixent® (dupilumab) chronic spontaneous urticaria Phase 3 program. Sanofi. February 18, 2022, 2022. Available at: https://www.sanofi.com/en/media-room/press-releases/2022/2022-02-18-06-00-00-2387700. Accessed 5/2/, 2023.

157. Rossavik E, Lam W, Wiens L. M003 novel use of dupilumab in a patient with idiopathic anaphylaxis. Ann Allergy Asthma Immunol 2020;125(5):S54–5.

158. Alvarado D, Maurer M, Gedrich R, et al. Anti-KIT monoclonal antibody CDX-0159 induces profound and durable mast cell suppression in a healthy volunteer study. Allergy. Aug 2022;77(8):2393–403.

159. Schanin J, Gebremeskel S, Korver W, et al. A monoclonal antibody to Siglec-8 suppresses non-allergic airway inflammation and inhibits IgE-independent mast cell activation. Mucosal Immunol 2021;14(2):366–76.

160. Korver W, Wong A, Gebremeskel S, et al. The Inhibitory Receptor Siglec-8 Interacts With FcεRI and Globally Inhibits Intracellular Signaling in Primary Mast Cells Upon Activation. Front Immunol 2022;13:833728.

161. Altrichter S, Staubach P, Pasha M, et al. An open-label, proof-of-concept study of lirentelimab for antihistamine-resistant chronic spontaneous and inducible urticaria. J Allergy Clin Immunol 2022;149(5):1683–90.e7.

162. Polloni L, Muraro A. Anxiety and food allergy: A review of the last two decades. Clin Exp Allergy 2020;50(4):420–41.

163. Weiss D, Marsac ML. Coping and posttraumatic stress symptoms in children with food allergies. Ann Allergy Asthma Immunol 2016;117(5):561–2.
164. O'Connell C, Shafran R, Bennett S. A systematic review of randomised controlled trials using psychological interventions for children and adolescents with medically unexplained symptoms: A focus on mental health outcomes. Clin Child Psychol Psychiatr 2020;25(1):273–90.
165. Lieberman P, Nicklas RA, Randolph C, et al. Anaphylaxis—a practice parameter update 2015. Ann Allergy Asthma Immunol 2015;115(5):341–84.
166. Roberts G, Vazquez-Ortiz M, Knibb R, et al. EAACI Guidelines on the effective transition of adolescents and young adults with allergy and asthma. Allergy 2020;75(11):2734–52.
167. National Institute of Allergy and Infectious Diseases. Cause of Unexplained Anaphylaxis. ClinicalTrials.gov Identifier: NCT00719719 Updated June 15, 2023. Available at: https://www.clinicaltrials.gov/study/NCT00719719. Accessed June 27, 2023.
168. Sharma J, Jindal AK, Banday AZ, et al. Pathophysiology of Hereditary Angioedema (HAE) Beyond the SERPING1 Gene. Clin Rev Allergy Immunol 2021; 60(3):305–15.
169. Bichon A, Bourenne J, Gainnier M, et al. Capillary leak syndrome: State of the art in 2021. Rev Med Interne 2021;42(11):789–96.
170. Bozzini MA, Milani GP, Bianchetti MG, et al. Idiopathic systemic capillary leak syndrome (Clarkson syndrome) in childhood: systematic literature review. Eur J Pediatr 2018;177(8):1149–54.
171. Heide R, van Doorn K, Mulder PG, et al. Serum tryptase and SCORMA (SCORing MAstocytosis) Index as disease severity parameters in childhood and adult cutaneous mastocytosis. Clin Exp Dermatol 2009;34(4):462–8.
172. Jiang Y, Yuan IH, Dutille EK, et al. Preventing iatrogenic gelatin anaphylaxis. Ann Allergy Asthma Immunol 2019;123(4):366–74.
173. Kwittken PL, Rosen S, Sweinberg SK. MMR vaccine and neomycin allergy. Am J Dis Child 1993;147(2):128–9.

# Monogenic Etiology of Hypertension

Vaishali Singh, MD[a],*, Scott K. Van Why, MD[a]

## KEYWORDS

- Monogenic hypertension • Renin • Aldosterone • Liddle syndrome
- Congenital adrenal hyperplasia • Apparent mineralocorticoid excess
- Gordon syndrome • Adolescent

## KEY POINTS

- Although rare, clinicians should have high suspicion of monogenic etiology of hypertension in patients with electrolyte abnormalities including hyper/hypokalemia or metabolic alkalosis/acidosis.
- The primary mechanism of monogenic hypertension involves excessive sodium retention leading to total body volume expansion.
- Besides renin and aldosterone levels as part of initial screening, genetic testing is most often the best method to reach a diagnosis of monogenic hypertension.
- Treatment of monogenic hypertension usually differs from conventional antihypertensive therapy.

## INTRODUCTION

Several monogenic etiologies of hypertension, which may present during adolescence, are now well defined. Those causes of hypertension, however, are exceedingly rare and thus may not be considered or recognized in an adolescent who is found to be hypertensive. The first step in the evaluation of an adolescent for hypertension is to define whether in fact the patient is hypertensive. The 2017 AAP clinical practice guidelines for management of hypertension in children and adolescents is used to define hypertension.[1] The current guideline that includes hypertension definition and staging leads to seamless interfacing with the 2017 AHA and American College of Cardiology (ACC) adult HTN guidelines for adolescents over 13 years of age (**Table 1**).

Before embarking on an evaluation for underlying cause of hypertension, verifying whether an adolescent is truly hypertensive is the first step. Accurate blood pressure measurement is fundamental in identification of hypertension. Manual, auscultatory

[a] Department of Pediatrics, Medical College of Wisconsin, Suite 510, 999 North 92nd Street, Milwaukee, WI 53226, USA

* Corresponding author. Department of Pediatrics, Medical College of Wisconsin, Suite 510, 999 North 92nd Street, Milwaukee, WI 53226.

E-mail address: vsingh@mcw.edu

Med Clin N Am 108 (2024) 157–172
https://doi.org/10.1016/j.mcna.2023.06.005
0025-7125/24/© 2023 Elsevier Inc. All rights reserved.

| Table 1 The 2017 AAP clinical practice guidelines for management of hypertension in children and adolescent over 13 y of age | |
|---|---|
| | For Children, Adolescents Aged ≥13 y |
| Normal BP | <120/<80 mm Hg |
| Elevated BP | 120–129/<80 mm Hg |
| Stage 1 HTN | 130–139/80–89 mm Hg |
| Stage 2 HTN | ≥140/90 mm Hg |

blood pressure is the most accurate, and the normative data are based on this method. An accurate reading depends on positioning and appropriate cuff size. Sitting relaxed and using a cuff with a bladder that covers a minimum 80% mid-arm circumference and 40% of arm length is optimal. A well calibrated oscillatory device can be used for initial screening, but abnormal findings should be then validated with auscultatory method as soon as is reasonable considering the context of the initial measurement. Blood pressure measurement should be done on the right arm. If blood pressure is found there to be elevated, four extremity readings should be obtained to evaluate for vascular anomalies, particularly, aortic coarctation.

It is common for patients to be anxious or stressed during a visit to a clinic, urgent care, or emergency department. That can result in transient elevation in blood pressure, not indicative of established hypertension. So, if the initial blood pressure reading is in the elevated blood pressure or stage 1 hypertension range, additional readings should be obtained on different days, over days to weeks following the initial measurements, to confirm the presence of hypertension. If there is concern that anxiety is affecting blood pressure assessment, 24-h ambulatory blood pressure monitoring (ABPM) can separate those with sustained hypertension from those with 'white coat hypertension.'

If blood pressure is severely high or associated with symptoms that suggest either accelerating symptomatic hypertension (hypertensive urgency or emergency) or accompanying serious systemic disease, more urgent assessment and evaluation than described above is needed. It is beyond the scope of this article to detail the symptoms and findings that indicate the need for urgent evaluation. In brief, accompanying headache, visual changes, dizziness, altered mental status, dyspnea, skin lesions, edema, gross hematuria, or other systemic symptoms indicate the need for prompt and full evaluation. For thorough discussion of this issue please see references.[2,3]

Monogenic causes of hypertension are not only rare, they also rarely if ever present as hypertensive urgency or emergency. So, with severe or symptomatic hypertension other etiologies need to be considered first and promptly. Thus, before describing the known monogenic forms of hypertension, we will outline the more common causes of hypertension for which a patient should first undergo evaluation before pursuing a diagnosis of a monogenic etiology.

## COMMON AND LESS COMMON CAUSES OF HYPERTENSION IN ADOLESCENTS

In contrast to adulthood where primary hypertension is widespread with progressive age, hypertension in childhood is uncommon and is usually from a cause other than primary hypertension. In adolescents hypertension usually is secondary to an identifiable cause and is most often from renal disease. Disease processes that cause hypertension in childhood typically manifest at different ages, with the major differences

**Box 1**
**Causes of hypertension in adolescents**

*Hypertension in Adolescents*

Common Causes
- Primary and obesity associated
- Parenchymal Renal Disease
  - Acute and chronic glomerulonephritis
    - Post-infectious glomerulonephritis
    - Systemic vasculitis with renal involvement (SLE, HSP, ANCA vasculitis)
    - Primary, idiopathic (IgA nephropathy, FSGS, crescentic glomerulonephritis)
  - Hemolytic Uremic Syndrome
  - Hereditary cystic kidney disease – PKD, MCKD, nephronophthisis
  - Sickle cell disease
  - Interstitial nephritis
- End stage kidney disease of unknown etiology
- Congenital urinary tract malformations – obstructive or cystic dysplasia, either isolated or syndromic
- Scarred kidney – congenital Ask-Upmark kidney or acquired from renal injury, for example, pyelonephritis
- Drug induced – therapeutic and illicit

Less Common Causes
- Vascular/Renal artery stenosis
  - Aortic coarctation
  - Fibromuscular dysplasia
  - Syndromic – Williams syndrome, neurofibromatosis, Turner syndrome, middle aortic syndrome
  - Tumor associated extrinsic compression – kidney tumor, neuroblastoma, lymphoma
  - Large vessel vasculitis – Takayasu, Moyamoya, polyarteritis nodosum
  - Trauma associated perirenal hematoma
- Neoplasia – Renal tumors, neuroblastoma, pheochromocytoma, infiltrative lymphoma
- Persistent or late onset hypertension from perinatal renal insult, prematurity associated.
- Neurologic
  - High intracranial pressure from head trauma, intracranial tumor, or pseudotumor cerebri
  - Secondary to seizure
  - Peripheral neuropathies – Guillain-Barre, poliomyelitis

Rare causes
- Monogenic
  - Liddle syndrome
  - Hyperaldosteronism – familial and glucocorticoid remedial
  - Congenital adrenal hyperplasia
  - Gordon syndrome – pseudohypoaldosteronism
  - Apparent mineralocorticoid excess (AME)
- Dysautonomia
- Endocrine
  - Thyroid disease
  - Cushing syndrome
  - Catecholamine secreting tumors
  - Hypercalcemia – Vitamin D intoxication, hyperparathyroidism, malignancy associated

*Abbreviations:* ANCA, anti-neutrophil cytoplasmic antibody; HSP, Henoch Schoenlein purpura; MCKD, multi-cystic dysplastic kidney; PKD, polycystic kidney disease; SLE, systemic lupus erythematosis.

being between infants and older children. Our discussion here will focus on causes of hypertension presenting during late childhood and adolescence.

### Hypertension in Adolescents

While much of childhood hypertension is discovered during evaluation for an acute illness or symptomatic hypertension, with progressive age hypertension becomes more often found incidentally during examination on a well-child visit. **Box 1** outlines common and less common causes of hypertension that present during adolescence.

### Common Causes

The younger the child or adolescent the more likely there will be an identifiable cause of elevated blood pressure, and thus secondary hypertension will be found with appropriate investigation. Primary hypertension, then, is a diagnosis of exclusion. When secondary hypertension has been ruled out (see Evaluation section below), primary hypertension is presumed when blood pressure elevation in an adolescent is not severe, is asymptomatic, is associated with obesity, and there is family history of early onset primary hypertension. Outside of that scenario, other identifiable causes of hypertension, as outlined below and in **Box 1**, need to be considered.

Acute and symptomatic hypertension in adolescents is most likely to be secondary to glomerular disease. Acute post-infectious glomerulonephritis is the most common cause of nephritis in childhood and early adolescence. Patients with systemic vasculitis with renal involvement, including lupus, Henoch-Schoenlein purpura and ANCA vasculitis, at presentation and during flares of the disease often have significant hypertension. Hemolytic uremic syndrome (HUS), both toxigenic and atypical forms, usually present earlier in childhood but can present during adolescence and routinely have associated hypertension during the episode. The hypertension from HUS may abate after the HUS episode resolves, but may persistent and become a long term sequela.

Patients with crescentic glomerulonephritis, whether idiopathic or secondary to other identifiable nephropathy, typically have significant and often severe hypertension at presentation. Primary idiopathic forms of glomerulonephritis such as IgA nephropathy and focal segmental glomerulosclerosis variably have hypertension as a presenting feature. Early onset hypertension in patients with sickle cell disease is usually associated with overt sickle cell nephropathy. Finally, drug induced hypertension is common in adolescence. Any adolescent presenting with severe and symptomatic hypertension, who does not have evident renal disease on initial testing and is not on a prescribed medication known to cause hypertension, should be evaluated for the possibility of other drug induced hypertension (see refs. 2,3).

### Less Common Causes

Vascular causes of hypertension, though usually identified earlier, on occasion present during adolescence. These include aortic coarctation or renal artery stenosis, both idiopathic or syndromic forms, that typically present with incidentally found severe hypertension that is asymptomatic.

Neoplastic disease that compromises the major renal vasculature can cause hypertension. Renal malignancies or lymphoma may cause hypertension by direct infiltration of normal renal parenchyma. Pheochromocytoma and neuroblastoma cause hypertension through elaboration of excessive catecholamines.

Neurologic injury or disease can have associated elevation in blood pressure. High intracranial pressure from head trauma, intracranial tumor, or pseudotumor cerebri often results in high blood pressure. Peripheral neuropathies such as from Guillain-Barre syndrome or poliomyelitis not uncommonly have hypertension from autonomic dysfunction in the acute phase of the disease. Blood pressure is often elevated during seizure activity and does not require anti-hypertensive treatment or specific evaluation if seizure alone is clearly the cause of the elevated blood pressure. However, since hypertensive crisis caused by several underlying diseases may present with new onset seizure, it must always be considered whether the finding of elevated blood pressure is the cause or effect of the seizure.

### Rare Causes

While well known to cause elevated blood pressure, endocrine causes of hypertension are rare in childhood. Other than catecholamine secreting tumors, endocrine causes of hypertension do not typically present as hypertension as the principal feature. More often high blood pressure is found when being evaluated for other signs or symptoms attributable to the underlying endocrine disorder.

## EVALUATION FOR MORE LIKELY CAUSES OF HYPERTENSION

Since monogenic causes of hypertension are rare, it is incumbent first to direct evaluation for the common and less common causes of hypertension in adolescence (outlined in **Box 1**). For a full description of necessary evaluation for most causes of hypertension in adolescents see references.[2,3] In brief, in all adolescents found to have hypertension, the initial approach is garnering a thorough history and physical examination. Not only does this direct to investigations likely to be fruitful in identifying the cause, it also identifies those patients in whom investigation must move quickly.

### Investigation for Common and Less Common Causes of Hypertension in Adolescents

**Fig. 1** outlines investigative paths that should be pursued first before considering monogenic causes of hypertension. Adolescents who present with symptomatic

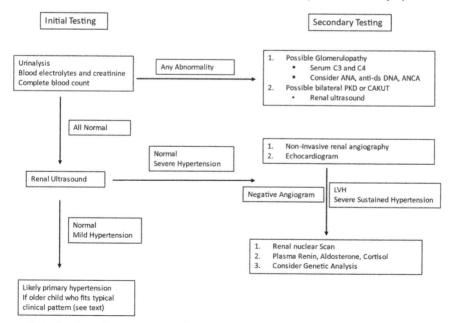

**Fig. 1.** Evaluation of more common forms of Adolescent Hypertension.

hypertension are likely to have acute glomerular disease. So initial investigation should be prompt and focus on those potential etiologies. If neurologic symptoms are a prominent feature of the presentation and brain imaging is unremarkable, drug ingestion needs to be considered. If acute glomerulopathy or toxic ingestion appear to be ruled out, renal imaging is then indicated. Renal ultrasound readily identifies congenital urinary tract abnormalities or cystic kidney diseases that cause hypertension.

If the more common etiologies of secondary hypertension have been ruled out with the initial investigations as above, the possibility of an underlying renovascular cause then needs to be explored. Aortic coarctation is simply ruled out on examination using 4-extremity blood pressure measurements. Vascular imaging using non-invasive abdominal CT or MR angiogram may reveal renovascular causes of hypertension.

Tachycardia and flushing at presentation suggest the possibility of a catecholamine secreting tumor or thyroid disease, in which thyroid function tests or blood and urine catecholamine studies reveal the etiology. If an endocrine cause other than thyroid disease is suspected, blood renin, aldosterone and cortisol levels are tested.

## MONOGENIC CAUSES OF HYPERTENSION

Monogenic hypertension is a category of secondary hypertension caused by pathogenic mutations in a single gene involved with renal and adrenal regulation of blood pressure and intravascular volume. Of the several forms of monogenic hypertension identified to date, essentially all have the same primary mechanism of hypertension wherein increased sodium retention causes total body volume expansion. This inappropriate volume expansion causes suppression of renin levels; hence, hyporeninemia is the cardinal feature of all forms of monogenic hypertension. The entities causing increased renal sodium retention can be separated into primary, monogenic defects in the renal tubule or monogenic abnormal endocrine (adrenal) signaling for inappropriate increase in renal sodium retention.

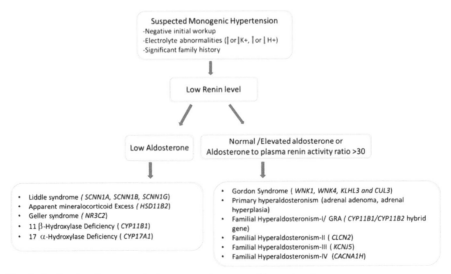

**Fig. 2.** Evaluation for suspected monogenic cause of hypertension.

## Investigation for Monogenic Forms of Hypertension

The prevalence of inherited forms of hypertension is unknown. Though monogenic hypertension is rare, it should be considered when common causes of hypertension have been ruled out. Electrolyte abnormalities are not always present, but abnormalities in serum K+ level or presence of metabolic alkalosis or acidosis should prompt consideration of inherited forms of hypertension. When considering a monogenic form of hypertension, blood renin and aldosterone levels should be obtained prior to any treatment. As mentioned, hyporeninemia is a universal finding in monogenic hypertension. An elevated aldosterone (ng/dL) to plasma renin activity (ng/ml/h) ratio suggests hyperaldosteronism even in the context of normal serum aldosterone level. A ratio greater than 30 is consistent with primary hyperaldosteronism. **Fig. 2** shows biochemical investigations that screen for and direct toward a diagnosis of specific forms of monogenic hypertension.

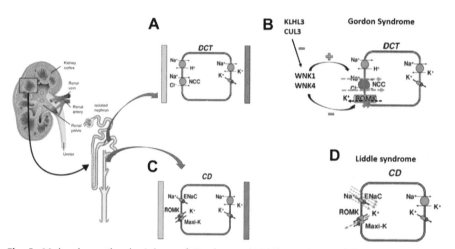

**Fig. 3.** Molecular pathophysiology of Gordon and Liddle syndrome. (*A*) Sodium reabsorption and potassium secretion at the level of the distal convoluted tubule. In the DCT WNK-1 and WNK-4 increase the activity of NCC, which reabsorbs Na+, and increase the internalization of ROMK channel, which secrets K+. WNK-1 also stimulates ENaC via SGK1 (not shown) in the CD. (*B*) In Gordon syndrome, mutation of WNK-1 and WNK-4 genes result in increased WNK activation resulting in increased Na + reabsorption by NCC, and decreased ROMK availability at the apical surface leading to decreased K+ secretion and hyperkalemia. KLHL3 and CUL3 encode for proteins that are part of a ubiquitin-protein ligase complex that degrades WNKs. Inactivating mutations in these genes result in increased availability of WNK-1 and WNK-4. (*C*) Sodium reabsorption and potassium secretion at the level of the collecting duct. In the CD segment of the nephron, aldosterone binds to MR which activates genomic and non-genomic signaling pathways to enhance ENaC, Na + absorption and K+ secretion by increasing the activity of ENaC, ROMK, and Na+/K + ATPase. (*D*) In Liddle syndrome, mutations of ENaC subunits decrease internalization and degradation of ENaC, and thus increases the number of functional ENaC at the apical surface of principal cells. This results in increased Na + absorption and hypertension accompanied with hypokalemia. CD, collecting duct; CUL3, cullin 3 gene; DCT, distal convoluted tubule; ENaC, epithelial sodium channel; KLHL3, Kelch-like 3 gene; NCC, sodium chloride cotransporter; ROMK, renal outer medullary potassium (K+) channel; WNK, with no lysine serine/threonine protein kinases gene.

The most effective method to make a diagnosis of a monogenic form of hypertension now is by genetic sequencing and analysis. With the advancement in molecular genetics and increased application broadly in medical practice, genetic testing has become less cost prohibitive and hence increasingly used in evaluation of the select subset of patients with hypertension as defined above.

## Monogenic Renal Tubule Defects

**Liddle syndrome** is an autosomal dominant disease caused by pathogenic variants of the amiloride sensitive epithelial Na + channel (ENaC) that constitutively increase sodium reabsorption in principal cells of the distal nephron.[4] ENaC is expressed in the apical membranes of the distal convoluted tubule (DCT), connecting tubule, and collecting duct (**Fig. 3**). Aldosterone upregulates the expression of ENaC channel via the mineralocorticoid receptor (MR) in principle cells.[5] Pathogenic variants in genes encoding either the β or γ subunits of ENaC have been identified in Liddle syndrome.[6,7] Under normal conditions both subunits of ENaC facilitate trafficking of ENaC away from the apical membrane for internalization and degradation. The pathologic variants then effectively cause unregulated gain of ENaC function due to impaired ENaC internalization and degradation, thus increasing the number of functional ENaC channels at the apical surface of principal cells.[8,9] Other mechanisms of pathologic variants of ENaC causing channel overactivity include insensitivity of ENaC to high intracellular Na + concentration or alteration in channel open probability.[9–11] Each variant, then, results in increased Na + reabsorption, plasma volume expansion and hypertension.[12]

Liddle syndrome appears to be the most common form of monogenic hypertension.[13] Hypertension can start in childhood and be significant, but commonly is asymptomatic. However, patients with Liddle syndrome who are either unrecognized or untreated are at significantly increased risk of developing early onset cardiovascular and peripheral vascular disease, including stroke.[14]

*Diagnosis*: While a definite diagnosis requires genetic testing, screening laboratory evaluation may show hypokalemic metabolic alkalosis. These findings result from the increased Na + reabsorption that creates a negative charge in the tubule lumen, thereby promoting secretion of K+ and H+ ions. Both serum renin and aldosterone levels typically are suppressed. Because of these features Liddle syndrome is also known as pseudohyperaldosteronism.

*Treatment*: Based on the pathophysiology of the disease, treatment of Liddle syndrome is with a combination of rigorous dietary sodium restriction along with direct inhibition of ENaC. The latter is accomplished with amiloride or triamterene, both which directly interfere with constitutive ENaC function.[14]

**Gordon syndrome**, also known as Pseudohypoaldosteronism Type II (PHAII), is caused by increased activity of the thiazide-sensitive sodium-chloride-cotransporter (NCC) located on the apical membrane of tubule cells in the distal nephron (see **Fig. 3**).[15] Autosomal dominant, pathogenic variants of kinases WNK-1 and WNK-4, which increase the activity of these kinases, were found to cause Gordon syndrome/PHAII.[16] Both kinases increase the activity of NCC, and WNK-1 also stimulates EnaC through a separate mechanism,[17] thus increasing sodium reabsorption through two pathways. In addition, both kinases also increase the internalization of the renal outer medullary potassium (ROMK) channel (see **Fig. 3**). The ROMK channel, when in the membrane, facilitates secretion of potassium into the tubule lumen. So pathogenic overactivity of the WNK kinases, resulting in increased internalization of ROMK channels, by reducing K+ secretion contributes to the hyperkalemia often found in Gordon syndrome.[18] Variants in KLHL3 and CUL3 also cause Gordon syndrome through a similar mechanism as both proteins are part of a complex that degrades WNKs.[16,19]

Characteristics of Gordon Syndrome/PHAII include hypertension, hyperkalemia, muscle weakness, short stature, dental abnormalities, and developmental delay.[16,19] The pattern of presentation is variable, with hyperkalemia and metabolic acidosis often manifest before onset of hypertension, the latter which may only be found late in adulthood.[20] Those with pathologic variants in CUL3 and KLHL3 commonly have a more severe phenotype compared with those with causal WNK-1 and WNK-4 variants.[16]

*Diagnosis*: Initial screening studies may reveal hyperkalemia and metabolic acidosis. Plasma renin activity is typically low. Aldosterone level may be normal or elevated at presentation, with high aldosterone likely stimulated by the hyperkalemia. As might be expected with increased constitutive activity of NCC, many PHAII/Gordon syndrome patients have hypercalciuria. Like other forms of monogenic hypertension, molecular genetic testing is ideal for diagnosis.

*Treatment*: Targeting the pathophysiology of this syndrome as described, treatment of Gordon syndrome is with a combination of diet restricted in Na+ and K+ along with administration of thiazide diuretics.[21]

**Geller syndrome** is caused by an autosomal dominant, activating pathogenic variant of the gene NR3C2, which encodes the mineralocorticoid receptor (MR). It appears that the pathophysiology of this disease includes increased sensitivity of the MR to non-mineralocorticoid steroids, including progesterone. Affected patients have constitutively active MR and accompanying overstimulation of tubular Na + reabsorption not only by aldosterone but also by cortisone and progesterone[22] (**Fig. 4**). For that reason, this syndrome is more likely to be recognized in females and has alternately been called "hypertension exacerbated by pregnancy." While hypertension is present and can be severe in nonpregnant patients, it typically worsens

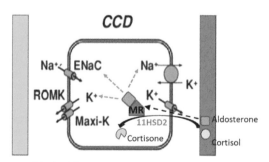

**Fig. 4.** The MR receptor binds aldosterone and cortisol. Although cortisol is more available systemically than aldosterone, it is quickly converted locally in the CCD to cortisone (inactive metabolite) by the 11β-HSD2 enzyme. This prevents overstimulation of MR. In AME, over stimulation of MR results from inactivating mutations of the HSD11B2 gene that make cortisol more available to the MR. In Geller syndrome, activating mutations in the gene NR3C2, which encodes the MR, results in a constitutively active MR and overstimulation of Na + absorption not only by aldosterone but also cortisone and progesterone. In familial glucocorticoid resistance, levels of cortisol are elevated due to glucocorticoid receptor resistance. The elevated cortisol levels then overwhelm the ability of the 11β-HSD2 enzyme to convert it to cortisone. This results in MR activation and excessive Na + absorption. 11HSD2, 11 beta-hydroxysteroid dehydrogenase enzyme type 2; AME, apparent mineralocorticoid excess; CCD, collecting duct; ENaC, epithelial sodium channel; MR, mineralocorticoid receptor; ROMK, renal outer medullary potassium channel.

during pregnancy since progesterone increases substantially during pregnancy. Geller syndrome can manifest at an early age and is accompanied by symptoms of mineralocorticoid excess. Spironolactone, much like progesterone, can stimulate the abnormal mineralocorticoid receptor instead of inhibiting it. Thus, that medication in contraindicated in Geller syndrome.

*Diagnosis*: Laboratory studies typically show normal or low blood K+ along with low renin and aldosterone levels. A clear diagnosis can be made by genetic testing for gene mutations in the mineralocorticoid receptor.

*Treatment*: Therapy includes salt restriction along with thiazide diuretics or an ENaC antagonist. Since paradoxically the mutated form of MR can also be stimulated by spironolactone, MR antagonists are contraindicated. In pregnant patients, delivery of the fetus ameliorates the symptoms.

**Apparent mineralocorticoid excess (AME)** is an autosomal recessive disease caused by inactivating mutation of 11b-hydroxysteroid dehydrogenase type2 enzyme (HSD11B2 gene). 11bHSD2 is expressed in renal tubule cells that have mineralocorticoid receptors and catalyzes conversion of cortisol to cortisone.[23] This conversion is critical to prevent overstimulation of the MR in renal tubule cells by cortisol because cortisone has 100-fold less binding affinity to MRs compared with cortisol. In AME, due to the inactivating mutation in HSD11B2, cortisol is not metabolized resulting in high local cortisol levels with binding to MR and resultant overstimulation of $Na^+$

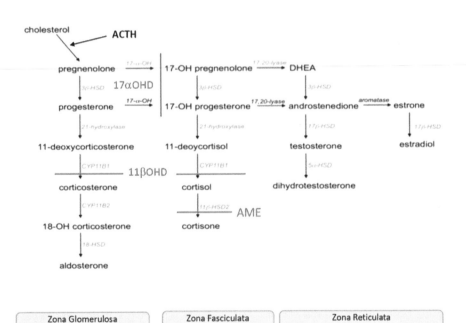

**Fig. 5.** Steroid synthesis pathway and steroid hormone-metabolizing enzymes that catalyze the synthesis or inactivation of the corresponding hormones (11β-OHD, 17α-OHD, AME; 11β-OHD, 11β-hydroxylase deficiency; 17α-OH, 17α-hydroxylase enzyme; 17α-OHD, 17α-hydroxylase deficiency; 11β-HSD2, 11β-hydroxysteroid dehydrogenase type 2; AME, apparent mineralocorticoid excess). (*From* Genes for blood pressure: an opportunity to understand hypertension. Georg B. Ehret and Mark J. Caulfield; Eur Heart J. 2013 Apr 1; 34(13): 951-961.)

reabsorption in the distal nephron. This leads to increased net negativity in the tubule lumen causing increased extrusion of H+ and K+ (see **Fig. 4**).

*Diagnosis:* Besides electrolyte abnormalities of hypokalemia and metabolic alkalosis, those with AME have low renin and low serum aldosterone levels. The hallmark of AME is elevated urinary cortisol to cortisone ratio (THF + 5aTHF to THE) in a 24 hr urine collection. In patients with milder phenotype, the urine steroid profile may be normal requiring genetic testing for a definitive diagnosis. It is important to distinguish AME from acquired suppression of 11b HSD2 caused by chronic licorice ingestion, in which case the symptoms resolve with discontinuation of the offending agent.

*Treatment*: Mineralocorticoid receptor antagonist such as spironolactone or eplerenone are the mainstay of therapy along with sodium restricted diet and potassium supplementation.

### Monogenic Abnormal Adrenal Signaling

Several monogenic causes of disordered adrenal steroid synthesis have been identified as causes of hypertension. **Fig. 5** summarizes steroid synthesis pathways that may be affected to cause hypertension through enhanced sodium retention.

**Congenital Adrenal Hyperplasia (CAH)** encompasses a group of autosomal recessive syndromes caused by defects in cortisol biosynthesis (see **Fig. 5**). Patients with 21hydroxylase deficiency, the most common cause of CAH, usually are not usually hypertensive. 11bβ hydroxylase deficiency (*11β OHD* or CAH type IV) and 17α hydroxylase deficiency (*17α-OHD* or CAH type V) are two subtypes known to cause monogenic hypertension. 11βOHD (CYP11B1) and 17αOHD (CYP17) deficiency both cause accumulation of upstream metabolites, deoxycortisol and deoxycorticosterone. Even though these metabolites have weak MR activity, their accumulation leads to significant MR activity and subsequent hypertension from excess Na $^+$ reabsorption in the distal nephron.[24] Both forms commonly manifest hypertension and hypokalemia.

*Diagnosis*: Like other CAH subtypes, 11OHD and 17OHD deficiency manifest abnormal sexual development. In 11OHD, increased levels of androgens lead to virilization in female infants and precocious puberty in males and females. Patients usually present with hypertension at an early age. 17OHD on the other hand leads to sex hormone deficiency, delayed sexual development and primary amenorrhea in girls and ambiguous genitalia in males. Correct diagnosis relies on clinical presentation and plasma/urine steroid profiles after ACTH stimulation. Genetic diagnosis of both conditions can be made by testing for mutations that either abolish or severely depress enzyme activity.

*Treatment*: Mineralocorticoid receptor antagonists are effective in treating the hypertension and hypokalemia in both conditions. In addition, use of exogenous glucocorticoids normalizes ACTH secretion and ACTH mediated build-up of cortisol precursors proximal to the enzymatic deficiency.

**Primary Aldosteronism (PA)** can result either from an aldosterone producing adenoma or bilateral adrenal hyperplasia.[25] Mutations in the KCNJ5 gene cause about 40% of aldosterone-producing adenomas. It is one of the more common causes of monogenic hypertension. Sporadic forms of hyperaldosteronism are more common than familial forms. In patients with a family history of hypertension who present with hypokalemia, the possibility of genetic causes of primary hyperaldosteronism should be considered. Genetically inherited forms of hyperaldosteronism are outlined below.

**Familial Hyperaldosteronism (FH)** includes a number of autosomal dominant, rare conditions that typically present with early onset hypertension. Four types of FH are known. Differentiating them from sporadic PA based upon biochemical and clinical profile can be challenging, but genetic analysis can be definitive.

*Familial Hyperaldosteronism type 1 (FH-1) or Glucocorticoid Remediable Aldosteronism (GRA):* FH1 or GRA is very rare, accounting for less than 1% of all PA patients. Aldosterone is synthesized by aldosterone synthase in the zona glomerulosa of the adrenal cortex, in normal conditions under control of angiotensin II. Cortisol is produced by 11β-hydroxylase in the zona fasciculata under control of adrenocorticotropic hormone (ACTH). The genes encoding aldosterone synthase and 11β hydroxylase are located adjacent to each other on chromosome 8. FH-1/GRA is caused by a hybrid/chimeric gene resulting from asymmetric crossover on chromosome 8q consisting of the regulatory region of the 11β-hydroxylase gene, CYP11B1, coupled with the structural region of the aldosterone synthase gene, CYP11B2.[26] This hybrid gene thus contains an ACTH-responsive promoter combined with an aldosterone synthase encoding region. The result is ACTH-dependent stimulation of aldosterone production that is independent of regulation by renin, angiotensin, K+ or Na + balance.[26,27] FH-1/GRA patients often present with hypertension early in childhood and may have significant cardiovascular morbidity. Complications can include thoracoabdominal aneurysm and cerebrovascular aneurysm or stroke.[28] Primary aldosteronism patients with significant family history of stoke or aneurysm thus should undergo genetic testing for FH-1/GRA. Patients with proven GRA should undergo vascular screening for aneurysms.

*Diagnosis*: Laboratory testing may show hypokalemia, but only in 50% of affected individuals, and some may display mild metabolic alkalosis. Plasma renin activity is typically suppressed while aldosterone levels are commonly increased. In some patients aldosterone level may be normal and only the aldosterone-to-renin ratio may be elevated. Other diagnostic tools used include a dexamethasone suppression test, urinary steroid profile (with an elevated 18-oxocortisol level), adrenal imaging, and adrenal vein sampling. However, current genetic testing with reported 100% sensitivity and specificity for identifying the FH-1/GRA chimeric gene has effectively eliminated the need for challenging studies to make the diagnosis.

*Treatment*: FH-1/GRA is effectively treated with low-dose glucocorticoid to downregulate ACTH-stimulated mineralocorticoid production.[29] If glucocorticoid administration alone is not sufficient, additional therapy includes an MR antagonist such as spironolactone, which blocks binding of aldosterone to the MR.

*Familial Hyperaldosteronism type 2 (FH-II):* FH-II is another monogenic, autosomal dominant abnormality of adrenal function that causes hypertension. The defect in FH-II appears in some patients to be caused by gain of function mutations of CLCN2 gene that encodes voltage gated chloride channel ClC-2.[30] This leads to increased membrane depolarization in the adrenal zone glomerulosa with resultant upregulation of aldosterone synthase and aldosterone production.[31]

*Diagnosis:* FH-II patients frequently have a family history of bilateral adrenal hyperplasia or adrenal adenoma. In contrast to FH-I/GRA, FH-II patients usually present in adolescence and in adulthood. FH-II is distinguished from FH-I/GRA in that, in contrast to GRA, aldosterone levels are suppressed by dexamethasone challenge in FH-II. Genetic testing for CLCN2 mutations may prove helpful.

*Treatment:* Mineralocorticoid receptor antagonists are the principal therapy, though unilateral adrenalectomy has been used.

*Familial Hyperaldosteronism type 3 (FH-III)* is another autosomal dominant, rare form of monogenic hypertension accounting for approximately 0.3% of PA patients. Pathogenic variants in KCNJ5, which encodes the inwardly rectifying K+ channel Kir3.4 cause FH-III in both familial and sporadic forms of primary hyperaldosteronism. KCNJ5 somatic mutations in the adrenal gland also account for about 40% of aldosterone producing adenomas. The KCNJ5 mutation affects the selectivity of the Kir3.4

pore resulting in membrane depolarization and increased CYP11B2 expression.[32,33] The latter, encoding for aldosterone synthase, then increases aldosterone production.

*Diagnosis*: Patients with FH-III can present with severe hypertension and hypokalemia and be found to have bilateral adrenal hyperplasia. Imaging of the adrenal glands is thus often helpful to make the diagnosis and to exclude development of a mass that requires surgical resection. FH-III mostly presents in adulthood, but on occasion can present in childhood. Genetic testing often provides the diagnosis. However, some are not germline mutations but rather somatic KCNJ5 mutations, and thus only detected in tissue from the adrenal gland.

*Treatment*: Similar to FH-II, medical treatment is with MR antagonists. Depending on the severity of the disease and whether an adrenal mass is found, adrenalectomy may be needed.

**Familial Hyperaldosteronism type 4 (FH-IV)** is a rare form of autosomal dominant FH with unclear prevalence. It is caused by germline mutation in CACNA1H, which encodes a subunit of a calcium channel Cav3.2 that is expressed in the adrenal zona glomerulosa. Gain-of-function mutations in CACNA1H increase calcium influx and increased aldosterone production.[34] The symptoms are comparable to other forms of FH. As in the other forms of familial hyperaldosteronism, genetic testing may be informative to provide specific diagnosis. Medical management is also similar to other FH with MR antagonists as the first line with consideration of adrenalectomy for more severe disease.

**Familial glucocorticoid resistance (GCCR)** is an autosomal dominant disease caused by variants in NR3C1, which encodes the glucocorticoid receptor (GR). Mutations in NR3C1 gene leads to inability of the GR to respond to cortisol, resulting in feedback activation of the hypothalamic-pituitary-adrenal axis with the augmentation of ACTH.[35] The result, then, is impaired suppression of cortisol synthesis. The elevated cortisol levels overwhelm the ability of 11b-HSD2 to convert cortisol to cortisone, thereby leading to MR activation and excessive renal $Na^+$ reabsorption with consequent hypertension (see **Fig. 4**).

*Diagnosis:* Clinical features may include virilization in females and pseudo precocious males, but there is no manifestation of Cushing syndrome due to GR resistance to cortisol. Typical laboratory studies in GCCR are significantly high plasma cortisol and ACTH levels along with high urinary free cortisol. In GCCR the abnormally high levels of cortisol do not decrease after adrenal suppression by dexamethasone.

*Treatment*: The hypertension in the disease is treated with MR antagonists. Dexamethasone is considered to suppress the secretion of ACTH to reduce over-production of mineralocorticoids and androgens.

## SUMMARY

Hypertension in an adolescent in uncommon and deserves evaluation for identifiable causes other than primary hypertension. Usual causes of hypertension found in this age group are most often from an acquired or congenital form of renal disease or a vascular etiology. If no such etiology is found, then exploration for rare causes of hypertension need be pursued, including for monogenic causes of hypertension. Several monogenic etiologies of hypertension are well defined, but are exceedingly rare and thus may not be recognized in a hypertensive adolescent unless considered. A few biochemical screening tests may provide clues toward a potential monogenic etiology of hypertension in such cases. Precise diagnosis of a monogenic cause of hypertension in most cases requires genetic analysis. Identifying a monogenic cause of hypertension is essential in those who have not been found to have more common identifiable causes of hypertension in adolescents, since treatment strategies for these rare conditions are specific and different from antihypertensive regimens for the other more common causes of hypertension in this age group.

## CLINICS CARE POINTS

- Hypertension in adolescents is uncommon and deserves evaluation for underlying etiology including blood tests and imaging to look for causes other than primary hypertension.
- Screening for monogenic hypertension should include serum electrolytes, renin and aldosterone levels.
- Single gene pathogenic mutations leading to increased sodium retention and volume expansion is the primary mechanism for monogenic hypertension.

## AUTHOR CONTRIBUTIONS

All the authors are responsible for the literature review, drafting and revision of the manuscript, and approved the final version of the manuscript.

## CONFLICT OF INTEREST STATEMENT

The authors declare no commercial or financial conflict of interest.

## REFERENCES

1. Clinical Practice Guideline for Screening and Management of High Blood Pressure in Children and Adolescents. Pediatrics 2017;140(3):e20171904. https://doi.org/10.1542/peds.2017-1904.
2. Van Why SK, Sreedharan R. Hypertension. In: Kliegman RM, editor. Nelson pediatric symptom-based diagnosis. 2nd Edition. Philadelphia: Elsevier; 2023. p. 190–202.
3. Van Why SK, Pan CG. Primary Causes of Hypertensive Crisis. Crit Care Clin 2022; 38(2):375–91.
4. Hansson JH, Nelson-Williams C, Suzuki H, et al. Hypertension caused by a truncated epithelial sodium channel gamma subunit: genetic heterogeneity of Liddle syndrome. Nat Genet 1995;11:76–82 [PubMed: 7550319].
5. Soundararajan R, Pearce D, Ziera T. The role of the ENaC-regulatory complex in aldosterone-mediated sodium transport. Mol Cell Endocrinol 2012;350:242–7 [PubMed: 22101317].
6. Shimkets RA, Warnock DG, Bositis CM, et al. Liddle's syndrome: heritable human hypertension caused by mutations in the beta subunit of the epithelial sodium channel. Cell 1994;79:407–14 [PubMed: 7954808].
7. Hiltunen TP, Hannila-Handelberg T, Petäjäniemi N, et al. Liddle's syndrome associated with a point mutation in the extracellular domain of the epithelial sodium channel gamma subunit. J Hypertens 2002;20:2383–90 [PubMed: 12473862].
8. Staub O, Dho S, Henry P, et al. WW domains of Nedd4 bind to the proline-rich PY motifs in the epithelial Na+ channel deleted in Liddle's syndrome. EMBO J 1996; 15:2371–80 [PubMed: 8665844].
9. Knight KK, Olson DR, Zhou R, et al. Liddle's syndrome mutations increase Na+ transport through dual effects on epithelial Na+ channel surface expression and proteolytic cleavage. Proc Natl Acad Sci U S A 2006;103:2805–8 [PubMed: 16477034].

10. Kellenberger S, Gautschi I, Rossier BC, et al. Mutations causing Liddle syndrome reduce sodium-dependent downregulation of the epithelial sodium channel in the Xenopus oocyte expression system. J Clin Invest 1998;101:2741–50 [PubMed: 9637708].

11. Anantharam A, Tian Y, Palmer LG. Open probability of the epithelial sodium channel is regulated by intracellular sodium. J Physiol 2006;574:333–47 [PubMed: 16690707].

12. Warnock DG. Liddle syndrome: an autosomal dominant form of human hypertension. Kidney Int 1998;53:18–24 [PubMed: 9452995].

13. Vehaskari VM. Heritable forms of hypertension. Pediatr Nephrol 2009;24:1929–37 [PubMed: 17647025].

14. Fan P, Zhang D, Pan XC, et al. Premature Stroke Secondary to Severe Hypertension Results from Liddle Syndrome Caused by a Novel SCNN1B Mutation. Kidney Blood Press Res 2020;45:603–11 [PubMed: 32698182].

15. O'Shaughnessy KM. Gordon Syndrome: a continuing story. Pediatr Nephrol 2015; 30:1903–8 [PubMed: 25503323].

16. Wilson FH, Disse-Nicodème S, Choate KA, et al. Human hypertension caused by mutations in WNK kinases. Science 2001;293:1107–12.

17. Xu BE, Stippec S, Chu PY, et al. WNK1 activates SGK1 to regulate the epithelial sodium channel. Proc Natl Acad Sci U S A 2005;102:10315–20 [PubMed: 16006511].

18. Kahle KT, Wilson FH, Leng Q, et al. WNK4 regulates the balance between renal NaCl reabsorption and K+ secretion. Nat Genet 2003;35:372–6 [PubMed: 14608358].

19. Boyden LM, Choi M, Choate KA, et al. Mutations in kelch-like 3 and cullin 3 cause hypertension and electrolyte abnormalities. Nature 2012;482:98–102 [PubMed: 22266938].

20. Gordon RD. Syndrome of hypertension and hyperkalemia with normal glomerular filtration rate. Hypertension 1986;8:93–102.

21. Gordon RD, Hodsman GP. The syndrome of hypertension and hyperkalaemia without renal failure: long term correction by thiazide diuretic. Scott Med J 1986;31:43–4 [PubMed: 3961473].

22. Geller DS, Farhi A, Pinkerton N, et al. Activating mineralocorticoid receptor mutation in hypertension exacerbated by pregnancy. Science 2000;289:119–23.

23. Gomez-Sanchez EP, Gomez-Sanchez CE. 11beta-hydroxysteroid dehydrogenases: a growing multi-tasking family. Mol Cell Endocrinol 2021;526:111210.

24. Peterson RE, Imperato-McGinley J, Gautier T, et al. Male pseudohermaphroditism due to multiple defects in steroid-biosynthetic microsomal mixed-function oxidases. A new variant of congenital adrenal hyperplasia. N Engl J Med 1985; 313:1182–91.

25. Zennaro MC, Boulkroun S, Fernandes-Rosa FL. Pathogenesis and treatment of primary aldosteronism. Nat Rev Endocrinol 2020;16:578–89 [PMID: 32724183].

26. Lifton RP, Dluhy RG, Powers M, et al. A chimaeric 11 beta-hydroxylase/aldosterone synthase gene causes glucocorticoid-remediable aldosteronism and human hypertension. Nature 1992;355:262–5 [PMID: 1731223].

27. Pascoe L, Curnow KM, Slutsker L, et al. Glucocorticoid-suppressible hyperaldosteronism results from hybrid genes created by unequal crossovers between CYP11B1 and CYP11B2. Proc Natl Acad Sci U S A 1992;89:8327–31 [ PMID: 1518866].

28. Al Romhain B, Young AM, Battacharya JJ, et al. Intracranial aneurysm in a patient with glucocorticoid-remediable aldosteronism. Br J Neurosurg 2015;29:715–7.

29. Stowasser M, Bachmann AW, Huggard PR, et al. Treatment of familial hyperaldosteronism type I: only partial suppression of adrenocorticotropin required to correct hypertension. J Clin Endocrinol Metab 2000;85:3313–8.
30. Scholl UI, Stölting G, Schewe J, et al. CLCN2 chloride channel mutations in familial hyperaldosteronism type II. Nat Genet 2018;50:349–54.
31. Stowasser M, Wolley M, Wu A, et al. Pathogenesis of Familial Hyperaldosteronism Type II: New Concepts Involving Anion Channels. Curr Hypertens Rep 2019;21: 31 [PMID: 30949771].
32. Choi M, Scholl UI, Yue P, et al. K+ channel mutations in adrenal aldosterone-producing adenomas and hereditary hypertension. Science 2011;331:768–72.
33. Monticone S, Hattangady NG, Nishimoto K, et al. Effect of KCNJ5 mutations on gene expression in aldosterone-producing adenomas and adrenocortical cells. J Clin Endocrinol Metab 2012;97. E1567–72 [PMID: 22628608].
34. Daniil G, Fernandes-Rosa FL, Chemin J, et al. CACNA1H Mutations Are Associated With Different Forms of Primary Aldosteronism. EBioMedicine 2016;13: 225–36.
35. Hurley DM, Accili D, Stratakis CA, et al. Point mutation causing a single amino acid substitution in the hormone binding domain of the glucocorticoid receptor in familial glucocorticoid resistance. J Clin Invest 1991;87:680–6.

# Adolescent Onset of Muscle Weakness

Meghan K. Konda, MD*, Matthew Harmelink, MD

## KEYWORDS

- Peripheral neurology • Neuropathy • Weakness • Muscle

## KEY POINTS

- Localization to categories of peripheral causes of muscle disease can be done relatively quickly and easily.
- Periclinical testing (laboratory, imaging, electrodiagnostic) can help further define the etiology.
- By defining the underlying etiology, referrals can be directed by urgency as well as to the appropriate specialist.
- Creatine kinase can be a helpful marker between the various diseases but as there are frequent exceptions, a normal creatine kinase cannot rule out muscle disease.

## INTRODUCTION

Adolescent onset of muscle weakness can be due to various causes including the central nervous system, non-neurologic systemic (ex. cardiac failure) and psychogenic causes. Thus, this article will focus on the peripheral etiologies of adolescent-onset muscle weakness. However, even with this narrowing, there are hundreds of potential disorders. Many of these have remarkably similar examination features which require paraclinical testing to confirm.

Additionally, for genetic causes, pathophysiology often starts before the clinical symptoms may become apparent. As such, the approach to adolescent patients should simultaneously exclude non-neuromuscular causes while evaluating neuromuscular etiologies. The inclusion of paraclinical testing: histopathology, electrophysiology, and even laboratory testing including a detailed physical examination, can often detect these subtle differences. Additionally, early symptoms traditionally thought to be adult diseases are now being diagnosed more frequently in adolescence with genetic testing being more readily available.

Department of Neurology, Section of Child Neurology, Medical College of Wisconsin, 9000 West Wisconsin Avenue CCC 540, Milwaukee, WI 53226, USA
* Corresponding author.
E-mail address: Mkonda@mcw.edu

Med Clin N Am 108 (2024) 173–187
https://doi.org/10.1016/j.mcna.2023.06.015
0025-7125/24/© 2023 Elsevier Inc. All rights reserved.

medical.theclinics.com

As such, this article will not be able to provide a comprehensive discussion but rather an introductory guide on the recognition and diagnosis of these diseases with further research. The goal will be to discuss common presentations of the classes of diseases and initial evaluations. Regarding treatments, there has been an explosion of treatments in research and in the clinics so this area will be avoided as well though the reader is advised to look up contemporary data as new treatments are arising frequently.

Finally, there will not be a discussion of any of the toxic, metabolic, systemic, and/or infectious causes of weakness as many of these are not specific to the adolescent age population.

A table to assist with the diagnosis and management of Neuromuscular emergencies is also provided here for reference (**Table 1**).

## DISCUSSION

The evaluation of muscle weakness onset in teenagers can be approached by various methods. Additionally, muscle weakness can be a primary muscle disease or can be secondary to connective tissue, neuromuscular junction, or nerve diseases (**Fig. 1**).

The best way to evaluate is to simultaneously review the timeline, course, and localization of symptoms. Practically speaking, obtaining the time-course is often the best initial step to frame the discussion followed by course (static, variable, progressive, improving). Finally, while historical information can help with localization, the neurologic examination is essential to helping define the disease.

Of note, one easy question to differentiate is to determine if there are any sensory phenomenon as pure motor diseases (myopathies, myotonias, dystrophies, neuromuscular junction disorders (NMJ), and motor nerve diseases) will have normal sensorium. Finally, screening for central nervous system disease involvement and systemic signs and symptoms can also help determine if the disease is mixed which will significantly differentiate the disease process as well. **Table 2** summarizes some of these features.

Additionally, further differentiation then between episodic weakness disorders and those which are static or progressive can further assist delineation. Obtaining laboratory testing such as serum creatine kinase can help differentiate between myopathic and dystrophic disorders. At that level of evaluation, an expert neuromuscular physician should be involved given the broad phenotypic overlaps and the need for interpreting variant results in the patient's context. An initial flow diagram can be seen in **Fig. 2**.

Later in discussion discussions of these categories will be discussed further.

### Neuropathies

#### Genetic neuropathies
Genetic neuropathies can show presenting symptoms at any age group largely based on the exact gene involved. The most common sub-set of sensorimotor polyneuropathies is often called Charcot-Marie-Tooth Diseases (CMT). This category is then further subdivided based on its inheritance (axonal, demyelinating, X-linked). While the physical examination cannot reliably determine the sub-type in every case, a family history often with mildly affected women and more severe men/boys is suggestive of X-linked CMT.[1] Overall, there are over 300 genes known to cause CMT. Electrodiagnostic testing is recommended as first-line testing in any patient clinically suspected of having genetic neuropathy. This helps confirm the diagnosis as well as the sub-type. Four genes: MP22, GJB1, MPZ and MFN2 make up 90% of all CMT.[2] Thus, directed testing can be done first prior to expanding to broad panels.

**Table 1**
Peripheral neuromuscular emergencies with presentation, diagnosis and management

| Emergencies | Presentation | Diagnosis | Management |
|---|---|---|---|
| Myasthenic Crisis | Oculobulbar weakness with ptosis, diplopia, and ophthalmoplegia, progressive respiratory failure | Serum antibodies, cold pack test on eyes, Forced Vital Capacity <60% | Respiratory support, IVIG/plasmapheresis |
| Malignant hyperthermia | Tachycardia, Supraventricular arrhythmia, masseter spasm and generalized stiffness | Temperature increases 1 degree Celsius per 15 min and muscle rigidity | Remove offending agents, respiratory support, dantrolene 2-10 mg/kg |
| AIDP | Acute ascending sensorimotor weakness over days with decreased FVC, +/− ataxia and ophthalmoplegia | Cerebral Spinal Fluid showing albuminocytologic dissociation, areflexia, lumbar MRI cauda equina enhancement. | Respiratory support and IVIG/plasmapheresis |
| Tick Paralysis | Viral prodrome followed by symmetric ascending weakness and paralysis. Travel or living in Northwestern USA. Bulbar and facial nerve involvement | Find the tick | Remove the tick and respiratory support |
| Rhabdomyolysis | Weakness, severe muscle pain, dark urine, and encephalopathy | Hyperkalemia, myoglobinuria, abnormal phosphate, and electrolytes | Fluids and pain relief. If due to snake bite then anti-venom and possible surgical debridement |
| Periodic Paralysis | Acute onset proximal limb weakness and hyporeflexia and trouble taking breaths | Potassium level and thyroid level. | Respiratory support Potassium normalizing therapy and observe |

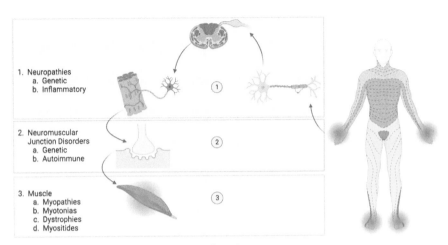

1. Neuropathies
   a. Genetic
   b. Inflammatory

2. Neuromuscular
   Junction Disorders
   a. Genetic
   b. Autoimmune

3. Muscle
   a. Myopathies
   b. Myotonias
   c. Dystrophies
   d. Myositides

**Fig. 1.** Localization of peripheral causes of weakness.

Adolescents will present with foot deformities, numbness/tingling in the feet as well as distal weakness. The physical examination may reveal extremity muscle weakness as well as the classic pes planus or pes cavus deformities, sensory ataxia, decreased deep tendon reflexes, distal muscle atrophy, and decreased sensation in the extremities.

As with many diseases, while most CMT's are length-dependent, there are variations of different patterns including those which may be upper extremity predominant.[3,4] For this reason, atypical neuropathy presentations should have a broad differential of both the autoimmune, toxic, and genetic etiologies. Additionally, there are pure motor and pure sensory sub-types as well (Hereditary Motor and Hereditary Sensory Neuropathy, respectively).

The current management of CMT is supportive care including appropriate bracing and surgical correction of foot deformities by a skilled multi-disciplinary center.[5]

Of the genetic neuropathies, a special note should be made toward 5q SMA type 3 or type 4 patients. In this disease, for which the infantile form is more well known, a small sub-set can present at a later age. Unlike most CMT diseases, these patients will present with pure motor proximal predominant weakness and commonly areflexia. It is important to differentiate 5q SMA from other motor neuropathies due to the development of multiple FDA-approved genetic modifying therapies that are effective in treatment. Given that these diseases do cause irreversible motor neuron disease, the earlier treatment is better. Most states in the US now screen for 5q SMA as part of their newborn screening so the incidence of undiagnosed adolescents will decrease significantly going forward.[6]

Juvenile amyotrophic lateral sclerosis (ALS) should also be identified early. A genetic predisposition is more often uncovered in juvenile ALS compared to the adult manifestation of the disease. Additionally, while the life-expectancy of an adult diagnosed with ALS averages 2 to 3 years, the prognosis for juvenile ALS can vary wildly from a more aggressive disease to a much milder form.[7] Current research is devoted to discovering treatments for some of the genetic forms while the standard of supportive care remains in the hands of multidisciplinary centers skilled with motor neuron diseases.

### Inflammatory neuropathies

There are various inflammatory neuropathies, many of which can be associated with systemic inflammation and thus will not be covered here. The primary inflammatory

**Table 2**
**Adolescent Weakness Overview with Examples and Typical Clinical Features**

| Category | Name | Inheritance | Weakness Distribution | Weakness Duration | Pain/Parenthesias | Key Associated Symptoms | Key Exam Findings | CK | Diagnostic Testing | Treatment |
|---|---|---|---|---|---|---|---|---|---|---|
| Neuropathy | Charcot-Marie-Tooth diseases | AR, DR, or X-linked | Symmetric, Distal | Slowly Progressive (Months to years) | Pain, numbness, and tingling distally | Foot deformities, high thin calves muscle atrophy of the feet | Sensory ataxia, decreased DTR, atrophy of extremities | Normal | EMG to differentiate sub-type then CMT genetic testing | Supportive care |
| Neuropathy | SMA 5q Type 3 | AR | Trunk, shoulder, Pelvic girdle Symmetric | Slowly Progressive (Months to years) | None | Pulmonary and bulbar weakness in some patients, difficulty climbing stairs | Hyporeflexia or Areflexia, predominant proximal weakness | Normal | Genetic Testing for SMN1 genetic changes | Disease modifying therapies exist but timeliness is important to treat |
| Neuropathy-inflammatory | Acute demyelinating polyradiculopathy (AIDP) | Acquired Autoimmune | Distal onset ascending Symmetric | Progressive over hours to days | Often in distal extremities | Previous illness 2 wk preceding, followed by difficult ambulation and weak grip, can develop respiratory failure | Hyporeflexia, decreased strength distal > proximal. May have bulbar signs, orphthalmoplegia, and decreased FVC% | Normal | CSF cell count and analysis showing Albuminocytologic dissociation. MRI with lumbosacral root enhancement | IVIG initially with consideration for plasmapheresis for severe cases |
| Neuropathy-inflammatory | Chronic demyelinating poly-radiculopathy (CIDP) | Acquired Autoimmune | Distal onset with some proximal weakness Symmetric | Slowly progressive for weeks to months | Less common than AIDP | Prolonged or worsening AIDP course. History of AIDP | Hyporeflexia or areflexia, strength decreased distal > proximal. | Normal | EMG showing conduction block and delayed peak latencies in motor ± sensory distribution, antibody panel, and CSF cell count and analysis | Steroids, IVIG as well as steroid sparing immuno-suppression |
| NMJ disorder-post-synaptic | Congenital Myasthenia gravis syndrome | AD and AR | Proximal weakness, ocular, bulbar and respiratory | Fluctuating worsening after activity may have fixed baseline weakness Often long-standing months to years | None | Ptosis, diplopia, neck and extremity weakness worse with exertion | Fatigable weakness in the strength testing | Normal | EMG/NCS with Repetitive nerve stimulation or single fiber EMG Genetic Testing to confirm subtype | Various by subtype Ex-Pyridostigmine, fluoxetine, liquid albuterol |
| NMJ disorder-post-synaptic | Autoimmune Myasthenia gravis syndrome | Acquired Autoimmune | Proximal, distal, facial Symmetric | Often days to months of symptoms, may be progressive since onset | None | Ptosis, diplopia, neck and extremity weakness worse with exertion | Fatigable weakness in the strength testing | Normal | EMG/NCS with Repetitive nerve stimulation or single fiber EMG Antibody Testing | Pyridostimine, steriods, autoimmune therapies, IVIG, remove offending agent, and supportive therapy. |

(continued on next page)

**Table 2**
*(continued)*

| Category | Name | Inheritance | Weakness Distribution | Weakness Duration | Pain/Parenthesias | Key Associated Symptoms | Key Exam Findings | CK | Diagnostic Testing | Treatment |
|---|---|---|---|---|---|---|---|---|---|---|
| Myopathy | CPT II deficiency and other carnitine deficiency/transport disorders | Autosomal Recessive | Proximal/ Generalized Symmetric | May have mild fixed weakness often with intermittent rhabdomyolysis | Cramping or pain after activity or triggers | Cardiomyopathy/ arrhythmias, seizures, exercise intolerance, muscle cramps with exertion, fatigue Triggers: illness, overheating, exertion, high fat meals, dehydration, and hunger/ fasting | Hepatomegaly, generalized weakness, normal strength, normal Neuro exam | ++ with rhabdomyolysis Nml/+ at baseline | EMG, EKG, and muscle biopsy | Low fat and high carbohydrate diet, triheptanoin, bezafibrate, and trigger avoidance |
| Myopathy | RYR1 | AD and AR | Proximal, Symmetric Or None | Variable course | None | Risk of malignant hyperthermia with heat or anesthesia +/- history of delayed motor development and slowly progressive weakness | Appendicular hypotonia and weakness, scapular winging, short stature, pes cavus, dysmorphisms, ptosis, strabismus | Normal To Mildly Elevated | EMG, muscle biopsy, and CK Genetic testing to confirm | Supportive care, avoid volatile anesthetics |
| Myopathy - metabolic | Pompe disease- Adolescent Onset | Autosomal Recessive | Proximal | Slowly progressive | Exercise Myalgias | May have early respiratory symptoms | Proximal Weakness worse in Hips, intact reflexes and sensation | Elevated when symptomatic | Creatine Kinase, Genetic Testing with/without enzyme activity | For symptomatic patients can consider enzyme replacement therapy |
| Myopathy - metabolic | McArdle disease | Autosomal Recessive | Typically no weakness as adolescence but can developed slowly progressive (over years) | None to slowly progressive | Exercise Myalgias | "Second wind" effect following exertion. Illness, cold temperatures, and exercise exacerbate weakness. | Normal | Elevated at Baseline | Creatine Kinase, Genetic Testing | Dietary and exercise modifications |
| Myotonia | Myotonic Dystrophy Type 1 | Autosomal Dominant | Distal Weakness | Slowly Progressive (months to years) | Myotonic Cramping Pains in hands and feet | Cardiac Arrythmias, Endocrine Abnormalities, Cognitive Impairments, Myotonia | As adolescents may have myotonia (not all mild cases will), distal weakness | Normal to Mild Elevations | EMG/NCS and Creatine Kinase with Genetic Testing being definitive | No overt treatment, medications for cramping and endocrine/cardiac disease |
| Myotonia | Myotonia Congenita | AD (Becker) and AR (Thomsen) | None to mild fixed proximal weakness | None | Myalgias and myotonia | None but some weakness with short exercise | Muscle hypertrophy, percussion myotonia | Normal to Mild Elevations | EMG/NCS and Creatine Kinase with Genetic Testing being definitive | Treatment of Cramping |

| Category | Disease | Inheritance | Weakness Pattern | Progression | Myalgias | Associated Symptoms | Exam Findings | CK Level | Diagnostic Testing | Treatment |
|---|---|---|---|---|---|---|---|---|---|---|
| Myotonia | Paramyotonia Congenita | Autosomal Dominant | Episodic exercise induced weakness as well as with cold lasting minutes to days | Fixed, non-progressive | Myalgias | Some patients with cardiac arrythmias | May not have myotonia at normal temperatures but arises when cooled | Mildly high | EMG/NCS and Creatine Kinase with Genetic Testing being definitive | Symptomatic Treatment |
| Myotonia | Myotonia Fluctuans and Permanens | Autosomal Dominant | No overt weakness but often stiffness or cramping | None | Myalgias | None | Myotonia without over weakness Not temperature affected | Elevated | EMG/NCS and Creatine Kinase with Genetic Testing being definitive | Symptomatic Treatment |
| Periodic Paralysis | Periodic Paralysis | Autosomal Dominant | Rarely Mild fixed weakness but with episodes of severe weakness lasting minutes to days | Typically not progressive but may have mild weakness develop over years | None | May have cardiac arrythmias in some sub-types | Normal exam between episodes with weakness during events | Normal | EMG/NCS will be normal between episodes but abnormal during an episode Genetic Testing | Modifying potassium can help as well as new disease genetic treatments are becoming available |
| Dystrophy | Becker | X-linked | Variable from mild proximal weakness to no weakness in adolescence | Slowly progressive over years, affects hip girdle before shoulder girdle | Myalgias with activities | Some patients with cognitive delays or autism, cardiac failure | Slowly progressive proximal weakness with calf hypertrophy | Very elevated (typically in the 1000s to >10,000 IU/ml) | Creatine Kinase and genetic testing | No overt treatments for this mild form though therapies are being researched |
| Dystrophy | Emery Dreifuss | Dominant, Recessive or X-Linked | Humeroperoneal Weakness | Progressive over years | None | Cardiac arrythmias can be severe | Humeroperoneal Weakness with frequent elbow contractures | Mildly elevated to 10x normal | Creatine Kinase and genetic testing | No overt treatment but supportive care and cardiac monitoring |
| Dystrophy | Limb Girdle Dystrophy | Dominant, Recessive or X-Linked | Proximal Symmetrical is typical but can be distal predominant forms | Progressive over years | None | Depending upon subtype can have cognitive, cardiac and other organs involved | Proximal Symmetrical is typical but can be distal predominant forms Calf atrophy or hypertrophy in some forms | Moderately to severely elevated | Creatine Kinase and genetic testing Muscle biopsy in rare cases | No overt treatments though multiple clinical trials for genetic modifying therapies are currently underway |
| Myositis | Dermatomyositis | Acquired Autoimmune | Proximal Symmetrical | Days to Weeks | Myalgias but rare | Heliotropic and extensor surface rash, Gotton's Papules, photosensitive skin | Proximal Weakness with rashes | Normal to elevated | Creatine Kinase, Muscle Biopsy and Muscle MRI | Corticosteroids, IVIG, Methotrexate |
| Myositis | Primary Polymyositis | Acquired Autoimmune | Proximal Symmetrical | Days to Weeks | Myalgias but rare | Rare extra-muscular symptoms | Proximal Weakness | Normal to elevated | Creatine Kinase, Muscle Biopsy and Muscle MRI | Corticosteroids, IVIG, Methotrexate |

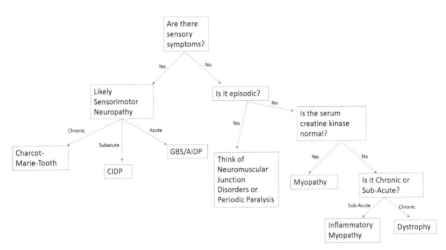

**Fig. 2.** Overview of diagnostic approach to an adolescent with weakness from peripheral causes.

neuropathies (such as multifocal motor neuropathy), outside of Guillain-Barre Syndrome (GBS) are rare in adolescence. The most common forms of inflammatory neuropathy in adolescence are the various sub-groups of GBS. Acute inflammatory demyelinating polyradiculoneuropathy (AIDP), the most common sub-type follows the classic pattern of acute ascending weakness with sensory phenomenon and hyporeflexia/areflexia. In this disease, antibodies attack the myelin of the predominantly proximal sensorimotor nerves resulting in the classic ascending length-dependent weakness. In many of these cases, early treatment with intravenous immunoglobulin (IVIG) can slow or halt the rate of demyelination, functional decline, and hasten recovery; IVIG has been shown to be more effective than plasmapheresis in treatment while corticosteroids remain ineffective.[8,9] While respiratory and bulbar failure are common in the classic AIDP, other variants such as ataxia, ophthalmoplegia, and facial weakness can be associated with other antibodies.

A chronic form of the AIDP, chronic inflammatory demyelinating polyradiculoneuropathy (CIDP), will typically have a slower onset of weeks to months, and is less likely to have respiratory features. In this set of diseases, corticosteroids are not contraindicated as they are with AIDP. However, given the chronic nature, transitioning to a steroid-sparing agent is important to prevent the adverse effects of long-term steroid treatment. Patients will often present with worsening or persistent weakness and areflexia in a sub-acute to chronic setting (>3 weeks).

In both the AIDP and CIDP variants, a lumbar puncture can demonstrate albuminocytologic dissociation while the lumbar MRI can demonstrate nerve root enchancement.[10] Electrodiagnostic testing can be helpful in the sub-acute phase if concerned for CIDP. However, the diagnosis of AIDP is often made clinically.

### Neuromuscular Junction Disorders

Moving distally from the nerves, diseases of the neuromuscular junction often present with episodic or fluctuating weakness. This makes the evaluation difficult as, unless the patient is examined during an episode, their examination may be normal. The patient often presents with worsening weakness after activity that improves with rest. Given the warmer temperature of the core, more proximal muscles tend to be affected.

On examination, using prolonged maneuvers such as holding upward gaze for 1 minute has been shown to demonstrate weakness in patients with myasthenia gravis.[11]

### Genetic neuromuscular junction disorders

Genetic neuromuscular junction diseases, called congenital myasthenia gravis, are less likely to present in adolescence. These diseases are due to mutations in the junction and often have presentations of mild fixed weakness with significant fluctuations though some rare patients can present with normal development prior to a flair.[12] These patients do not have positive antibody testing and do not necessarily respond to immunotherapy due to the genetic nature of the disease. Nevertheless, pyridostigmine among other medications can help patients depending on their genetic variant.

### Acquired neuromuscular junction disorders

While most people think acquired myasthenia gravis is a chronic autoimmune disease, which is mostly true, there are some rare exposures which can lead to a transient phenomenon. This is an ever-expanding list but should be verified when considering an acquired neuromuscular junction disorder in the differential diagnosis.[13]

Patients that have no offending agent, as is with most cases, will present with variable weakness, sometimes in addition to an acquired fixed weakness. Weakness tends to be proximal and may affect bulbar, ocular, and respiratory functioning as well. The hallmark feature of NMJ disorders on the examination is the fatigability of the muscle. For example, having a patient lookup for 1 minute can result in worsening ptosis when asked to return to a neutral gaze.[12]

When this disease is suspected, sending antibody testing and considering prescribing acute therapies is warranted when this disease is suspected. The traditional antibodies considered are also expanding, so consulting with a local neuromuscular physician and/or testing lab is desirable in order to be succinct in testing. While the sensitivity is reported to be 85% to 90% in myasthenia gravis, negative testing should not be used to exclude this disease.[14] In those patients, electrodiagnostic testing is helpful to confirm the diagnosis.

Pyridostigmine, an acetylcholinesterase inhibitor, can temporarily improve strength but considering underlying disease treatment is also appropriate. Initiation with corticosteroids is often the first step in management during the diagnostic evaluation while testing is pending. Be aware that there can be some mild worsening with corticosteroids in the first few weeks after initiation and so should not be administered to a tenuous patient. Rather, in acute or refractory cases, the use of intravenous immunoglobulins (IVIG) is reasonable while initiation with a longer-acting steroid-sparing agent is being considered.[15]

Finally, in the adult population there is literature to support thymectomy. In children, there is not strong evidence, but post-pubescent presentations are likely to have similar physiology to adults and can be considered in that group. Regardless, for generalized myasthenia gravis, imaging of the thymus is warranted at diagnosis and periodically after to watch for a thymoma.[15]

### Primary Muscle Diseases

#### Myopathies

**Genetic myopathies.** The myopathies are a diverse group of diseases that mostly affect muscles. Myopathies can frequently initially present in the adolescent age group given they are often static. However, patients with milder myopathies can have long-standing symptoms but only present for medical care as an adolescent when their growth increases and/or functional level (eg, ability to play sports) compared to their peers widens.

We will note that there is a sub-group of myopathies which have baseline normal strength but have an increased risk of rhabdomyolysis when placed under heightened metabolic demands. This sub-group is often comprised of patients with an underlying genetic metabolic disease.

One of the more common diseases is Carnitine palmitoyltransferase II (CPT II) deficiency (myopathic form). While the infantile form often presents with a severe phenotype of seizures, hypotonia, and developmental delay, the myopathic form often has normal baseline creatine kinase levels, mild weakness to normal strength but recurrent episodes of rhabdomyolysis. Treatment consists of staying hydrated, decreasing heat exposure, increasing carbohydrate intake, reducing fat intake, and considering supplementing with triheptanoin.[16]

Another group of common muscle diseases is RYR1-related myopathies. This group has a broad spectrum of disease onset and severity which ranges from neonatal hypotonia to normal strength with increased malignant hyperthermia risk due to volatile anesthetics. These patients also often have normal creatine kinase, a very mild to normal examination but have an increased risk of rhabdomyolysis and/or malignant hyperthermia. As such, their evaluation can be difficult and any patient who has recurrent rhabdomyolysis with or without underlying neuromuscular symptoms should be evaluated for an underlying myopathy etiology that increases their risk for future episodes of rhabdomyolysis or malignant hyperthermia.[17]

Pompe's disease is a glycogen storage disease defined by an alpha-glucosidase deficiency and has 2 very different phenotypes. The infantile form has features of cardiac failure and hypotonia at or shortly after birth. The late-onset form can present with mild proximal weakness and early respiratory symptoms with a slow decline. In these cases, creatine kinase may be normal pre-symptomatically but will often rise during the onset of symptoms. Additionally, there are now enzyme replacement therapies which can slow the progression of symptomatic patients.[18] Therefore, early recognition can be beneficial.

McArdle's disease can present in this age group as episodic rhabdomyolysis with or without baseline weakness. In this disease, due to a glycogen phosphorylase deficiency, patients can present with exercise intolerance, the classic second-wind phenomenon, and often present with periodic exertional rhabdomyolysis.[19] What differentiates this disease from others, however, is baseline creatine kinase is elevated in patients with McArdle's disease.

**Myotonias.** Myotonic diseases are by nature an interesting group of disorders. Adolescents may initially present with the typical cramping symptoms. Myotonias are defined by delayed skeletal muscle relaxation exacerbated by voluntary movement. While myotonic dystrophy type I is the most common disease, patients can present with other sub-types. Unlike myotonic dystrophy which is a multi-organ disease secondary to DMPK trinucleotide repeat expansions, the other myotonic diseases are often due to ion channelopathy disorders.

In myotonic disorders, the type of cramping can vary by the type of channel affected. For example, sodium channelopathies have earlier onset, get worse with repetitive exercise, have marked muscle pain, and have facial stiffness/myotonia.

Myotonic Dystrophy, type 1 has anticipation in inheritance. This is the most prevalent neuromuscular disease in adults but can present in adolescence. Juvenile disease is characterized by facial weakness without ophthalmoplegia, cognitive delay, percussion myotonia, and cardiac conduction defects. Facial weakness can include dysphagia, ptosis, hatchet face, and temporal wasting. Patients, or their older family members, may also have cataracts, ptosis, hypogonadism, hypoventilation, and OSA or sleep hypoventilation. Patients will have normal to mildly elevated creatine kinases levels but can have endocrine abnormalities (low testosterone, type 1 diabetes and/or thyroid abnormalities). Their pattern of weakness is typically distal predominant though proximal muscles may also be involved as the patient ages.

Myotonia congenita is divided into either dominant or recessive forms. The dominant form, Thomsen myotonia congenita, is mild whereas the recessive form, Becker myotonia congenita, is more severe. The age of onset for both is between infancy and adulthood. Common features are mild myotonia that decreases with repeated activity (warm up phenomenon), muscle hypertrophy, distal weakness with exercise, and functional proximal weakness (climbing stairs and getting up from seated positions). Given this, patients often have been reported as "lazy" throughout their childhood.

The clinical examination demonstrates patients who appear very muscular and often are described as looking like "bodybuilders" in childhood. Definitive diagnosis is made through genetic testing of the CLCN1 gene. Although there are no curative treatments, symptomatic treatment with drugs such as carbamazepine, mexiletine, and lamotrigine may reduce muscle cramping.

Paramyotonia is another disease caused by autosomal dominant sodium or chloride channel variants. The initial presentation may be similar to myotonia congenita. However, patients with paramyotonia have worsening myotonia with activity (paradoxic myotonia) and with cold exposure. Patients may report that when they eat cold foods or drink cold beverages their weakness worsens.

**Myotonia fluctuans and myotonia permanens.** These diseases are both caused by autosomal dominant mutations in the SCN4A sodium channel gene. In myotonia fluctuans, AD missense mutation of SCN4$\alpha$ decreases inactivation of the channel. While there is no baseline weakness, patients experience myotonia minutes to an hour after exercise or after eating high-potassium foods.

This is contrary to myotonia permanens in which the problems with the SCN4A gene results in a decreased electrical threshold of the channel. In these patients, their myotonia is constant and severe leading to possible muscle hypertrophy on physical examination. Their symptoms are also worsened with activity and potassium-rich foods.

**Periodic paralysis.** The periodic paralysis diseases are similar to the myotonic diseases in that channels are effected. However, whereas myotonic disorders are a result of a lack of ability to inactivate the channel, the periodic paralysis diseases are due to impaired channel function.

These diseases can be sub-classified based upon their relative potassium levels during attacks. The overall incidence of these combined diseases is about 1 in 1,000,000 for both hypokalemic (CACNA1S mutation) and hyperkalemic (SCN4A mutation) periodic paralysis and 1 in 1,000,000 for Anderson-Tawil syndrome (KCNJ2 mutation).

In this group of diseases, patients often have no weakness or abnormalities at baseline between the episodes but during a spell will have proximal predominant weakness. This weakness can vary from mild symptoms to being fully paralyzed. Often, the respiratory muscles are not affected. Spells can be spontaneous but also can be provoked by illness, carbohydrate-dense meals, activity, or cold exposures. Individuals are also at increased risk of malignant hyperthermia and may have difficulty regaining strength after surgeries requiring general anesthesia.

There is no curative treatment, but identification can guide them to find appropriate diet and activity modifications which can help prevent further spells. Additionally, depending upon the genotype, there are some symptom-based treatments beyond potassium management such dichlorphenamide and acetazolamide.

For both the periodic paralysis and non-dystrophic myotonias, there is a very nice in-depth review by Stunnenberg and colleagues.[20]

**Dystrophies.** Muscular dystrophies are a varied group of diseases which are often associated with progressive weakness due to ongoing damage and poor regrowth of skeletal muscle. Genetic dystrophies are associated with wide variations of gene mutations and phenotypes depending on the genetic variant.

Historically, dystrophinopathy was divided into Duchenne's and Becker's phenotypes. As new drugs are developed to modulate the course of this disease, there will be patients who would have been previously more severe but now have milder symptoms in adolescence. Here we will focus on the undiagnosed patients. Those with a prior diagnosis on genetic modifying therapies are likely already in a specialized center.

X-linked dystrophies can present in adolescence if they have milder variations. These patients may have mild proximal muscle weakness, cramping after activity, and possibly severe myositis. The importance in the diagnosis is not only for understanding and modifying exercise, but also for future family planning and more importantly to monitor for the cardiac and pulmonary effects that go along with this disease. Of note, because dystrophin is globally expressed, x-linked dystrophies can be associated with ADHD, compulsive type behaviors, and anxiety.

On examination, patients will have proximal muscle weakness typically in the hips before they start developing in the shoulders and will describe a slow progressive nature of their symptoms over months and years. Women may be asymptomatic carriers for the disease due to x-linked inactivation. Unlike their male counterparts who tend to have elevated creatine kinase levels, women who are affected may not. Female patients may have early heart disease, intellectual disabilities and/or the muscle symptoms as dictated by the amount of in-active to active X-chromosomes which carry the dystrophin variant. For this reason, any woman who is presenting with symptomology of having symptoms similar to men with Becker's dystrophinopathy, should be evaluated for a dystrophin variant.

The dystrophies also include the category of the limb girdle muscular dystrophies (LMGD). Theis larger group of muscle diseases are much more varied in their presentation and are based upon the gene that is found to be defective. This group typically demonstrated more proximal than distal weakness with elevated creatine kinase and may or may not have multisystem involvement. These diseases are less common than the dystrophinopathies. An elevated creatine kinase should raise suspicion for limb girdle dystrophy.

The importance of diagnosing these diseases is best demonstrated by discussing Emory Dreyfus muscular dystrophy. This disease is caused by multiple genes including EIN and LMNA. Some of the subtypes can cause severe cardiac arrhythmias which often require preventative pacemakers for arrhythmias and bradycardias. Genetic confirmation of this disease subset and understanding the variant phenotype is incredibly important for the patients with LMGD. Additionally, the progression of symptoms can vary from very rapidly progressive with Duchenne phenotype or can be mild, slower, and without risk of losing ambulation.

Another important muscle disease of adolescence is facioscapulohumeral muscular dystrophy type 1. This disease is caused by complex multi-gene genetics but has a more frequent incidence than the non-dystrophinopathy LGMD with an incidence of 1 in 8500 to 15,000. Clinical features include asymmetric facial and scapular weakness with the earliest features being scapular and biceps weakness. This is contrary to the LGMD-type disease in which patients often have features of leg involvement sooner. Additionally, patients have difficulty closing their eyes and are unable to use straws or blow-up balloons. Their creatine kinase levels are often normal to only mildly elevated. While there is no definitive cure, knowing the patient's phenotype can help direct appropriate management.

## INFLAMMATORY/IMMUNE

Inflammatory myositis can occur in adolescents and is often described as a sub-acute onset with elevated creatine kinase, proximal weakness, and potentially other systemic features. Certainly, weakness can be associated with more systemic inflammatory diseases such as lupus, which causes secondary myositis, but primary myositis should also be considered. In any adolescent with sub-acute muscle weakness, consider myositis. As part of that evaluation, screening for primary systemic rheumatologic diseases is warranted.

While most patients have elevated creatine kinase, not all patients present in this manner and the level depends upon the extent of the inflammation. Additionally, patients with dermatomyositis can present without the classic dermatologic features. As such, neuroimaging of the muscle as well as a muscle biopsy is often warranted in these patients to help differentiate the sub-type and direct treatment. Steroids and/or IVIG remain the first-line treatments with the early addition of steroid-sparing agents such as methotrexate and/or other immunosuppressive agents. A definitive diagnosis is important to obtain.

One should be wary to ensure that mimickers such as dysferlinopathy, a genetic limb-girdle muscular dystrophy, is not treated with immunosuppression. The slowly progressive asymmetric weakness associated with dysferlinopathy can help distinguish it from inflammatory myopathies.

## SUMMARY

Adolescent weakness can present from a variety of peripheral causes. In general, broad categories can be determined based on the pattern of weakness with specific treatments based on the exact disease found. As such, identification of a concerning cause of weakness and referral to a skilled pediatric neuromuscular center is warranted. In addition, understanding the presentations can also help direct the urgency of the referral. This urgency is likely to change, however, as etiologic treatments are being rapidly developed for multiple diseases. Included in **Table 2** is a summary of the example diseases discussed in this article.

## CLINICS CARE POINTS

- Localization to categories of peripheral causes of muscle disease can be done relatively quickly and easily
- Periclinical testing (laboratory, imaging, electrodiagnostic) can help further define the etiology
- By defining the underlying etiology, referrals can be directed by urgency as well as to the appropriate specialist
- Creatine kinase can be a helpful marker between the various diseases but as there are frequent exceptions, a normal creatine kinase cannot rule out muscle disease

## DISCLOSURE

Dr M. Harmelink is a consultant for Sarepta Therapeutics as well as Encoded Therapetics. He has participated in advisory boards for Biogen, Sarepta, Novartis, and PTC.
He is a speaker for Sarepta Therapeutics. He participates as a local Site PI for trials run
by Sarepta, Biogen, Novartis, Genetech, Capricor, as well as Muscular Dystrophy
Association.

## REFERENCES

1. Panosyan FB, Laura M, Rossor AM, et al, Inherited Neuropathies Consortium—
   Rare Diseases Clinical Research Network (INC-RDCRN). Cross-sectional analysis of a large cohort with X-linked Charcot-Marie-Tooth disease (CMTX1).
   Neurology 2017;89(9):927–35.
2. Murphy SM, Laura M, Fawcett K, et al. Charcot-Marie-Tooth disease: frequency of
   genetic subtypes and guidelines for genetic testing. J Neurol Neurosurg Psychiatry 2012;83(7):706–10.
3. Turčanová Koprušáková M, Grofik M, Kantorová E, et al. Atypical presentation of
   Charcot-Marie-Tooth disease type 1C with a new mutation: a case report. BMC
   Neurol 2021;21:293.
4. Kulkarni Shilpa, Sayed Rafat, Garg Meenal, et al. Atypical presentation of
   Charcot-Marie-Tooth disease 1A: A case report. Neuromuscul Disord : NMD
   2015;25. https://doi.org/10.1016/j.nmd.2015.09.002.
5. Yiu EM, Bray P, Baets J, et al. Clinical practice guideline for the management of
   paediatric Charcot-Marie-Tooth disease. J Neurol Neurosurg Psychiatry 2022;
   93(5):530–8.
6. Hale K, Ojodu J, Singh S. Landscape of Spinal Muscular Atrophy Newborn
   Screening in the United States: 2018-2021. Int J Neonatal Screen 2021;7(3):33.
7. Lehky T, Grunseich C. Juvenile Amyotrophic Lateral Sclerosis: A Review. Genes
   2021;12(12):1935.
8. Elahi Erum, Ashfaq Muhammad, Nisa Bader, et al. Plasma Exchange Versus
   Intravenous Immunoglobulin in Children with Guillain Barré Syndrome. Journal
   of the Dow University of Health Sciences 2019;13:133–7.
9. Hughes RA, Brassington R, Gunn AA, et al. Corticosteroids for Guillain-Barré syndrome. Cochrane Database Syst Rev 2016;10(10):CD001446.
10. Althubaiti F, Guiomard C, Rivier F, et al. Prognostic value of contrast-enhanced
    MRI in Guillain-Barré syndrome in children. Arch Pediatr 2022;29(3):230–5.
11. Mihara M, Hayashi A, Fujita K, et al. Fixation stability of the upward gaze in pa-
    tients with myasthenia gravis: an eye-tracker study. BMJ Open Ophthalmol
    2017;2(1):e000072.
12. Harmelink MM. A case Description of a novel Mutation of SCN4A in a child Pre-
    senting with congenital myasthenia gravis (conference presentation.) UCI Neuro-
    muscular Colloquium, Irvine, California.
13. Sheikh S, Alvi U, Soliven B, et al. Drugs That Induce or Cause Deterioration of
    Myasthenia Gravis: An Update. J Clin Med 2021;10(7):1537.
14. Chung IY, Sheth SJ, Wells KK, et al. The Usefulness of Anti-acetylcholine Recep-
    tor Binding Antibody Testing in Diagnosing Ocular Myasthenia Gravis. J Neuro
    Ophthalmol 2021;41(4):e627–30.
15. Narayanaswami P, Sanders DB, Wolfe G, et al. International Consensus Guidance
    for Management of Myasthenia Gravis: 2020 Update. Neurology 2021;96(3):
    114–22.

16. Lehmann D, Motlagh L, Robaa D, et al. Muscle Carnitine Palmitoyltransferase II Deficiency: A Review of Enzymatic Controversy and Clinical Features. Int J Mol Sci 2017;18:82.
17. Snoeck M, van Engelen BG, Küsters B, et al. RYR1-related myopathies: a wide spectrum of phenotypes throughout life. Eur J Neurol 2015;22(7):1094–112.
18. Cupler EJ, Berger KI, Leshner RT, et al. Consensus treatment recommendations for late-onset Pompe disease. Muscle Nerve 2012;45:319–33.
19. Llavero F, Arrazola Sastre A, Luque Montoro M, et al. McArdle Disease: New Insights into Its Underlying Molecular Mechanisms. Int J Mol Sci 2019;20:5919.
20. Stunnenberg BC, LoRusso S, Arnold WD, et al. Guidelines on clinical presentation and management of nondystrophic myotonias. Muscle Nerve 2020;62: 430–44.

# Hemophagocytic Lymphohistiocytosis in Adolescents and Young Adults
## Genetic Predisposition and Secondary Disease

Alejandra Escobar Vasco, MD[a,b], Julie-Ann Talano, MD[a,b],
Larisa Broglie, MD, MS[a,b],*

## KEYWORDS

- Hemophagocytic lymphohistiocytosis (HLH) • Familial HLH • Secondary HLH
- Primary immunodeficiency • Adolescents • Young adults

## KEY POINTS

- Hemophagocytic lymphohistiocytosis (HLH) is a disorder of impaired immune regulation that results in extreme hyperinflammation and is fatal without treatment.
- Adolescents and young adults have been typically diagnosed with secondary HLH. However, genetic variants associated to familial disease and primary immunodeficiency should also be consider in this patient population.
- Maintaining a high index of suspicion in patients with hyperinflammation, will allow prompt diagnosis and treatment, preventing morbidity and mortality associated with the disease.

## INTRODUCTION

Hemophagocytic lymphohistiocytosis (HLH) is a disorder of impaired immune regulation that results in extreme hyperinflammation, subsequent tissue infiltration, and multiorgan failure. It is ultimately fatal if not appropriately diagnosed and treated.[1]

As HLH can have a genetic cause, HLH is often considered a diagnosis of infants; however, patients can present with symptoms of HLH into adolescence and even adulthood. Familial HLH is caused by genetic mutations affecting the function of cytotoxic T lymphocytes (CTLs) and natural killer cells (NK), resulting in hyperinflammation. Recent data shows that around 25% of all cases of HLH, regardless of age of onset, have a genetic mutation that classifies it as familial disease.[2] Secondary HLH may occur in the

[a] Medical College of Wisconsin, 8701 Watertown Plank Road, MFRC 3018, Milwaukee, WI 53226, USA; [b] Division of Hematology/Oncology/Blood and Marrow Transplantation, Department of Pediatrics, Medical College of Wisconsin, 8701 Watertown Plank Road, MFRC 3018, Milwaukee, WI 53226, USA
* Corresponding author. 8701 Watertown Plank Road, MFRC 3018, Milwaukee, WI 53226.
*E-mail address:* lbroglie@mcw.edu

Med Clin N Am 108 (2024) 189–200
https://doi.org/10.1016/j.mcna.2023.05.019
0025-7125/24/© 2023 Elsevier Inc. All rights reserved.
medical.theclinics.com

absence of genetic predisposition, triggered by infections, malignancies, rheumato-logic disorders or immune deficiency which can often also present in adolescence.[3]

HLH presentation in adolescents, therefore, can pose a particular clinical diagnostic challenge due to the nonspecific nature of the clinical manifestations of this disease and significant overlap with other systemic inflammatory syndromes. Establishing the diagnosis of HLH and assigning the correct etiology has significant management implications, for prompt treatment is needed to prevent the significant morbidity and mortality associated with hyperinflammation. Maintaining a high index of suspicion in children of all ages is imperative to reach this goal.

Here we discuss an example clinical case of an adolescent and consider (1) the diagnostic criteria for HLH, (2) the possible etiologies and pathophysiology driving HLH, and (3) the management of the disease.

## PATIENT PRESENTATION

A 15-year-old, previously healthy male presents with bloody diarrhea and is diagnosed with E. Coli gastroenteritis. Despite supportive management, he rapidly evolves to septic shock. He has persistent fever and laboratory work up demonstrates pancyto-penia, low fibrinogen, and significantly elevated ferritin levels. Despite supportive management and antibiotic therapy, he continues to have unmodulated systemic hyperinflammation, multiorgan dysfunction, and clinical deterioration.

## CLINICAL CRITERIA DEFINING HEMOPHAGOCYTIC LYMPHOHISTIOCYTOSIS

As seen in this example case, the patient presents with acute infection and has rapid clinical deterioration. Identifying that this patient has an ongoing hyperinflammatory state with HLH driving the clinical picture, is the priority. In 1991, the Histiocyte Society presented the first set of diagnostic guidelines for HLH. Following the results of the first prospective international treatment protocol (HLH-94), the guidelines for diagnosis have subsequently been revised.[4] Clinical criteria include fever, splenomegaly, cyto-penias, hypertriglyceridemia and/or hypofibrinogenemia, hemophagocytosis on bi-opsy, decreased natural killer (NK)-cell function, elevated ferritin, and elevated soluble IL-2 receptor levels (also known as sCD25) (**Box 1**).[4,5] These criteria reflect inherited susceptibility to HLH (NK function), immune activation (ferritin and sIL-2R), and immunopathology (hemophagocytosis, splenomegaly, and disseminated intra-vascular coagulation) that reflect the essence of this disease process. Although pa-tients with a variety of inflammatory conditions can display immune activation, normal cytotoxic immune regulatory mechanisms tend to dampen immune activation before unusual or paradoxic immunopathology develops. The combination of acute systemic immune activation and the specific findings on immunopathology is largely what distinguishes HLH from other inflammatory disorders.[6]

Once HLH is suspected, a multidisciplinary team should guide additional evaluation based on history and risk factors. Recommended work up should include evaluation for secondary HLH as well and rapid screening for genetic causes of HLH no matter the age of the patient. Multidisciplinary teams caring for patients with HLH should be familiar with commercially available genetic panels to test for HLH. Rapid turnover times and lower prices make these panels a useful and timely tool to help with the diagnosis of HLH and plan for optimal treatment. In the absence of rapidly available genetic testing, low/absent NK cell function and markers of impaired cytotoxicity (decreased expression of perforin, SAP, XIAP, or mobilization of CD107a), have been shown to be effective screening tools for familial HLH.[6–9]

---

**Box 1**
**Diagnostic criteria for HLH**

1. Molecular diagnosis with a pathogenic mutation in HLH-causing gene

2. Clinical and laboratory criteria (must meet at least 5 of the 8 criteria)
    Fever
    Splenomegaly
    Cytopenias: Affecting greater than 2 of the 3 lineages in the peripheral blood
    • Hemoglobin less than 9 g/dL (in infants <4 weeks: hemoglobin <10 g/dL)
    • Platelets less than 100 × 103/mL
    • Neutrophils less than 1.0 × 103/mL
    Hypertriglyceridemia (fasting triglycerides >265 mg/dL) and/or hypofibrinogenemia
    (Fibrinogen <150 mg/dL)
    Hemophagocytosis in bone, spleen, or lymph nodes with no evidence of malignancy
    Low or absent NK cell activity (per local laboratory reference)
    Ferritin greater than 500 mcg/L
    sCD25 (Soluble IL-2 receptor) >2400 pg/mL

Henter et al. HLH-2004: Diagnostic and Therapeutic Guidelines for Hemophagocytic Lympho-histiocytosis. 2007.[4]

---

## ETIOLOGIES DRIVING HEMOPHAGOCYTIC LYMPHOHISTIOCYTOSIS IN ADOLESCENTS AND YOUNG ADULTS
### Secondary Hemophagocytic Lymphohistiocytosis

Secondary HLH accounts for the majority of HLH in both pediatric and adult patients. The pathophysiology of nongenetic (secondary) HLH is not fully understood, however multiple potential mechanisms have been proposed to contribute. These include (1) abnormal cytokine production, in the setting of infection, or underlying autoimmunity or malignancy, (2) abnormal immune activation or antigen persistence related to malignancies, and (3) immune derangements caused by immunosuppression or chemotherapy (**Box 2**).[8,10]

---

**Box 2**
**Common causes of secondary HLH**

Rheumatologic disease
    Juvenile Idiopathic Arthritis
    Systemic Lupus Erythematosus
    Kawasaki Disease
    Inflammatory bowel disease

Infections
    Epstein Barr Virus (EBV)
    Cytomegalovirus (CMV)
    Parvovirus B-19
    Herpes simplex virus (HSV)
    HIV
    Tuberculosis
    Malaria
    Leishmaniasis

Malignancy
    Leukemia
    Lymphoma

Infection-associated HLH is the most common cause of secondary disease with Epstein Barr virus (EBV) being the most frequently associated infection, however other viruses, bacteria, and fungi have also been associated with HLH. A thorough clinical history, including travel history, and exam will help guide the infectious work up.[11] Malignancy as a trigger of HLH is rare in the pediatric population and when present, it generally affects older children (school age and adolescents).[12] Similar to the adult population, leukemia and lymphoma are the most common triggering malignancies and despite aggressive treatment, it continues to be associated with a poor prognosis.[12]

Macrophage Activation Syndrome (MAS) was initially described as a complication of rheumatologic disorders, especially juvenile idiopathic arthritis (JIA).[13] Patients with this syndrome share clinical and laboratory findings of HLH and, in recent years, it has become clearer that MAS and secondary HLH represent a spectrum of the same clinical entity. Even though secondary HLH includes different triggering mechanisms other than rheumatologic disorders, some authors continue to use the term MAS exclusively in the setting of rheumatological disease.[14]

In Japan, researchers developed a nationwide survey of HLH in all ages, to try to clarify epidemiology and clinical outcomes of HLH. This cohort consisted of 567 patients, of which 60% were pediatric patients and 40% adults (>18 years of age). The most frequent subtype was EBV-associated HLH, followed by other infections or lymphoma-associated HLH. Familial HLH was diagnosed almost exclusively in infants, and lymphoma-associated HLH occurred almost exclusively in adult patients. HLH associated with autoimmune disease occurred in a similar proportion of pediatric and adult patients (10% of pediatric patients, 8.5% of adult patients). Infection-associated HLH (particularly EBV-driven) occurred with a substantially higher frequency in pediatric patients (68% of patients <15 year old).[8]

### Familial Hemophagocytic Lymphohistiocytosis, Defects in Cytotoxicity

Even though adolescents and young adults have been typically diagnosed with secondary HLH because of older age and association with concomitant conditions, many of the genetic changes found in familial HLH are also reported in the older patient population.[15,16]

Familial HLH was originally described as a clinical presentation in the first 2 years of life, with or without a positive family history. However, since the first familial HLH-related gene map was reported by Stepp and colleagues in 1999,[17] there are increasing reports of "late onset" familial HLH and genetic testing has become the gold standard for diagnosis of familial disease in the HLH-2004 diagnostic guidelines of the Histiocyte Society.[4,10,18]

Familial HLH is often the result of a defect in the function of CTLs or NK cells; their normal function is to identify cells infected with a virus or with malignant changes and destroy them through perforin-dependent and death-receptor-dependent pathways. Perforin-dependent cytotoxicity induces apoptosis of a target cell through a pathway in which cytotoxic granules are generated, delivered to the cell surface, extruded from the cell, and then introduced into the target cell through a perforin-mediated channel.[4] HLH results from the inability of activated CTLs to clear antigen presenting targets, causing uncontrolled expansion of T-cell and macrophage populations that leads to a marked increase in the amount of cytokines in the blood (**Fig. 1**).[6] This delineates how congenital inborn errors of immunity that lead to either impaired perforin synthesis or function, or its dysregulated release, result in primary HLH. This includes familial HLH, that specifically describes mutation in PRF1-dependent cytotoxic pathway, pigmentary disorders that have compromise of granule trafficking,

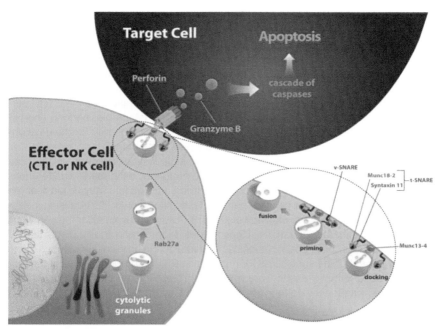

**Fig. 1.** Mechanism of cytotoxic function. (*Obtained from* Jordan MB, et al. How I treat hemophagocytic lymphohistiocytosis. Blood. 2011.[6])

X-linked lymphoproliferative (XLP) disorders, and Epstein Barr Virus (EVB)-susceptibility disorders (**Table 1**).[18,19]

To better understand the late presentation (at an older age) of familial disease, authors have explored differences in the gene pathogenic variants, the pathogenic variant patterns, and the presence of a trigger. Miao and colleagues[19] described that most of

| Table 1 | |
|---|---|
| **Classification of primary HLH** | |
| **Primary HLH** | **Genetic Mutation** |
| Familial HLH | FHLH1: Unknown. Linked to chromosome 9q21.3–2 |
| | FHLH2: PRF1 mutation |
| | FHLH3: UNC13D/MUNC13–4 |
| | FHLH4: STX11 |
| | FHLH5: STXBP2 |
| Pigmentary disorder associated with HLH | Griscelli syndrome type 2: RAB27 A |
| | Chediak-Higashi syndrome: LYST |
| | Hermansky-Pudlak syndrome type 2: AP3B1 |
| XLP-1 and XLP-2 | SH2D1A |
| | XIAP |
| | NLRC4 |
| | CDC42 |
| EBV Susceptibility disorders | MAGT1 |
| | ITK |
| | CD27 |
| | CD70 |

the variants present in pediatric-onset FHLH2 are nonsense and frameshift mutations in PRF1. On the contrary, missense mutations are much more prevalent in late-onset HLH and suggest that these gene mutations may partially damage, rather than completely eliminate, the function of the affected proteins.[19] Similarly, Trizzino and colleagues[20] described the presence of biallelic mutation or compound heterozygous mutations that encodes for a partial PRF1 protein that may retain part of the cytotoxicity and delay the onset of the disease. Risma and colleagues[21] described the class I perforin mutation with partial maturation and reduced, but detectable, perforin and NK function. This mutation, named A91 V, confers genetic susceptibility for the development of HLH but is not enough to trigger the disease on its own.

In 2011, Zhang and colleagues[15] published a single institution cohort of 1531 patients evaluated for genetic testing for primary HLH and they described the differences in frequency and nature of the mutations in children and adults. They report that the highest frequency (44%) of positive genetic testing in known HLH-causing genes was noted in infants (0–1 year old); however, 14% of adult patients older than 18 years were also found to harbor mutations in these genes. Mutations in adult patients tended to be missense and splice site mutations as opposed to the nonsense mutations found in younger patients. The specific A91 V mutation in PRF1, comprised 48% of the mutations in adults. Similar results were noted in 252 adolescent and adult patients in China, where mutations were found in 14% of adolescent patients and 5.1% of adult patients.[22]

Adolescents and young adults presenting with HLH have been found to have not only pathogenic mutations on familial HLH genes but also mutations in genes associated with primary immunodeficiencies and immune regulation, with some patients developing HLH as the primary clinical manifestation of disease.

### Primary Immunodeficiency and Disorders of Primary Immune Regulation

With improved understanding of the role of NK and T cells in the pathophysiology of HLH, new reports of patients with a variety of primary immune deficiency disorders (PID), particularly T cell deficiencies, have been reported to develop HLH, usually as a complication of infection (**Table 2**).[23] Similarly acquired T cell deficiency like in HIV and patients on immunosuppressive therapies have been reported to develop secondary HLH.[24,25]

Bode and colleagues,[26] on behalf of the Histiocyte Society and the Inborn Errors Working Party of the European Society for Blood and Marrow Transplantation (EBMT), report an international cohort of 63 patients with PID other than genetic disorders of cytotoxicity or XLP, who fulfilled the current clinical criteria for HLH. Of this patient population, 57% presented with HLH prior to the diagnosis of PID. Patients with T-cell deficiencies and chronic granulomatous disease (CGD) had infection as a trigger for HLH, supporting the theory that uncontrolled pathogen replication is a major risk factor for this hyperinflammatory syndrome. On the contrary, HLH was not found to be reported in other phagocyte defects other than CGD, postulating the hypothesis that this disease possesses a genetic predisposition to hyperinflammatory syndromes.[26]

Interestingly in the above-mentioned cohort, they described 3 patients with X-linked SCID that developed HLH, suggesting that this syndrome can develop despite the severe deficiency of T and NK cells. Although this is a rare occurrence in patients with a high incidence of infections, this report mandates further evaluation of their genetic makeup and additional evaluation of other players in the immune system capable of inducing cytokine storm.[26]

Similarly, Chinn and colleagues,[2] reported 122 patients evaluated at Texas Children's hospital with a diagnosis of HLH. This cohort of patients were pediatric patients

**Table 2**
**Primary immunodeficiency syndromes that are associated with HLH**

| Primary Immune Deficiency | Genetic Mutation |
|---|---|
| Severe combined immunodeficiency (SCID) | ILR2G |
| | RAG-1 |
| | IL7RA |
| | CD3E |
| Combined immunodeficiency | 22q11 (DiGeorge syndrome) |
| | WAS (Wiskott-aldrich syndrome) |
| | DKC1 |
| | CD27 |
| | ATM (Ataxia Telangiectasia) |
| Chronic granulomatous disease (CGD) | CGD (p91) |
| | CGD (p47) |
| | CGD (p22) |
| | CGD (DHR) |
| Others | FAS (ALPS) |
| | STAT1 GOF |
| | BTK (X-linked agammaglobulinemia) |
| | PNP (Purine nucleoside phosphorylase deficiency) |

from diverse ethnic backgrounds and a median age of disease presentation of 6.1 year old. They performed genetic testing in 101 patients and their results demonstrated that the genetic mechanisms for HLH go beyond the currently described causes of familial HLH. The authors introduce the concept of dysregulated immune activation or proliferation (DIAP) to include genetic mutation in genes with a role in immune regulation that can manifest with HLH. Based on these genetic results they grouped their patients in one of the 5 categories: (1) Familial HLH, with biallelic mutation in genes previously described in this group, present in 19% and monoallelic mutations on 35%, (2) Primary immune deficiency disorders in 16% of patients, (3) DIAP in 8%, (4) Those having other candidate defects in 5%, and (5) No genetic explanation in 17%. This cohort adds supporting evidence that patients classify as having secondary disease should be considered for genetic testing to evaluate possible immune deficiency or dysregulation syndrome.[2]

## TREATMENT

Once a diagnosis of HLH is made, a multidisciplinary team should guide additional evaluation based on history and risk factors (**Fig. 2**).[6,11] Therapy should be started as soon as possible; when patients are critically ill, early initial treatment with steroids can be considered while awaiting the results of diagnostic studies.[6]

When treating familial HLH, the principal goal of induction therapy is to suppress the life-threatening inflammatory process that underlies HLH, followed by allogeneic hematopoietic cell transplantation (HCT) to correct their genetic defect. For secondary disease, in addition to controlling the hyperinflammatory state, it is also critical to search for and treat the underlying triggers of HLH.[11]

The first international treatment protocol for HLH was organized by the Histiocyte Society (HLH-94 protocol) and includes an 8-week induction therapy with dexamethasone, etoposide, and intrathecal methotrexate for patients with central nervous system (CNS) disease. At the end of 8 weeks, patients are either weaned off therapy or transitioned to continuation therapy, which is intended only as a bridge to HCT. This protocol resulted in an overall 3-year survival of 51%.[27,28]

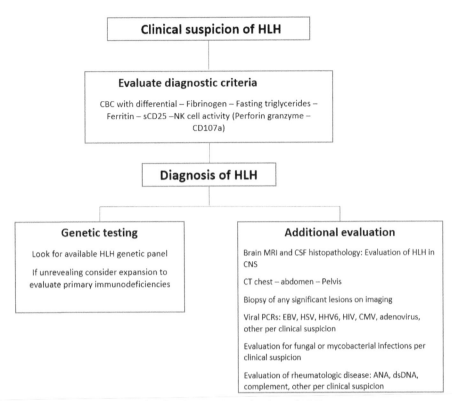

**Fig. 2.** Proposed algorithm for the diagnostic evaluation of HLH.

In 2004 the Histiocyte Society developed the 2004-HLH treatment protocol that included the early administration of cyclosporin to the HLH-94 protocol. Results of the study demonstrated increase toxicity from cyclosporin with no improvement in survival and so early administration of this medication is currently not recommended.[4] However, this study demonstrated that, with steroids and etoposide, approximately 53% of patients can be expected to achieve a complete response at 2 months, and approximately 32% of patients can be expected to achieve a partial response.[4,29] Several single-center studies have evaluated the use of alternative immunotherapy for the first-line treatment of HLH, however given the small number of patients, experts continue to recommend etoposide and dexamethasone the standard front-line therapy for this disease.[30]

Patients with relapsed or refractory disease represent a challenge for clinicians, with no current standardized treatment guidelines and a high mortality rate. With increased knowledge of the cytokine profile of patients with HLH and the availability of medications that specifically target some of these inflammation mediators, different therapy combinations have been studied for these patients. Interferon-$\gamma$ is a known key player of the hyperinflammation seen in familial HLH. Elevated levels have been shown to correlate with disease activity and preclinical studies demonstrated that blocking this cytokine improved symptomatology and survival.[31,32] Emapalumab is an IFN-$\gamma$-targeted monoclonal antibody that has demonstrated safety and efficacy with response in 63% of patients in an initial study by Locatelli and colleagues.[33] This data supported the use of emapalumab in HLH and in 2018, this medication became the first Food and Drug Administration (FDA)–approved treatment for adult and pediatric patients who can't tolerate conventional therapy or those with refractory, recurrent, or progressive familial HLH.[14,34,35]

Other immunomodulators that have been studied in HLH include alemtuzumab (CD52-targeted monoclonal antibody), anakinra (recombinant IL-1 antagonist), ruxolitinib (JAK1/2 inhibitor), and tocilizumab (IL-6 targeted monoclinal antibody). All have shown promising responses when included as part of treatment for secondary HLH (especially secondary to autoimmune disease), in relapse or refractory HLH, as bridging therapy to HCT and even as part of the HCT conditioning regimen. Large scale studies are required to determine the safety and efficacy of these medications in the treatment of HLH.[36–39]

For patients with secondary HLH, treatment is targeted to the underlying process. While steroids can help calm ongoing inflammation, antimicrobial treatment is indicated in the setting of a known infectious trigger. For patients with autoimmune diseases and malignancy, HLH can present in 2 different settings: (1) infection in the setting of disease treatment (immune modulation or chemotherapy), or (2) active oncologic or rheumatologic disease requiring treatment escalation. In a patient with a compromised immune system and infection, holding medications to allow immune reconstitution is necessary to control the infectious trigger and calm the inflammatory response.[40] When HLH occurs with acute flairs of autoimmune disease or at the time of diagnosis of leukemia or lymphoma, treating the primary disease (with the use of immune modulators or chemotherapy) will allow control of HLH.

## PATIENT DIAGNOSIS AND MANAGEMENT (CONTINUED)

In our example patient, given the severe inflammation and rapid clinical deterioration, HLH was considered. Soluble IL2 receptor levels were obtained and found to be significantly elevated. The patient met the diagnostic criteria of HLH and therapy per HLH-94 with dexamethasone and etoposide was started while continuing supportive care and antibiotic therapy. The patient was proven to be refractory to treatment and continued to develop multiorgan dysfunction. Emapalumab was started with dramatic response. The patient's hyperinflammation improved and he started to recover from organ dysfunction. While managing his acute HLH flair, next-generation sequencing for familial HLH genes was sent and demonstrated a pathogenic variant in UNC13D. The patient was referred for allogeneic HCT.

Additionally, the patient's sister was found to harbor the same mutation in UNC13D. While undergoing evaluation for transplant, she developed an HLH flair secondary to infection that was controlled with HLH-94 therapy. Following control of her symptoms, she underwent allogeneic HCT.

## SUMMARY

HLH is a rare disease which is fatal without treatment and maintaining a high index of suspicion in patients with evidence of hyperinflammation is of utmost importance. With increasing knowledge of the genetic bases of the disease and the understanding that familial HLH is not a disease exclusive of infants, adolescents with HLH should undergo genetic evaluation for familial HLH. Primary immune deficiencies and dysregulation disorders should also be considered simultaneously with evaluation for other secondary causes. Prompt diagnosis and initiation of treatment is needed to prevent morbidity and mortality related to the hyperinflammation of HLH.

## CLINICS CARE POINTS

- HLH is a clinical diagnosis made using criteria specified in the 1994 diagnostic guidelines. Once diagnosis is made genetic testing for familial HLH and/or immunodeficiency variants should be consider no matter age of diagnosis and send early in the course of disease.

- Management of patient with HLH should include a multidisciplinary team with expertise in this disease and its cause (either familial or secondary). Early initiation of therapy using the HLH-94 protocol and/or management of primary triggers is of outmost importance to prevent mortality.

- Treatment team should be familiar with new available immunomodulating medications with evidence in the treatment of HLH, specially in the case of refractory disease.

## DISCLOSURE

The authors have no financial conflicts of interest to disclose.

## REFERENCES

1. Usmani GN, Woda BA, Newburger PE. Advances in understanding the pathogenesis of HLH. Br J Haematol 2013;161(5):609–22.
2. Chinn IK, Eckstein OS, Peckham-Gregory EC, et al. Genetic and mechanistic diversity in pediatric hemophagocytic lymphohistiocytosis. Blood 2018;132(1):89–100.
3. Chesshyre E, Ramanan AV, Roderick MR. Hemophagocytic Lymphohistiocytosis and Infections: An Update. Pediatr Infect Dis J 2019;38(3):e54–6.
4. Henter JI, Horne A, Aricó M, et al. HLH-2004: Diagnostic and therapeutic guidelines for hemophagocytic lymphohistiocytosis. Pediatr Blood Cancer 2007;48(2):124–31.
5. Henter JI, Elinder G, Ost A. Diagnostic guidelines for hemophagocytic lymphohistiocytosis. The FHL Study Group of the Histiocyte Society. Semin Oncol 1991;18(1):29–33.
6. Jordan MB, Allen CE, Weitzman S, et al. How I treat hemophagocytic lymphohistiocytosis. Blood 2011;118(15):4041–52.
7. Voskoboinik I, Smyth MJ, Trapani JA. Perforin-mediated target-cell death and immune homeostasis. Nat Rev Immunol 2006;6(12):940–52.
8. Ishii E, Ohga S, Imashuku S, et al. Nationwide survey of hemophagocytic lymphohistiocytosis in Japan. Int J Hematol 2007;86(1):58–65.
9. Bryceson YT, Pende D, Maul-Pavicic A, et al. A prospective evaluation of degranulation assays in the rapid diagnosis of familial hemophagocytic syndromes. Blood 2012;119(12):2754–63.
10. Wysocki CA. Comparing hemophagocytic lymphohistiocytosis in pediatric and adult patients. Curr Opin Allergy Clin Immunol 2017;17(6):405–13.
11. Canna SW, Marsh RA. Pediatric hemophagocytic lymphohistiocytosis. Blood 2020;135(16):1332–43.
12. Huang Z, Jia Y, Zuo Y, et al. Malignancy-associated hemophagocytic lymphohistiocytosis in children: a 10-year experience of a single pediatric hematology center. Hematology 2020;25(1):389–99.
13. Hadchouel M, Prieur AM, Griscelli C. Acute hemorrhagic, hepatic, and neurologic manifestations in juvenile rheumatoid arthritis: possible relationship to drugs or infection. J Pediatr 1985;106(4):561–6.

14. Henderson LA, Cron RQ. Macrophage Activation Syndrome and Secondary Hemophagocytic Lymphohistiocytosis in Childhood Inflammatory Disorders: Diagnosis and Management. Paediatr Drugs 2020;22(1):29–44.

15. Zhang K, Jordan MB, Marsh RA, et al. Hypomorphic mutations in PRF1, MUNC13-4, and STXBP2 are associated with adult-onset familial HLH. Blood 2011;118(22):5794–8.

16. zur Stadt U, Rohr J, Seifert W, et al. Familial hemophagocytic lymphohistiocytosis type 5 (FHL-5) is caused by mutations in Munc18-2 and impaired binding to syntaxin 11. Am J Hum Genet 2009;85(4):482–92.

17. Stepp SE, Dufourcq-Lagelouse R, Le Deist F, et al. Perforin gene defects in familial hemophagocytic lymphohistiocytosis. Science 1999;286(5446):1957–9.

18. Jin Z, Wang Y, Wang J, et al. Primary hemophagocytic lymphohistiocytosis in adults: the utility of family surveys in a single-center study from China. Orphanet J Rare Dis 2018;13(1):17.

19. Miao Y, Zhu HY, Qiao C, et al. Pathogenic Gene Mutations or Variants Identified by Targeted Gene Sequencing in Adults With Hemophagocytic Lymphohistiocytosis. Front Immunol 2019;10:395.

20. Trizzino A, zur Stadt U, Ueda I, et al, Histiocyte Society HLH Study group. Genotype-phenotype study of familial haemophagocytic lymphohistiocytosis due to perforin mutations. J Med Genet 2008;45(1):15–21.

21. Risma KA, Frayer RW, Filipovich AH, et al. Aberrant maturation of mutant perforin underlies the clinical diversity of hemophagocytic lymphohistiocytosis. J Clin Invest 2006;116(1):182–92.

22. Wang Y, Wang Z, Zhang J, et al. Genetic features of late onset primary hemophagocytic lymphohistiocytosis in adolescence or adulthood. PLoS One 2014;9(9):e107386.

23. Faitelson Y, Grunebaum E. Hemophagocytic lymphohistiocytosis and primary immune deficiency disorders. Clin Immunol 2014;155(1):118–25.

24. Bhatia S, Bauer F, Bilgrami SA. Candidiasis-associated hemophagocytic lymphohistiocytosis in a patient infected with human immunodeficiency virus. Clin Infect Dis 2003;37(11):e161–6.

25. Frederiksen JK, Ross CW. Cytomegalovirus-associated hemophagocytic lymphohistiocytosis in a patient with myasthenia gravis treated with azathioprine. Blood 2014;123(15):2290.

26. Bode SF, Ammann S, Al-Herz W, et al. Inborn Errors Working Party of the EBMT. The syndrome of hemophagocytic lymphohistiocytosis in primary immunodeficiencies: implications for differential diagnosis and pathogenesis. Haematologica 2015;100(7):978–88.

27. Henter JI, Samuelsson-Horne A, Aricò M, et al. Treatment of hemophagocytic lymphohistiocytosis with HLH-94 immunochemotherapy and bone marrow transplantation. Blood 2002;100(7):2367–73.

28. Trottestam H, Horne A, Aricò M, et al. Chemoimmunotherapy for hemophagocytic lymphohistiocytosis: long-term results of the HLH-94 treatment protocol. Blood 2011;118(17):4577–84.

29. Bergsten E, Horne A, Aricó M, et al. Confirmed efficacy of etoposide and dexamethasone in HLH treatment: long-term results of the cooperative HLH-2004 study. Blood 2017;130(25):2728–38.

30. Mahlaoui N, Ouachée-Chardin M, de Saint Basile G, et al. Immunotherapy of familial hemophagocytic lymphohistiocytosis with antithymocyte globulins: a single-center retrospective report of 38 patients. Pediatrics 2007;120(3):e622–8.

31. Buatois V, Chatel L, Cons L, et al. Use of a mouse model to identify a blood biomarker for IFNγ activity in pediatric secondary hemophagocytic lymphohistiocytosis. Transl Res 2017;180:37–52.e2.

32. Henter JI, Elinder G, Söder O, et al. Hypercytokinemia in familial hemophagocytic lymphohistiocytosis. Blood 1991;78(11):2918–22.

33. Locatelli F, Jordan MB, Allen C, et al. Emapalumab in Children with Primary Hemophagocytic Lymphohistiocytosis. N Engl J Med 2020;382(19):1811–22.

34. Summerlin J, Wells DA, Anderson MK, et al. A Review of Current and Emerging Therapeutic Options for Hemophagocytic Lymphohistiocytosis. Ann Pharmacother 2022. https://doi.org/10.1177/10600280221134719. 10600280221134719.

35. US Food and Drug Administration. FDA approves first treatment specifically for patients with rare and life-threatening type of immune disease. Available at. https://www.fda.gov/drugs/fda-approves-emapalumab-hemophagocytic-lymphohistiocytosis. Accessed March 30, 2023.

36. Marsh RA, Allen CE, McClain KL, et al. Salvage therapy of refractory hemophagocytic lymphohistiocytosis with alemtuzumab. Pediatr Blood Cancer 2013;60(1):101–9.

37. Mehta P, Cron RQ, Hartwell J, et al. Silencing the cytokine storm: the use of intravenous anakinra in haemophagocytic lymphohistiocytosis or macrophage activation syndrome. Lancet Rheumatol 2020;2(6):e358–67.

38. Wang J, Wang Y, Wu L, et al. Ruxolitinib for refractory/relapsed hemophagocytic lymphohistiocytosis. Haematologica 2020;105(5):e210–2.

39. Dufranc E, Del Bello A, Belliere J, et al. TAIDI (Toulouse Acquired Immune Deficiency and Infection) study group. IL6-R blocking with tocilizumab in critically ill patients with hemophagocytic syndrome. Crit Care 2020;24(1):166.

40. Biank VF, Sheth MK, Talano J, et al. Association of Crohn's disease, thiopurines, and primary epstein-barr virus infection with hemophagocytic lymphohistiocytosis. J Pediatr 2011;159(5):808–12.

# Severe, Refractory Seizures

## New-Onset Refractory Status Epilepticus and Febrile Infection-Related Epilepsy Syndrome

Ross Carson, MD[a], Coral M. Stredny, MD[b],*

KEYWORDS

• NORSE • FIRES • Epilepsy • Seizure • Refractory status epilepticus

KEY POINTS

- NORSE (new-onset refractory status epilepticus) is a presentation characterized by new-onset refractory status epilepticus with no underlying structural lesion, toxic insul, or metabolic abnormality.
- Prompt recognition of NORSE is important because early treatment may be associated with better outcomes in the acute phase.
- Autoimmune and inflammatory, infectious, and genetic etiologies should be thoroughly investigated before assigning the diagnosis of cryptogenic NORSE as the treatment and prognosis may differ.
- First-line immunotherapies for cryptogenic NORSE are steroids, IVIg, and/or plasma exchange. Second-line immunotherapies may include anakinra or tocilizumab. Long-term treatment involves epilepsy management, cognitive and motor rehabilitation, and ongoing support and therapies in school/work.
- The prognosis of NORSE is variable, but many survivors will have cognitive impairment, and most will have epilepsy.

## INTRODUCTION

New-onset refractory status epilepticus (NORSE) is a presentation of fulminant seizures without apparent underlying structural, metabolic, or toxic etiology. Febrile infection-related epilepsy syndrome (FIRES) is a subcategory of NORSE in which patients have a preceding fever. NORSE/FIRES may be due to autoimmune, infectious, or genetic causes, and remain cryptogenic in up to half of cases. In cryptogenic cases, an aberrant innate immune system is felt to be at play, including interleukin (IL)-1 and IL-6

[a] Department of Neurology, Boston Children's Hospital, Harvard Medical School, Boston, MA, USA; [b] Division of Epilepsy and Clinical Neurophysiology, Program in Neuroimmunology, Department of Neurology, Boston Children's Hospital, Harvard Medical School, 300 Longwood Avenue, Boston, MA 02115, USA
* Corresponding author. Boston Children's Hospital, 300 Longwood Avenue, Fegan 11, Boston, MA 02115.
E-mail address: coral.stredny@childrens.harvard.edu

pathways. Recent consensus guidelines outline proposed diagnostic pathways and empiric treatment, with some special considerations for the pediatric and adolescent populations. These syndromes are associated with significant morbidity and mortality, often leading to cognitive impairment and chronic epilepsy in survivors. Hence, early recognition of NORSE/FIRES is important for the timely initiation of targeted immunotherapy which may improve outcomes, although further studies are needed in this regard.

## DEFINING NEW-ONSET REFRACTORY STATUS EPILEPTICUS AND FEBRILE INFECTION-RELATED EPILEPSY SYNDROME
### New-Onset Refractory Status Epilepticus

In a 2018 consensus statement, NORSE was defined as "a clinical presentation" of refractory status epilepticus without an underlying structural lesion or metabolic/toxic cause.[1] It is important to emphasize that NORSE is not a single entity but rather a presentation of a variety of underlying diseases. NORSE includes patients with viral and autoimmune encephalitis (AE), even if an autoantibody is identified or infectious testing is positive within the first few days of presentation, and those with a history of resolved epilepsy. NORSE may also be the initial presentation of a genetic epilepsy syndrome. If a cause cannot be identified despite extensive testing, NORSE is considered "cryptogenic" or "NORSE of unknown etiology."[1]

### Febrile Infection-Related Epilepsy Syndrome

FIRES is defined as a subcategory of NORSE requiring the onset of fever 1-14 days before seizure onset.[1] While it is typically discussed as a clinical presentation in school-aged children, its definition is not limited by age and includes adolescents and adults. Timing of the febrile period was added to differentiate from febrile seizures, which will more typically have fever onset within 24 hours of seizure onset. Febrile SE compared to FIRES is also more common in younger patients, particularly those less than 2 years of age. Identifying this subcategory may be important for prognostication as cryptogenic FIRES may have a different response rate to initial therapies and prognosis compared to cryptogenic NORSE.[2,3]

### Status Epilepticus

Refractory status epilepticus (RSE) is defined as seizures continuing after the administration of two intravenous anti-seizure medications (ASMs) which may include a benzodiazepine. SE becomes super-refractory if the duration continues for 24 hours after the introduction of anesthesia with continuous infusion(s), there is recurrence while receiving continuous infusion(s), or there is recurrence with the downtitration of continuous infusion(s).[1] Most cases of NORSE include super-refractory status epilepticus (SRSE).[4] In many instances, refractory or super-refractory SE is prolonged, which by definition lasts more than 1 week in duration.[1]

## PATHOPHYSIOLOGY

In at least half of cases, NORSE/FIRES has an identifiable cause, but the remaining are cryptogenic. Evidence suggests that cryptogenic NORSE/FIRES is driven by an aberrant innate immune system, including IL-1 and IL-6 pathways.[5] Increased IL-1 and IL-6 signaling are pro-convulsant in animal models and have been implicated in drug-resistant epilepsy.[6] It is hypothesized that a nonspecific systemic infection and/or genetic susceptibility activates the innate immune system that then leads to neuroinflammation and epileptogenicity. Inflammation from seizures themselves further propagates this process, as well as malfunction of the "off switch" or antagonist anti-inflammatory pathways.[7]

As evidence of such, cerebrospinal fluid (CSF) and serum proinflammatory cytokines and chemokines, including interferon (IFN) $\gamma$, IL-1$\beta$, IL-6, C-X-C motif ligand (CXCL)8, CXCL9, and CXCL10, are elevated in patients with NORSE/FIRES.[8–11] When compared to other types of RSE, CSF IL-1$\beta$ and serum CXCL8, macrophage inflammatory protein (MIP)-1$\alpha$, and C-C motif ligand (CCL)2 were higher in NORSE in one study. While this highlights the concept that patients with established epilepsy and RSE also exhibit elevated CSF/serum proinflammatory cytokines, unique characteristics were seen in patients with NORSE.[11]

In addition to cytokine profiles, genetic sequencing in patients diagnosed with FIRES demonstrated a significant association between the RN2 allele of the gene encoding the IL-1 receptor compared to controls,[12] as well as non-coding genetic variants with altered isoform expression in this gene.[13] Patients were found to have a functional deficiency in IL-1 receptor antagonist (IL-1Ra), which could lead to unrestricted IL-1 driven inflammation.[13] Taken together, evidence suggests a model in which a triggered and unchecked innate immune response causes the release of pro-convulsant cytokines leading to inflammation and RSE (**Fig. 1**).

## RECOGNIZING NEW-ONSET REFRACTORY STATUS EPILEPTICUS AND FEBRILE INFECTION-RELATED EPILEPSY SYNDROME
### Epidemiology

Although consensus definitions suggest no age restriction, NORSE is often described in adults and FIRES in children in the existing literature. NORSE has a bimodal age of onset at 28.5 and 65.5 years; comparatively, the median age of onset in FIRES is 8 years.[14,15] In the childhood and adolescent population, males are predominantly affected, and in adults, females are predominantly affected.[14–16] While likely underreported, the incidence approximates 1/1,000,000 children and adolescents in one German study,[17] and NORSE accounts for up to 20% of pediatric RSE cases.[2]

### Clinical Presentation

The history of presenting illness usually includes a non-specific viral prodrome, particularly in FIRES (**Table 1**). This is most commonly an upper respiratory infection, and less often gastroenteritis.[14] In a study of children with NORSE, 61% had prodromal symptoms including preceding febrile illness (35%) and headache (32%).[2] In a similar adult study including patients as young as 18 years of age, 60% had prodromal symptoms which included confusion (45%), fever (34%), headache (22%), gastrointestinal illness (22%), and behavioral changes (16%), amongst others.[14] In both studies, prodromal symptoms usually started between 1 and 14 days prior to presentation.[2,14]

In terms of seizure presentation, most patients have new-onset focal seizures which increase in frequency and severity, evolving into SE over the course of hours to days.[18] The majority (90%) will have their first seizure prior to presentation to the hospital.[14] Focal onset seizures with progression to bilateral tonic clonic seizures are common.[15] NORSE should be strongly considered if SE continues after the administration of multiple intravenous ASMs and first-line immunotherapies.[3]

### Electroencephalogram

Ictal onsets are often unilateral or bilateral independent; generalized and multifocal onset are also reported.[14] Fronto-temporal foci are most common.[15] In a single center case series of 7 patients with FIRES, 4 characteristic EEG findings were noted: delta-

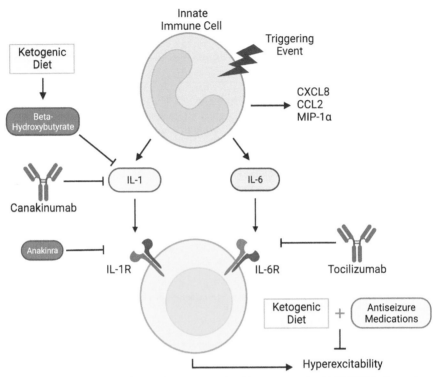

**Fig. 1.** Summary of molecular mechanisms involved in cryptogenic NORSE/FIRES: Current understanding of the pathophysiology suggests that a triggering event, often a nonspecific illness, causes inappropriate activation of the innate immune system yielding the release of numerous pro-inflammatory cytokines, including IL-1 and IL-6. Other cytokines/chemokines are released including CXCL8, CCL2, and MIP-1 which have been correlated with disease severity.[11] Propagation of this proinflammatory cascade and under activation of anti-inflammatory mechanisms leads to neuronal hyperexcitability and ultimately refractory seizures, which are treated with ASMs and ketogenic diet as well as targeted immunomodulation. The ketogenic diet generates beta-hydroxybutyrate which inhibits IL-1. Anakinra is an inhibitor of IL-1R and canakinumab is a monoclonal antibody that binds IL-1. Tocilizumab is a monoclonal antibody that acts as an IL-6R antagonist.[7,27] Created with BioRender.com.

beta complexes resembling extreme delta brush, gradual increase in seizure burden, focal fast activity at ictal onset, and seizures of shifting laterality.[18]

### Magnetic Resonance Imaging

MRI abnormalities are found in the majority of pediatric (55%) and adult (62%) cases, including T2 hyperintensities in the neocortex, mesial temporal lobe, basal ganglia, and claustrum as well as leptomeningeal enhancement.[2,14,15,19] Serial MRIs often reveal diffuse atrophy and increased T2/FLAIR hyperintensities over time.[2,14,15]

### Cerebrospinal Fluid

CSF is abnormal in 34% to 74% of large pediatric or adult cohorts.[2,14,15] Elevated protein and pleocytosis are seen, often less than 10 cells/mm³ but up to approximately 200 cells/mm³.[14] Higher protein levels are reported in NORSE (median 48 mg/dL,

| Table 1 Early identifying features of NORSE/FIRES | |
|---|---|
| Prodromal Phase | Prodromal illness most often with upper respiratory or GI symptoms<br>Fever<br>Headache[2,14] |
| Seizures | Focal seizures that evolve into SE over hours to days<br>Refractory to ASMs and first-line immunotherapy[18] |
| EEG | Unilateral or bilateral independent fronto-temporal ictal onsets[14,15]<br>Delta-beta complexes<br>Focal fast activity at ictal onset<br>Seizures of shifting laterality[18] |
| MRI | Neocortical, mesial temporal lobe, basal ganglia, claustrum T2/FLAIR hyperintensities<br>Leptomeningeal enhancement[2,14,15,19] |
| CSF | Mild pleocytosis ($\sim$10 cells/mm$^3$)<br>Moderate protein elevation[16] |

interquartile range [IQR] 24), while a higher degree of pleocytosis (median 10 cells/mm$^3$, IQR 28) is seen in FIRES.[16] Oligoclonal bands are positive in some.[2,14,15]

## Serum and Cerebrospinal Fluid Cytokine Analyses

As detailed above, certain proinflammatory cytokines and chemokines are elevated in patients with NORSE compared to controls and other causes of RSE.[11] CSF neopterin, a marker of T-cell and IFN$\gamma$-mediated inflammation, has also been found to be elevated in NORSE. Beyond this, some patients with FIRES meet diagnostic criteria for hemophagocytic lymphohistiocytosis (HLH); in critically ill patients, this diagnostic overlap should be considered, including monitoring ferritin, cytopenias, and evidence of multisystem dysfunction.[20]

## Brain Biopsy

Pathology is abnormal in approximately 80% of cases, with gliosis, neuronal loss, and perivascular T-cell-mediated inflammation being the most common features. Biopsy established a definitive diagnosis in 10% in a recent review, including infections and vasculitis.[21]

## DIFFERENTIAL DIAGNOSIS

A broad differential exists when considering the underlying etiology in NORSE/FIRES, including inflammatory and autoimmune encephalitis, infectious encephalitis, and genetic/metabolic conditions.[22] As such, diagnostic testing to rule out identifiable and treatable causes should be pursued with an algorithm recently proposed by expert consensus.[23] Ultimately, a cause is identified in up to half of patients, although rates are lower in children. AE is the most frequent cause in adults, and infectious etiologies are more common in children. Notably, however, a recent systematic review highlighted that such workups are often largely incomplete, with infectious, autoimmune, and genetic testing reported in only 80%, 60%, and 20% of cases, respectively, suggesting cryptogenic NORSE/FIRES may be overreported.[24]

## Autoimmune and Inflammatory

Autoimmune and inflammatory etiologies represent the most common identifiable cause of NORSE in the adult population, with anti-N-methyl-D-aspartate receptor

encephalitis (NMDARE) being the most frequent.[24] Some other reported autoantibodies in prior series have now been identified to be nonspecific (eg, voltage-gated
potassium channel (VGKC) without leucine-rich glioma inactivated 1 (LGI1) or
contactin-associated protein-like 2 (CASPR2) positivity).[25] In general, AE is less often
reported as an etiology in children with NORSE/FIRES, and this discrepancy may be at
least in part due to reporting bias.[22]

Importantly, cryptogenic NORSE/FIRES tends to be a monosymptomatic presentation predominated by seizures alone. This can be helpful in differentiating from
NORSE/FIRES secondary to AE, as the latter is almost always polysymptomatic
with neuropsychiatric symptoms, movement disorder, or dysautonomia in addition
to seizures. This has recently been captured in a score with high sensitivity (94%)
and specificity (100%) for differentiating cryptogenic NORSE from NORSE secondary
to antibody-positive AE in children and adults, in which a patient with $\geq$ 5/6 of the
following has a high likelihood of cryptogenic etiology: fever, previously healthy, refractory to ASMs, absence of psychiatric/behavioral symptoms, no movement disorder, and symmetric MRI changes.[26] Additionally, other systemic disease-specific
patterns may suggest conditions such as systemic lupus erythematosus, and history
of malignancy may point to a paraneoplastic syndrome.[22]

Appropriate workup may include CSF and serum autoimmune encephalopathy
panels including anti-myelin oligodendryocyte glycoprotein (MOG), anti-thyroid antibodies, erythrocyte sedimentation rate (ESR), C-reactive protein (CRP), ferritin, antinuclear antigen (ANA), and anti-neutrophilic cytoplasmic antibody (ANCA). Further
autoantibodies can be considered based on initial results and/or presence of systemic
rheumatologic symptoms. In many cases, immunoglobulins and cell subtypes are sent
prior to initial immunotherapy. CSF and serum cytokine panels are often sent but may
not return in time to guide initial treatment.[23]

### Infectious

Viral encephalitis is the most common etiology among children and adolescents.[24]
Other infectious causes include bacterial and very rarely parasitic and fungal infections.
Early clinical clues to suggest an infectious etiology include fever, rash, respiratory or
gastrointestinal involvement, and history of immunosuppression.[22]

It is important to consider empiric coverage of bacterial meningoencephalitis and
Herpes simplex virus (HSV) while obtaining appropriate workup. Initial studies may
include CSF and blood cultures as well as testing for HSV-1/2, human immunodeficiency virus (HIV), syphilis, SARS-CoV-2, arbovirus panel, and an infectious meningoencephalitis panel or metagenomic next generation sequencing. Regional endemic
pathogens, season-specific pathogens, travel history, recent exposures, and immunologic status can further inform the selection of diagnostic studies.[23,27]

### Genetic and Inborn Errors of Metabolism

While less common, genetic causes should be considered, especially in younger children.[24] NORSE/FIRES may represent an initial presentation of a genetic epilepsy,
including *SCN1A*, *PCDH19*, *DNM1L*, and *POLG*, amongst others.[24,28] Early clinical
clues suggesting genetic etiology are a history of developmental delay, intellectual
disability, and congenital dysmorphisms or brain malformations. Symptoms such as
migraine, strokes, regression, visual and hearing impairment may be seen in mitochondrial disorders.[22]

Initial investigations may include whole exome sequencing, mitochondrial genome
sequencing, and/or chromosomal microarray, in addition to serum, urine, and CSF
small molecule evaluation. The utility of performing comprehensive metabolic workup

in adolescents and young adults is debated but should be considered in patients who did not receive newborn screening or have characteristic features, including a strong family history of metabolic disease.[22,23]

## ACUTE TREATMENT
### Antiseizure Medications and Continuous Infusions

Initial treatment of RSE is typically per institutional protocol, including the escalation of ASMs and continuous infusions (eg, midazolam, pentobarbital, and ketamine) and often induction of burst suppression coma. There are no studies comparing the efficacy of different ASMs.[22]

### Ketogenic Diet

The high-fat, low-carbohydrate ketogenic diet is an established treatment for drug-resistant epilepsy that causes ketosis, often measured by levels of beta-hydroxybutyric acid. Evolving evidence has suggested that the ketogenic diet helps to treat seizures through direct anti-inflammatory effects, including the ability of beta-hydroxybutyric acid to decrease the release of IL-1β through the inhibition of inflammasome assembly.[29] In a cohort of 9 patients with FIRES treated with the ketogenic diet, introduction led to seizure cessation in the majority within 1 week of initiation.[30] A literature review also demonstrated positive effects of the ketogenic diet in 67% of patients with cryptogenic NORSE and 54% with cryptogenic FIRES.[3] A recent systematic review summarized the use of ketogenic diet in 72 children with SRSE, with SE cessation in 60% approximately 6 days after initiation.[31] These results have led to a consensus that ketogenic diet should be initiated in the first week of treatment of NORSE/FIRES and should be continued in prolonged and severe cases.[23]

### First-Line Immunotherapy: Steroids, Intravenous Immunoglobulin, and Plasma Exchange

Consensus guidelines suggest that steroids and/or IVIg be started within 72 hours of seizure onset, after ruling out bacterial infection and HSV/Varicella zoster virus (VZV).[23] A review of the literature demonstrates that steroids and IVIg provide positive effects in 38% and 30% of patients with cryptogenic NORSE, respectively, and 17% and 5% of patients with cryptogenic FIRES, respectively.[3] Additionally, plasma exchange was beneficial in 40% of patients with cryptogenic NORSE and 11% of patients with cryptogenic FIRES,[3] but is often a less favorable option given the requirement of a central line, removal of essential medications including ASMs, and delaying the administration of second-line immunotherapy.

First-line immunotherapy appears more effective in adults than children, which may be due to the higher incidence of antibody-mediated disease in adults.[3,22] Delaying immunotherapy has been associated with worse outcomes in AE,[32] and further studies are needed to better assess this in NORSE/FIRES secondary to AE.[22]

### Second Line Immunotherapies

#### Interleukin-1 blockade: anakinra and canakinumab

Anakinra is an IL-1Ra used to treat several inflammatory diseases. Expert consensus suggests initiating within 1 week if cryptogenic rather than antibody-mediated NORSE/FIRES is suspected and seizures remain refractory despite first-line immunotherapy.[23] An international retrospective case series found that earlier anakinra administration was associated with decreased intensive care unit (ICU) and hospital length of stay and duration of mechanical ventilation in 25 children with FIRES. In this study, at least a 50% seizure reduction was seen within 1 week of anakinra initiation in 11 of 15 patients. Side effects in the series include cytopenias and drug reaction with eosinophilia and systemic symptoms (DRESS), although the latter may be associated with several other medications patients are simultaneously receiving. Infections were not significantly increased and necessitated anakinra discontinuation in only one patient.[33] Use of anakinra has now been reported in over 60 cases, with the suggestion of efficacy in approximately 60%; while overall well-tolerated, the slight majority experience infections.[4] Notably all studies in NORSE/FIRES are retrospective and uncontrolled, and as such, further comparative and controlled studies are needed to understand efficacy, safety profile, and long-term outcomes.

Canakinumab is a monoclonal antibody that binds and neutralizes IL-1β. One case reports an adolescent with refractory seizures after anakinra treatment, who had a 90% reduction in seizure burden after the initiation of canakinumab.[34] While this medication fits well into the understood pathophysiology of NORSE, further research and experience is needed before it is recommended for broader use. Its larger size may prohibit the degree of blood–brain barrier penetration seen with anakinra.[35]

### Interleukin-6 blockade: tocilizumab

Tocilizumab is a monoclonal antibody targeting the IL-6 receptor. In a study of 7 adults with NORSE and ongoing seizures refractory to immunotherapy including rituximab, 6 patients experienced SE cessation within a median of 3 days from tocilizumab initiation and a range of 2 to 10 days.[8] Additionally, children presenting with FIRES, including one refractory to anakinra, experienced seizure cessation and improvement temporally associated with the initiation of tocilizumab.[36,37] Other reports document seizure control after tocilizumab in adolescents and young adults with elevated IL-6, suggesting a potential role for targeted immunotherapy based on cytokine testing, but further investigation is needed.[38,39] Due to relatively less evidence and potentially greater infectious risk, tocilizumab is generally considered if anakinra is ineffective.

### B cell depletion: rituximab

Rituximab is a monoclonal antibody targeting CD20 often used in AE, which is a common underlying etiology of NORSE, particularly in the adult population.[22,32] In cases of cryptogenic NORSE, only one in three patients responded to rituximab.[3] Consensus guidelines suggest that rituximab be used in the treatment of NORSE when an auto-antibody is positive or suspected.[23]

### Intrathecal dexamethasone

A recent series of 6 patients with FIRES assessed the use of intrathecal dexamethasone. All were able to wean continuous infusions and half experienced a decrease in seizure burden by 50%, with 2 being seizure free in short-term follow-up. Earlier administration correlated with decreased length of stay and duration of mechanical ventilation. CSF CXCL10 and neopterin decreased after administration. No significant side effects were reported.[10] Given isolated reports thus far, this has not been included in consensus treatment guidelines at this time.

## CHRONIC TREATMENT

Most patients require chronic treatment with ASMs, with lack of evidence regarding the most effective medications in NORSE/FIRES. One series found cannabidiol initiation was associated with an improvement in seizure burden in 6 of 7 patients with FIRES.[40] Currently, it is not recommended as a first-line ASM, but can be considered as an additional medication in the chronic phase of the disease.[5,23] Expert consensus recommends that if the ketogenic diet is effective acutely, it should be continued for a minimum of 3 months thereafter. If seizures are medically refractory, additional therapies such as vagus nerve stimulation or epilepsy surgery are often considered.[23]

In addition, some patients require ongoing immunotherapy, with recommendation to continue effective immunotherapy for at least 3 months following the acute phase, or restart previously effective immunotherapy if seizures worsen. If immunotherapy was not trialed in the acute phase, anakinra and tocilizumab may be considered in the chronic phase if seizures worsen.[23] There is otherwise currently little evidence to guide immunomodulation in the chronic phase of NORSE, but experience in this area is increasing, including a series noting decreased seizure frequency in 3out of 5 patients treated with anakinra and improvement in an additional patient after switching to tocilizumab.[41]

Due to prolonged ICU stays and hospitalization, patients typically require intensive rehabilitation in the post-acute phase. Neuropsychologic evaluations help determine appropriate therapies and accommodations in school/work if able to return. Most patients benefit from an individualized education plan with frequent re-evaluations to ensure appropriate ongoing support.[23]

## PROGNOSIS

Prognosis remains poor, although most large cohorts reported thus far did not receive second-line immunotherapy. In pediatric cohorts, mortality rates range from 10% to 23% with the majority going on to have epilepsy (>90%), and the minority return to cognitive baseline (cognitive and/or functional decline in 66%–77% of survivors).[2,15,42] A study in 125 adults with NORSE demonstrated a 22% mortality rate, with fair to poor functional outcomes in 60%, and 90% of surviving patients remaining on ASMs.[14] Larger studies are needed in the current era, but a small cohort of 6 patients preliminarily suggests that cognitive outcomes may not be significantly improved despite treatment with anakinra, showing cognitive impairment in all and ongoing decline in 3 patients who had repeat testing.[43]

Variables which correlate with a poor prognosis in the pediatric population include young age, prolonged burst suppression coma, SRSE, non-convulsive SE, and diffuse cortical edema.[2,15,42] Normal MRI has been associated with better outcomes in children.[2] Early leptomeningeal enhancement, subsequent hippocampal sclerosis, duration of SE, and status epilepticus severity score were associated with worse outcomes in adults.[14,44] In a study of 92 children with NORSE (90% FIRES), etiology, duration of SE, and use of methylprednisolone or IVIg were not statistically associated with prognosis, but other cohorts suggest an earlier time to treatment with anakinra or intrathecal dexamethasone may be associated with better short-term outcomes.[10,33,42]

Cytokines may be predictive of outcomes. A decrease in CSF cytokines has been seen after treatment with anakinra and intrathecal dexamethasone and associated with clinical improvement.[10,45] In proteomic analysis, increased CSF IL-6 and CXCL8 associated with more severe disease.[46] Finally, elevation of certain cytokines/chemokines may predict worse outcomes that are sustained for at least several months after discharge from the ICU, including serum IL-6, CCL2, and MIP-1$\alpha$.[11] As such, while further work is needed, these may serve as biomarkers to indicate risk of severe disease and lower threshold to escalate therapy.

While early immunomodulation and decreased duration of anesthetics are associated with better short-term outcomes in some initial studies, more data is needed to assess the long-term effectiveness of immunotherapy in a larger cohort. Although no randomized control trials exist, one systematic review suggests a trend toward better long-term outcomes in patients who received immunotherapy (first- and second-line) than those who did not (41% vs 30%), but this was relatively marginal and not statistically significant.[47]

## SUMMARY

NORSE and FIRES represent presentations of new-onset refractory SE in often previously healthy individuals for which an underlying etiology is identified in only about 50%. Autoimmune and infectious encephalitis are most common in adults and children, respectively. Identifying the presentation relies on recognizing the typical clinical and diagnostic features to embark on early and appropriate targeted immunomodulation. While initial studies are encouraging, larger, controlled studies with long-term follow-up are needed to understand the safety and efficacy of targeting innate immune system dysfunction in these patients, as well as further elucidating biomarkers of disease that may be predictive of outcome.

## CLINICS CARE POINTS

- Early and broad diagnostic evaluation is essential to identify a potential underlying etiology and provide prompt, targeted treatment
- While undergoing diagnostic evaluation, expert consensus guidelines support early initiation of first-line immunotherapy with steroids and/or IVIg and ketogenic diet
- Prognosis generally remains poor with most developing epilepsy and some degree of cognitive decline, and the effect of early, targeted immunomodulation on long-term outcomes in a larger cohort requires further study

## DISCLOSURE

C.M. Stredny receives grant support from the Pediatric Epilepsy Research Foundation, United States. She is a member of the Medical and Scientific Advisory Board of the NORSE Institute. All treatments discussed represent off-label uses.

## REFERENCES

1. Hirsch LJ, Gaspard N, van Baalen A, et al. Proposed consensus definitions for new-onset refractory status epilepticus (NORSE), febrile infection-related epilepsy syndrome (FIRES), and related conditions. Epilepsia 2018;59(4):739–44.
2. Sculier C, Barcia Aguilar C, Gaspard N, et al. Clinical presentation of new onset refractory status epilepticus in children (the pSERG cohort). Epilepsia 2021; 62(7):1629–42.
3. Gaspard N, Hirsch LJ, Sculier C, et al. New-onset refractory status epilepticus (NORSE) and febrile infection-related epilepsy syndrome (FIRES): State of the art and perspectives. Epilepsia 2018;59(4):745–52.
4. Sculier C, Gaspard N. New-onset refractory status epilepticus and febrile infection-related epilepsy syndrome. Curr Opin Neurol 2023;36(2):110–6.
5. Koh S, Wirrell E, Vezzani A, et al. Proposal to optimize evaluation and treatment of Febrile infection-related epilepsy syndrome (FIRES): A Report from FIRES workshop. Epilepsia Open 2021;6(1):62–72.
6. Vezzani A, French J, Bartfai T, et al. The role of inflammation in epilepsy. Nat Rev Neurol 2011;7(1):31–40.

7. van Baalen A, Vezzani A, Hausler M, et al. Febrile Infection-Related Epilepsy Syndrome: Clinical Review and Hypotheses of Epileptogenesis. Neuropediatrics 2017;48(1):5–18.

8. Jun JS, Lee ST, Kim R, et al. Tocilizumab treatment for new onset refractory status epilepticus. Ann Neurol 2018;84(6):940–5.

9. Sakuma H, Tanuma N, Kuki I, et al. Intrathecal overproduction of proinflammatory cytokines and chemokines in febrile infection-related refractory status epilepticus. J Neurol Neurosurg Psychiatry 2015;86(7):820–2.

10. Horino A, Kuki I, Inoue T, et al. Intrathecal dexamethasone therapy for febrile infection-related epilepsy syndrome. Ann Clin Transl Neurol 2021;8(3):645–55.

11. Hanin A, Cespedes J, Dorgham K, et al. Cytokines in New-Onset Refractory Status Epilepticus Predict Outcomes. Ann Neurol 2023. https://doi.org/10.1002/ANA.26627.

12. Saitoh M, Kobayashi K, Ohmori I, et al. Cytokine-related and sodium channel polymorphism as candidate predisposing factors for childhood encephalopathy FIRES/AERRPS. J Neurol Sci 2016;368:272–6.

13. Clarkson BD, LaFrance-Corey RG, Kahoud RJ, et al. Functional deficiency in endogenous interleukin-1 receptor antagonist in patients with febrile infection-related epilepsy syndrome (FIRES). Ann Neurol 2019. https://doi.org/10.1002/ana.25439. Published online.

14. Gaspard N, Foreman BP, Alvarez V, et al. New-onset refractory status epilepticus: Etiology, clinical features, and outcome. Neurology 2015;85(18):1604–13.

15. Kramer U, Chi CS, Lin KL, et al. Febrile infection-related epilepsy syndrome (FIRES): pathogenesis, treatment, and outcome: a multicenter study on 77 children. Epilepsia 2011;52(11):1956–65.

16. Nausch E, Schaffeldt L, Tautorat I, et al. New-onset refractory status epilepticus (NORSE) and febrile infection-related epilepsy syndrome (FIRES) of unknown aetiology: A comparison of the incomparable? Seizure 2022;96:18–21.

17. Van Baalen A, Hausler M, PleckoStartinig B, et al. Febrile infection-related epilepsy syndrome without detectable autoantibodies and response to immunotherapy: A case series and discussion of epileptogenesis in FIRES. Neuropediatrics 2012;43(4):209–16.

18. Farias-Moeller R, Bartolini L, Staso K, et al. Early ictal and interictal patterns in FIRES: The sparks before the blaze. Epilepsia 2017;58(8):1340–8.

19. Meletti S, Giovannini G, dOrsi G, et al. New-Onset Refractory Status Epilepticus with Claustrum Damage: Definition of the Clinical and Neuroimaging Features. Front Neurol 2017;8(MAR). https://doi.org/10.3389/FNEUR.2017.00111.

20. Farias-Moeller R, LaFrance-Corey R, Bartolini L, et al. Fueling the FIRES: Hemophagocytic lymphohistiocytosis in febrile infection-related epilepsy syndrome. Epilepsia 2018;59(9):1753–63.

21. Hanin A, Cespedes J, Huttner A, et al. Neuropathology of New-Onset Refractory Status Epilepticus (NORSE). J Neurol 2023. https://doi.org/10.1007/S00415-023-11726-X.

22. Sculier C, Gaspard N. New onset refractory status epilepticus (NORSE). Seizure 2019;68:72–8. https://doi.org/10.1016/j.seizure.2018.09.018.

23. Wickstrom R, Taraschenko O, Dilena R, et al. International consensus recommendations for management of New Onset Refractory Status Epilepticus (NORSE) including Febrile Infection-Related Epilepsy Syndrome (FIRES): Summary and Clinical Tools. Epilepsia 2022. https://doi.org/10.1111/EPI.17391.

24. Lattanzi S, Leitinger M, Rocchi C, et al. Unraveling the enigma of new-onset re-fractory status epilepticus: a systematic review of aetiologies. Eur J Neurol 2022;29(2):626–47.
25. Van Sonderen A, Schreurs MWJ, De Bruijn MAAM, et al. The relevance of VGKC positivity in the absence of LGI1 and Caspr2 antibodies. Neurology 2016;86(18): 1692–9.
26. Yanagida A, Kanazawa N, Kaneko J, et al. Clinically based score predicting cryp-togenic NORSE at the early stage of status epilepticus. Neurology(R) neuroimmu-nology & neuroinflammation 2020;7(5). https://doi.org/10.1212/NXI.0000000000 000849.
27. Koh S, Wirrell E, Vezzani A, et al. Proposal to optimize evaluation and treatment of Febrile infection-related epilepsy syndrome (FIRES): A Report from FIRES work-shop. Epilepsia Open 2021;6(1):62–72.
28. Varughese RT, Karkare S, Poduri A, et al. Child Neurology: Initial Presentation of PCDH19-Related Epilepsy With New-Onset Refractory Status Epilepticus and Treatment With Anakinra. Neurology 2022;99(5):208–11. https://doi.org/10.1212/ WNL.0000000000200855.
29. Koh S, Dupuis N, Auvin S. Ketogenic diet and Neuroinflammation. Epilepsy Res 2020;167. https://doi.org/10.1016/J.EPLEPSYRES.2020.106454.
30. Nabbout R, Mazzuca M, Hubert P, et al. Efficacy of ketogenic diet in severe re-fractory status epilepticus initiating fever induced refractory epileptic encepha-lopathy in school age children (FIRES). Epilepsia 2010;51(10):2033–7.
31. Schoeler NE, Simpson Z, Zhou R, et al. Dietary Management of Children With Super-Refractory Status Epilepticus: A Systematic Review and Experience in a Single UK Tertiary Centre. Front Neurol 2021;12. https://doi.org/10.3389/FNEUR. 2021.643105.
32. Titulaer MJ, McCracken L, Gabilondo I, et al. Treatment and prognostic factors for long-term outcome in patients with anti-NMDA receptor encephalitis: an observa-tional cohort study. Lancet Neurol 2013;12(2):157–65.
33. Lai YC, Muscal E, Wells E, et al. Anakinra usage in febrile infection related epilepsy syndrome: an international cohort. Ann Clin Transl Neurol 2020;7(12):2467–74.
34. DeSena AD, Do T, Schulert GS. Systemic autoinflammation with intractable epi-lepsy managed with interleukin-1 blockade. J Neuroinflammation 2018;15(1). https://doi.org/10.1186/S12974-018-1063-2.
35. Sjostrom EO, Culot M, Leickt L, et al. Transport study of interleukin-1 inhibitors us-ing a human in vitro model of the blood-brain barrier. Brain Behav Immun Health 2021;16. https://doi.org/10.1016/J.BBIH.2021.100307.
36. Stredny CM, Case S, Sansevere AJ, et al. Interleukin-6 Blockade With Tocilizumab in Anakinra-Refractory Febrile Infection-Related Epilepsy Syndrome (FIRES). Child Neurol Open 2020;7. https://doi.org/10.1177/2329048X20979253. 232904 8X2097925.
37. Cantarin-Extremera V, Jimenez-Legido M, Duat-Rodriguez A, et al. Tocilizumab in pediatric refractory status epilepticus and acute epilepsy: Experience in two patients. J Neuroimmunol 2020;340:577142. https://doi.org/10.1016/j.jneuroim. 2019.577142.
38. Kwack DW, Kim DW. The Increased Interleukin-6 Levels Can Be an Early Diag-nostic Marker for New-Onset Refractory Status Epilepticus. J Epilepsy Res 2022;12(2):78–81. https://doi.org/10.14581/JER.22015.
39. Goh Y, Tay SH, Litt Yeo LL, et al. Bridging the Gap: Tailoring an Approach to Treat-ment in Febrile Infection-Related Epilepsy Syndrome. Neurology 2023. https:// doi.org/10.1212/WNL.0000000000207068.

40. Gofshteyn JS, Wilfong A, Devinsky O, et al. Cannabidiol as a Potential Treatment for Febrile Infection-Related Epilepsy Syndrome (FIRES) in the Acute and Chronic Phases. J Child Neurol 2017;32(1):35–40. https://doi.org/10.1177/08830738166 69450.

41. Aledo-Serrano A, Hariramani R, Gonzalez-Martinez A, et al. Anakinra and tocilizu-mab in the chronic phase of febrile infection-related epilepsy syndrome (FIRES): Effectiveness and safety from a case-series. Seizure 2022;100:51–5. https://doi.org/10.1016/J.SEIZURE.2022.06.012.

42. Wu J, Lan X, Yan L, et al. A retrospective study of 92 children with new-onset re-fractory status epilepticus. Epilepsy Behav 2021;125. https://doi.org/10.1016/J.YEBEH.2021.108413.

43. Shrestha A, Wood EL, Berrios-Siervo G, et al. Long-term neuropsychological out-comes in children with febrile infection-related epilepsy syndrome (FIRES) treated with anakinra. Front Neurol 2023;14. https://doi.org/10.3389/FNEUR.2023.1100551.

44. Kim HJ, Lee SA, Kim HW, et al. The timelines of MRI findings related to outcomes in adult patients with new-onset refractory status epilepticus. Epilepsia 2020; 61(8):1735–48. https://doi.org/10.1111/EPI.16620.

45. Kenney-Jung DL, Vezzani A, Kahoud RJ, et al. Febrile infection-related epilepsy syndrome treated with anakinra. Ann Neurol 2016;80(6):939–45. https://doi.org/10.1002/ana.24806.

46. Wang D, Wu Y, Pan Y, et al. Multi-proteomic Analysis Revealed Distinct Protein Profiles in Cerebrospinal Fluid of Patients Between Anti-NMDAR Encephalitis NORSE and Cryptogenic NORSE. Mol Neurobiol 2023;60(1):98–115. https://doi.org/10.1007/S12035-022-03011-1.

47. Cabezudo-Garcia P, Mena-Vazquez N, Ciano-Petersen NL, et al. Functional out-comes of patients with NORSE and FIRES treated with immunotherapy: A system-atic review. Neurologia 2022. https://doi.org/10.1016/J.NRLENG.2022.03.004.

# Later Onset Congenital Central Hypoventilation Syndrome

Louella Amos, MD

## KEYWORDS

- Later onset congenital central hypoventilation syndrome • Adolescent • PHOX2B

## KEY POINTS

- Increased recognition of the clinical features of congenital central hypoventilation syndrome (CCHS) has led to the discovery of older children with later onset congenital central hypoventilation syndrome.
- Molecular genetic testing for variants in the PHOX2B gene has contributed to this increased identification of individuals with later onset CCHS and asymptomatic family members at risk for developing symptoms.
- Children with CCHS or later onset CCHS will eventually transition to adult primary care providers and subspecialists who will need to understand the pathophysiology and multidisciplinary nature of their lifelong disease.

## INTRODUCTION

Congenital central hypoventilation syndrome (CCHS) is a rare genetic disorder of the autonomic nervous system with the hallmark presentation of hypoxemic, hypercapnic respiratory failure due to abnormal central respiratory control. Mellins and colleagues described the first case report of CCHS in 1970.[1] Since then, approximately 3000 cases have been identified; however, this number is a believed to be an underestimation due to undiagnosed CCHS in individuals who have died from the disease or who have a mild phenotype that has not yet been recognized.[2] The estimated incidence is 1 in 200,000 live births.[3] Diagnosis of CCHS most often occurs during the first month of life. Later onset CCHS (LOCCHS) is defined as diagnosis of CCHS in those older than 1 month. With increased recognition of this congenital disease over the past 20 years and the advent of *PHOX2B* (paired homeobox 2B) genetic testing, LOCCHS has been diagnosed in older children, adolescents, and adults with milder disease phenotype.[4]

Medical College of Wisconsin, Children's Wisconsin, 9000 West Wisconsin Avenue, Milwaukee, WI 53226, USA
*E-mail address:* lamos@mcw.edu

Med Clin N Am 108 (2024) 215–226
https://doi.org/10.1016/j.mcna.2023.05.021
0025-7125/24/© 2023 Elsevier Inc. All rights reserved.

### Clinical Manifestations

The autonomic dysfunction associated with CCHS affects multiple organ systems.[4]

- Respiratory: children exhibit shallow breathing and alveolar hypoventilation with more profound respiratory insufficiency during sleep. They may develop morning headaches and hypersomnia due to hypercapnia. During wakefulness they may be cyanotic without dyspnea.
- Cardiovascular: undiagnosed CCHS with chronic hypoxemia can lead to pulmonary hypertension and right heart failure. Arrhythmias seen in CCHS such as bradycardia, prolonged sinus pause, and brief asystole may present as dizziness or syncope. More subtle manifestations include blood pressure dysregulation and reduced heart rate variability.
- Endocrine: aberrant glycemic control and hyperinsulinism may result in hypoglycemia.
- Gastrointestinal (GI): Hirschsprung disease more commonly presents in the neonatal period but has been diagnosed in late infancy and older children with CCHS. Other GI manifestations include chronic constipation and esophageal dysmotility.
- Ophthalmologic: ophthalmologic examination may reveal pupillary abnormalities (eg, dilated pupils with minimal response to light), anisocoria, convergence insufficiency, and/or strabismus.
- Neurocognitive: chronic hypoxemia and hypercapnia results in cognitive impairment and other neurologic sequelae such as seizures. Hypoglycemia may also cause seizures.
- Oncologic: children with *PHOX2B* nonpolyalanine repeat mutations (NPARMs) have increased risk for neural crest tumors (45%–50%), such as neuroblastomas, ganglioneuromas, and ganglioneuroblastomas, and usually present at an earlier age (mean age of 9 months) than non-CCHS–associated tumors.
- Nonspecific symptoms: temperature dysregulation and profuse sweating are other signs of dysautonomia associated with CCHS. Children may have "boxy" facies characterized by a broad, rectangular facial structure with midface hypoplasia.

### Clinical Manifestations Specific to Later Onset Congenital Central Hypoventilation

Children with LOCCHS present beyond the neonatal period usually because they have a milder respiratory phenotype and do not have ventilatory failure at birth that is characteristic of neonatal CCHS.[2,4] Breath-holding contests and near-drowning incidents associated with underwater swimming can expose the aberrant central respiratory drive in children with LOCCHS. Respiratory illness may trigger alveolar hypoventilation in children with LOCCHS due to their inadequate ventilatory response to hypoxemia and hypercapnia associated with the illness. They may also have recurrent pneumonias and prolonged recovery from severe respiratory illnesses due to an inability to wean from ventilatory support. Treatment of obstructive sleep apnea in affected children may reveal persistent hypoxemia and hypercapnia. Anesthesia also unmasks LOCCHS, as resumption of spontaneous breathing postoperatively typically relies on ventilatory response to carbon dioxide (CO2), which will not occur until the child is fully awake.

### Genetics

If there is clinical suspicion for LOCCHS, molecular genetic testing for heterozygous pathogenic variants in *PHOX2B* can confirm the diagnosis.[4] *PHOX2B* encodes a highly conserved transcription factor essential for the transcription of dopamine beta-hydroxylase and tyrosine hydroxylase, which are enzymes needed for the synthesis of norepinephrine. *PHOX2B* is critical for neural crest differentiation and the development of the autonomic nervous system. Therefore, clinically significant alterations in this gene adversely affect downstream proteins, thereby causing multisystem autonomic dysfunction.[5,6] There are 2 polyalanine repeat regions in exon 3 of *PHOX2B*, and expansion mutations in the second region are associated with CCHS (**Fig. 1**). There are normally 20 alanine repeats in this region. Polyalanine repeat mutations (PARMs) are the most common genetic variants. Children and adults diagnosed with LOCCHS commonly have 24 or 25 PARMs, whereas neonates with CCHS and those with more severe phenotype often have more than or equal to 26 PARMS.[4,7–9] NPARMs such as missense, nonsense, and frameshift variants are less common and have been associated with both neonatal CCHS and LOCCHS[9–12] (**Table 1**).

Genetic testing:

1. *PHOX2B* screening for PARMs and frameshift NPARMs of the second polyalanine repeat region using gel electrophoresis
2. *PHOX2B* sequence analysis to detect PARMs and NPARMs
3. *PHOX2B* duplication/deletion analysis—when PARMs or NPARMs are not detected with the first 2 steps despite clinical signs of CCHS

### Inheritance

A de novo *PHOX2B* pathogenic variant most commonly causes CCHS; however, autosomal dominant inheritance with variable penetrance has been seen in familial cases.[13,14] Genetic counseling helps guide further testing and provides prognostic information, particularly with pregnancy and family planning. Family members of a child with LOCCHS should undergo genetic testing, even if they are asymptomatic, due to the possibility of developing symptoms in the future and risk of passing along a pathogenic variant to their children.[15] Somatic or germline mosaicism may explain the absence of symptoms in a parent with the pathogenic variant, and it is important to keep in mind that this parent's other family members are at risk for disease.[9] Approximately 10% to 25% of children with CCHS have an asymptomatic parent with the same *PHOX2B* variant.[16] Affected children with LOCCHS have a 50% chance of passing their pathogenic variant on to their offspring.

Family history may reveal family members or relatives diagnosed with sudden infant death syndrome (SIDS), sudden unexplained death of childhood, syncope, breath-holding, cyanotic spells, or requiring nocturnal noninvasive ventilatory support.

### Evaluations

Once a child is diagnosed with LOCCHS, they should undergo further diagnostic testing to assess the severity of disease, which includes the following:[2,4,17,18]

- Polysomnography to evaluate multiple variables during wakefulness and sleep, such as an electrocardiogram, pulse oximetry, capnography, airflow, thoracoabdominal respiratory effort, and correlation of these variables with sleep stage.

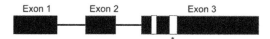

**Fig. 1.** *PHOX2B* gene and the 2 polyalanine repeat regions in exon 3 highlighted in white. The asterisk identifies the 20 polyalanine repeat region where the expansion mutations associated with CCHS occur.

**Table 1**
**Genotype-phenotype correlation[2,4]**

| Phenotype | 20/24, 20/25 PARM | 20/26 PARM | 20/27 PARM | NPARM |
|---|---|---|---|---|
| Hypoventilation | Asleep | Asleep ± awake | Asleep ± awake | Asleep ± awake |
| Cardiac arrhythmia | Possible—can develop with age | Yes | Yes | No |
| Hirschsprung disease | Rare | Yes | Yes | Yes |
| Severe constipation | Yes | Yes | Yes | Yes |
| Neural crest tumors | No | No | No | Yes |

Sleep-related hypoventilation is defined as having a $Pco_2$ greater than 55 mm Hg for at least 10 minutes or having an increase in $Pco_2$ of at least 10 mm Hg greater than baseline/awake $Pco_2$ and greater than 50 mm Hg for at least 10 minutes[19] (**Fig. 2**; *AASM scoring manual version 3*).

- Respiratory responsiveness to physiologic challenges (hypercarbia, hypoxemia)
- Blood gas measurements during wakefulness and sleep to assess for hypercapnia
- Serum bicarbonate as a marker of severity and chronicity of the hypoventilation
- Hemoglobin and hematocrit to monitor for polycythemia associated with chronic hypoxemia
- Sevety-two hour Holter monitoring for episodes of sinus pause or asystole
- Echocardiogram screening for signs of pulmonary hypertension or right heart failure due to chronic hypoxemia
- Cardiopulmonary exercise challenge test particularly in children or teenagers interested in organized sports

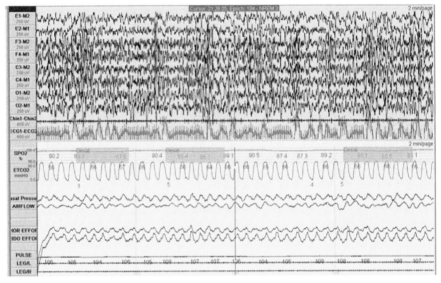

**Fig. 2.** A 2-minute epoch from an overnight polysomnogram performed on a 6-year-old child with LOCCHS. The child is in NREM 3 sleep, the SPO2 is in the 80s, and the end tidal CO2 is in the 60s. Despite hypoxemia and hypercapnia, she maintains a monotonous respiratory rate of 20 breaths per minute, which does not compensate for her abnormal oximetry and capnography.

- GI consultation if there is concern about esophageal dysmotility or chronic constipation
- Screening for neural crest tumors in children with NPARMs: urine catecholamines (homovanillic acid and vanillylmandelic acid), chest radiograph (mediastinal evaluation), abdominal ultrasound (adrenal and abdominal evaluation)
- Complete ocular examination by an ophthalmologist to evaluate for associated ophthalmologic abnormalities
- Neurocognitive assessment
- Comprehensive autonomic testing (if available)

### Treatment

- Respiratory:[2,4,17,18]

Chronic mechanical ventilation provides children with LOCCHS the life sustaining treatment of their central hypoventilation. Neonates with CCHS often require invasive ventilation via tracheostomy due to respiratory failure at birth and their need for 24-hour ventilatory support. Children with LOCCHS may also need invasive ventilation if they are unable to wean off continuous ventilatory support after a severe respiratory illness, if nocturnal noninvasive ventilation (NIV) via mask interface inadequately treats their hypoventilation, or if they do not tolerate nocturnal NIV. More commonly, however, nocturnal NIV can sufficiently support children with LOCCHS who do not exhibit hypoventilation during wakefulness. Ventilator settings should maintain the SPO2 greater than or equal to 95% and $Pco_2$ 35 to 45 mm Hg, and sleep study titration orders should explicitly state these respiratory parameters for the sleep lab respiratory therapists titrating the ventilator settings. When the SPO2 decreases to less than 95% during sleep, the $Pco_2$ will simultaneously increase, signifying insufficient ventilatory support, which requires intervention. Oxygen saturations continue to decrease and do not recover until an adjustment is made to the ventilator settings, mask/tracheostomy leak is addressed as a contributing factor, or until the child is awoken.

For those requiring 24-hour mechanical ventilation, diaphragmatic pacing can help maintain ventilation during wakefulness and liberate them from the ventilator during the day, thereby optimizing their quality of life. Children with LOCCHS usually do not undergo diaphragmatic pacer placement because they usually only require nocturnal ventilatory support.

Respiratory stimulants such as caffeine and acetazolamide do not restore the deficient central respiratory drive in children with CCHS. Progesterone augments ventilation in pregnant women by increasing the central chemosensitivity to CO2. A case report of 2 women with CCHS showed improved ventilation and chemosensitivity on the oral contraceptive progestin medication, desogestrel.[20] Other studies have not yet replicated this effect, but it suggests the possible benefit of progestin medications for oral contraception in adolescent and adult women with CCHS.

- Cardiovascular:

Children with evidence of bradycardia, prolonged sinus pause, or asystole require pacemaker placement and long-term follow-up with Pediatric Cardiology.

- Endocrine:

Children with LOCCHS do not usually present with the abnormal glycemic control and severe hypoglycemia that neonates with CCHS may have. Endocrine management may include the use of diazoxide and frequent glucose monitoring with intervention as needed to maintain normal glucose levels.

- GI:

Hirschsprung disease (HD) or large bowel dysmotility may manifest as severe, chronic constipation, warranting evaluation in any patient with CCHS with suggestive symptoms regardless of age. Rectal suction biopsy is the gold standard for diagnosing HD although anorectal manometry may also detect abnormalities characteristic of HD. Treatment of HD involves surgical resection of the affected gut and dietary modifications.

- Ophthalmologic:

Early recognition and treatment of refractive error, convergence insufficiency, and strabismus helps minimize the risk for learning difficulties and permanent visual impairment due to amblyopia.

- Neurocognitive:

Recognition and treatment of the underlying hypoxia or hypercapnia will help minimize the cognitive impairment. It is important to monitor the glucose levels to prevent hypoglycemic seizures.

- Oncologic:

Early referral to Pediatric Oncology for children at risk for neural crest tumors (NPARMs) may facilitate surveillance (**Table 2**) and timely treatment of the tumor if discovered.

## Differential Diagnosis

### Rapid-onset obesity with hypothalamic dysfunction

Rapid onset obesity with hypothalamic dysfunction (ROHHAD), hypoventilation, and autonomic dysregulation is a rare disorder characterized by rapid weight gain (up to 40 lbs.) over 4 to 6 months between ages 2 and 7 years and hypothalamic abnormalities such as elevated prolactin, hypothyroidism, diabetes insipidus or syndrome of inappropriate antidiuretic hormone secretion, and/or growth hormone insufficiency. Children eventually develop chronic respiratory insufficiency/failure with hypoxia and hypercapnia, and some develop neural crest tumors. Approximately 40% of patients with ROHHAD may have a neural crest tumor such as a ganglioneuroma or ganglioneuroblastoma. The autonomic dysfunction in ROHHAD includes temperature dysregulation, bradycardia, pupillary abnormalities, and decreased pain perception. ROHHAD was initially known as "late onset central hypoventilation with hypothalamic dysfunction" but was renamed in 2007 to ROHHAD. To date, there is no known cause for ROHHAD, which is diagnosed based on clinical presentation, diagnostic evaluations, and negative molecular genetic testing for CCHS.

### Other

Other disorders that can present with sleep-related hypoventilation include neuromuscular disease, intracranial abnormalities such as a posterior fossa tumor or Chiari malformation, and Prader Willi syndrome (PWS). Neurologic examination, pulmonary function testing, and other diagnostic testing (electromyography, muscle biopsy) can differentiate neuromuscular disorders from CCHS. MRI brain can identify posterior fossa abnormalities that would cause aberrant central control of breathing. As

**Table 2**
Surveillance[4,17,18]

| System | PHOX2B Variant | Test | Frequency |
|---|---|---|---|
| Respiratory | All | Comprehensive physiologic testing of SPO2, CO2, and cardiorespiratory monitoring during wakefulness and sleep; CBC evaluating for polycythemia; HCO3 evaluating for chronic hypoventilation | < 2 year old: every 6 mo<br>≥ 2 year old: yearly and as needed at shorter intervals |
| Cardiology | All | 72-h Holter monitoring, echocardiogram, and blood pressure | Yearly |
| Gastroenterology | All | Clinical history and examination evaluating for constipation | Yearly |
| Ophthalmology | All | Comprehensive ocular testing | Yearly |
| Neuropsychology | All | Comprehensive neurocognitive testing | < 3 year old: every 6 mo<br>≥ 3 year old: yearly |
| Oncology | 20/28–20/33 PARMs, NPARMs | Chest and abdominal imaging, urine catecholamines | < 2 year old: every 6 mo<br>2–7 years old: yearly<br>> 7 year old: per pediatric oncology protocol<br>*tumor surveillance is not usually recommended after age 10* |
| Dentistry | All on NIV | Examination for maxillary retrusion or development of midface hypoplasia | Yearly |

an adjunct to clinical evaluation, genetic testing definitively distinguishes other genetic disorders such as PWS from CCHS.[21]

## Special Considerations

### Exercise

Children and adolescents with LOCCHS can participate in sports and moderate exercise, but they need to take frequent breaks, particularly with intense activity because they have an altered perception of dyspnea due to hypoxia or hypercapnia. Interestingly, mechanoreceptors sensing movement in the extremities may stimulate breathing in children with CCHS and help them maintain adequate ventilation during exercise.[22–25] Cardiopulmonary exercise challenge testing may provide information about their ventilatory and cardiovascular response to intense activity. They can engage in closely supervised swimming but with limited submersion time underwater due to the lack of hypoxia-induced dyspnea.

### Air travel

Most commercial aircrafts pressurize the cabin to 7000 to 8000 feet altitude, which results in an $Fio_2$ less than 21%. Children with LOCCHS do not increase their minute ventilation in response to the relative decrease in $Fio_2$, may require ventilatory support while in flight, and therefore will need to bring their ventilators onto the airplane. Supplemental oxygen alone may help their oxygenation but would not treat their hypercapnia. In addition, portable oxygen concentrators are not approved for use in children, and personal oxygen tanks cannot be taken on airplanes, resulting in challenges to air travel.

### Anesthesia

Preoperative planning for procedures can help prevent postoperative complications. Anesthesia staff reviewing patient charts before procedures should familiarize themselves with the intrinsic ventilatory abnormalities in children with LOCCHS, which may alter the anesthetic agents chosen for the procedure and method of emergence from anesthesia used after the procedure. Short-acting medications, such as propofol, and regional anesthesia when possible are preferred due to the effect all anesthetic agents have on central respiratory drive and wakefulness.

### Alcohol/substance abuse

Parents and medical providers must counsel adolescents regarding the dangers of alcohol use and other recreational drugs that are known respiratory depressants. This awareness should continue into adulthood when they are of legal age to consume alcohol.

### Transition

As children and adolescents with LOCCHS age, they will eventually need to see adult primary care and subspecialists. Young adults often do not seek medical care regularly; however, those with LOCCHS need at least annual visits with their primary care providers and subspecialists. The medical providers and subspecialists who care for adolescents and young adults with LOCCHS need to be aware of the risk for sudden death, the lifelong need for chronic ventilatory support, and the multisystem involvement in this disease, which requires organized, multidisciplinary management. Early discussion regarding transition during early adolescence, identifying potential medical providers for this transition, and even making an appointment with these providers before official transition may facilitate the process and decrease the anxiety that is often associated with transition of care from pediatric to adult providers.

## CASE PRESENTATION

A 10-year-old female patient presents to the local emergency room with upper respiratory infection symptoms, cyanosis, and increased lethargy. Her SPO2 on room air is 50%, so she is placed on 4LPM oxygen, which increases her SPO2 to 90%. Her $P_{CO_2}$ on a capillary blood gas (CBG) is 45 mm Hg. Pediatric transport transfers her to the nearest pediatric intensive care unit (ICU) and en route she desaturates to the 80s on oxygen, but saturations improve with cough and deep breathing. On arrival to the pediatric ICU, her saturations are 97% on 4LPM oxygen. She remains on supplemental oxygen overnight, and the next morning, she is obtunded and $P_{CO_2}$ on the CBG is 160 mm Hg. Her chest radiograph exhibits bilateral pulmonary edema and an enlarged cardiac silhouette. Her echocardiogram shows elevated right ventricular pressures with flattening of the interventricular septum. On further questioning, family history reveals a sibling who died suddenly as a toddler due to "SIDS." Her mother states that she has always had "apneas" during sleep and that she is often difficult to wake in the morning. She is extubated to bilevel positive airway pressure and eventually tolerates weaning off positive pressure during the day. Overnight diagnostic polysomnography off noninvasive ventilation shows no obstructive sleep apnea but persistent hypoxemia and hypercapnia with end tidal CO2 in the 60s throughout most of the night with a $P_{CO_2}$ of 60 mm Hg on the morning capillary blood gas. Molecular genetic testing for CCHS reveals a *PHOX2B* 20/25 PARM.

## DISCUSSION

This case illustrates one of the potential clinical presentations of LOCCHS.

- Older child with a respiratory illness
- Profound hypoxia, which clinically manifests as cyanosis and lethargy rather than dyspnea
- High normal $P_{CO_2}$ during wakefulness but severe hypercapnia during sleep causing her obtunded mental status the next morning
- Signs of increased pulmonary and right ventricular pressures on echocardiogram due to severe hypoxemia on presentation, which may have been present for several days or longer before presentation
- Diagnostic polysomnography shows sleep-related hypoventilation throughout the night
- Molecular genetic testing reveals a 20/25 PARM in *PHOX2B*
- Sudden unexplained death in a toddler sibling, suggesting that other family members may have CCHS and the same *PHOX2B* variant

## SUMMARY

Diagnosis of CCHS no longer occurs solely during the neonatal period. Increased recognition of the clinical presentation has led to the diagnosis of LOCCHS in older children, adolescents, and adults who did not exhibit the hallmark symptom of hypoxemic, hypercapneic respiratory failure at birth. Molecular genetic testing for *PHOX2B* variants in individuals with LOCCHS most commonly uncovers a 20/24 PARM, 20/25 PARM, or NPARM. As in neonates with CCHS, a multidisciplinary approach to treatment optimizes the management of and surveillance for potential multiorgan complications associated with LOCCHS. As adolescents with LOCCHS transition to adulthood, adult medical providers should also acknowledge the importance of multidisciplinary management, regular surveillance, and anticipatory guidance for young adults with LOCCHS as they take over their care.

## CLINICS CARE POINTS

- Since the advent of *PHOX2B* genetic testing, approximately 3000 cases of neonatal CCHS and LOCCHS have been reported.
- External factors such as a respiratory illness, anesthesia, or treatment of obstructive sleep apnea may unmask hypoxemic, hypercapneic respiratory failure in older children and adolescents with LOCCHS.
- Definitive diagnosis requires molecular genetic testing for *PHOX2B* variants.
- Parents and family members of the affected child should also undergo genetic testing due to potential for autosomal dominant inheritance with variable penetrance within the family. Asymptomatic family members with the PHOX2B variant may develop LOCCHS symptoms in the future. Genetic counseling can provide guidance regarding testing and family planning.
- Symptomatic children with LOCCHS often require nocturnal ventilatory support, either invasively through a tracheostomy or noninvasively using a mask interface.
- Long-term management includes, but is not limited to, yearly polysomnography on nocturnal ventilatory support, Holter monitor recording for cardiac arrhythmias, and clinical surveillance for other system involvement (suh as GI dysmotility, endocrine, ocular abnormalities, or autonomic dysregulation).
- It is important to provide anticipatory guidance regarding aspects of adolescent life, including the management of respiratory illnesses, exercising with moderation, and the dangers of alcohol or recreational substance use.
- Transition to adult medicine will require a primary care provider as the medical home and referral to adult subspecialists due to the multisystem involvement in LOCCHS. Early discussion with the family, collaborative identification of potential adult medical providers, and transition during a period of medical stability will streamline the handoff and decrease the potential anxiety associated with this milestone.

## DISCLOSURE

The author has no commercial or financial conflicts of interest related to this article and there was no funding.

## REFERENCES

1. Mellins RB, Balfour HH Jr, Turino GM, et al. Failure of automatic control of ventilation (Ondine's curse). Report of an infant born with this syndrome and review of the literature. Medicine (Baltim) 1970;49:487–504.
2. Weese-Mayer D.E., Rand C.M., Khaytin I., et al., Congenital central hypoventilation syndrome. 2004 (Updated 2021 Jan 28). In: GeneReviews® [Internet]. Seattle (WA): University of Washington, Seattle; 1993-2004.
3. Trang H, Dehan M, Beaufils F, et al. The French congenital central hypoventilation syndrome registry: general data, phenotype and genotype. Chest 2005;127:72–9.
4. Weese-Mayer DE, Berry-Kravis EM, Ceccherini I, et al. An official ATS clinical policy statement: congenital central hypoventilation syndrome: genetic basis, diagnosis, and management. Am J Respir Crit Care Med 2010;181:626–44.
5. Pattyn A, Morin X, Cremer H, et al. The homeobox gene Phox2b is essential for the development of autonomic neural crest derivatives. Nature 1999;399:366–70.
6. Pattyn A, Goridis C, Brunet JF. Specification of the central noradrenergic phenotype by the homeobox gene Phox2b. Mol Cell Neurosci 2000;15:235–43.

7. Kasi AS, Kun SS, Keens TG, et al. Adult with PHOX2B Mutation and late onset congenital central hypoventilation syndrome. J Clin Sleep Med 2018;14:2079–81.

8. Magalhães J, Madureira N, Medeiros R, et al. Late-onset congenital central hypoventilation syndrome and a rare PHOX2B gene mutation. Sleep Breath 2015;19: 55–60.

9. Trochet D, de Pontual L, Straus C, et al. PHOX2B germline and somatic mutations in late-onset central hypoventilation syndrome. Am J Respir Crit Care Med 2008; 177:906–11.

10. Loghmanee DA, Rand CM, Zhou L, et al. Clinical features of subjects with non-polyalanine repeat mutations (NPARM) in the PHOX2B gene. Pediatr Res 2008; E-PAS2008:6356.

11. Ditmer M, Turkiewicz S, Gabryelska A, et al. Adolescent Congenital Central Hypoventilation Syndrome: An Easily Overlooked Diagnosis. Int J Environ Res Public Health 2021;18:13402.

12. Matera I, Bachetti T, Puppo F, et al. PHOX2B mutations and polyalanine expansions correlate with the severity of the respiratory phenotype and associated symptoms in both congenital and late onset central hypoventilation syndrome. J Med Genet 2004;41:373–80.

13. Berry-Kravis EM, Zhou L, Rand CM, et al. Congenital central hypoventilation syndrome: PHOX2B mutations and phenotype. Am J Respir Crit Care Med 2006;174: 1139–44.

14. Parodi S, Bachetti T, Lantieri F, et al. Parental origin and somatic mosaicism of PHOX2B mutations in congenital central hypoventilation syndrome. Hum Mutat 2008;29:206.

15. Hino A, Terada J, Kasai H, et al. Adult cases of late-onset congenital central hypoventilation syndrome and paired-like homeobox 2B-mutation carriers: an additional case report and pooled analysis. J Clin Sleep Med 2020;16: 1891–900.

16. Bachetti T, Parodi S, Di Duca M, et al. Low amounts of PHOX2B expanded alleles in asymptomatic parents suggest unsuspected recurrence risk in congenital central hypoventilation syndrome. J Mol Med 2011;89:505–13.

17. Trang H, Samuels M, Ceccherini I, et al. Guidelines for diagnosis and management of congenital central hypoventilation syndrome. Orphanet J Rare Dis 2020;15:252.

18. Kasi S, Li H, Harford K, et al. Congenital Central Hypoventilation Syndrome: Optimizing Care with a Multidisciplinary Approach. J Multidiscip Healthc 2022;15: 455–69.

19. Troester MM, Quan SF, Berry RB, et al. For the American academy of sleep medicine. *The AASM manual for the Scoring of Sleep and associated events: rules, Terminology and technical specifications.* IL: American Academy of Sleep Medicine; 2023. Version 3. Darien.

20. Straus C, Trang H, Becquemin M, et al. Chemosensitivity recovery in Ondine's curse syndrome under treatment with desogestrel. Respir Physiol Neurobiol 2010;171:171–4.

21. Cielo C, Marcus CL. Central Hypoventilation Syndromes. Sleep Med Clin 2014 Mar 1;9:105–18.

22. Gozal D, Marcus CL, Ward SL, et al. Ventilatory responses to passive leg motion in children with congenital central hypoventilation syndrome. Am J Respir Crit Care Med 1996;153:761–8.

23. Gozal D, Simakajornboon N. Passive motion of the extremities modifies alveolar ventilation during sleep in patients with congenital central hypoventilation syndrome. Am J Respir Crit Care Med 2000;162:1747–51.
24. Paton JY, Swaminathan S, Sargent CW, et al. Ventilatory response to exercise in children with congenital central hypoventilation syndrome. Am Rev Respir Dis 1993;147:1185–91.
25. Shea SA, Andres LP, Shannon DC, et al. Ventilatory responses to exercise in humans lacking ventilatory chemosensitivity. J Physiol 1993;468:623–40.

# Chronic Recurrent Multifocal Osteomyelitis

Bridget A. Rafferty, MD, MPH, MFA[a], Pooja Thakrar, MD[b],*

## KEYWORDS

- Chronic recurrent multifocal osteomyelitis • CRMO • CNO • Bone pain
- Whole-body MRI

## KEY POINTS

- Children with chronic recurrent multifocal osteomyelitis (CRMO) typically present with nonspecific bone pain at a single site.
- CRMO is an autoinflammatory disorder thought to be triggered by an imbalance between pro- and antiinflammatory cytokines.
- Early recognition and treatment of CRMO can help to obviate debilitating skeletal deformities and chronic pain.

## INTRODUCTION

Chronic recurrent multifocal osteomyelitis (CRMO) is an idiopathic condition for which no consensus definition exists. As its name suggests, the disease manifests as inflammatory bone lesions, often in multiple sites and frequently with a relapsing and remitting course. Various categorizations of CRMO have been attempted, but none have been fully adopted within the pediatric community. In particular, because some patients present with a single lesion and have no subsequent manifestations, the name *chronic nonbacterial osteomyelitis* (CNO) has been more recently suggested, with CRMO reserved for the more severe form of the disease (**Box 1**). Patients initially present with focal bone pain and soft tissue swelling, leading to evaluation for a musculoskeletal pathology. Radiographs are often unremarkable. Persistent and/or migratory pain then leads to further testing to assess for leukocytosis or elevated inflammatory markers. Often, multidisciplinary evaluation by specialties including infectious disease, oncology, rheumatology, and pediatric radiology is undertaken before the diagnosis is reached. CRMO is estimated to evade diagnosis by an average of 15 months to 2 years, as recognition of the disease is challenging due to its vague symptoms and obscure nature, and it becomes a diagnosis of exclusion.[1,2]

[a] Medical College of Wisconsin, 8701 W. Watertown Plank Road, Milwaukee, WI 53226, USA;
[b] Medical College of Wisconsin/Children's Wisconsin, 9000 W. Wisconsin Avenue, MS-721, Milwaukee, WI 53226, USA
* Corresponding author.
*E-mail address:* pthakrar@childrenswi.org

Med Clin N Am 108 (2024) 227–239
https://doi.org/10.1016/j.mcna.2023.05.022
0025-7125/24/© 2023 Elsevier Inc. All rights reserved.

> **Box 1**
> **Historical names for chronic nonbacterial osteomyelitis and associated diseases in the chronic nonbacterial osteomyelitis spectrum**
>
> Chronic multifocal symmetric osteomyelitis
>
> Chronic nonbacterial osteomyelitis (CNO)
>
> Chronic recurrent multifocal osteomyelitis (CRMO)
>
> Clavicular hyperostosis and acne arthritis
>
> Diffuse sclerosing osteomyelitis
>
> Nonbacterial osteitis (NBO)
>
> Pustulotic arthro-osteitis
>
> Symmetric multifocal osteomyelitis
>
> Synovitis, acne, pustulosis, hyperostosis, osteitis (SAPHO) syndrome

### Symptoms/Presentation

CRMO typically presents with bone pain and tenderness at a single affected site, which may be accompanied by overlying soft tissue swelling, erythema, and decreased range of motion. The onset of the disease is often insidious with vague symptoms. Although systemic signs such as fever, weight loss, and malaise may be present, they are uncommon. In addition, the typical findings of bone pain and soft tissue swelling, particularly in active children, may initially be attributed to sequelae of physical activity. Presentation for medical care may therefore be delayed, occurring days to years after initial symptom onset.

Patients are most often brought to initial attention with unifocal bone pain that characteristically affects the limbs, sacroiliac joints, or spine, although symptoms may instead reflect involvement of smaller bones, including the mandible, clavicle, scapula, sternum, ribs, or bones of the hands and feet.[3–6] Many will have additional clinically silent lesions that are discovered only after imaging is performed.[5,7] Other patients will become symptomatic at additional sites within a short period of time, cycling through relapses in a variety of locations, often in a symmetric pattern.[4,6,8–10] There is also a subset of patients with comorbidities involving other systems, including the skin, gastrointestinal tract, or joints.[2]

Classic areas of involvement by CRMO, including the clavicle and mandible, may guide the provider to the diagnosis. CRMO is the most common disease to affect the medial clavicle.[8] Unfortunately, CRMO more often involves the metaphyses of the long bones of the lower extremities (in particular, the tibia and femur), the pelvis, and the spine. Nevertheless, when the clavicle or mandible is involved, the unusual location should prompt suspicion for CRMO, particularly when unifocal and in the absence of trauma.

There is overlap between CRMO and other autoimmune conditions such that up to half of patients with CRMO develop associated skin, joint, or gastrointestinal manifestations.[8,11–13] Cutaneous involvement may be with psoriasis, palmoplantar pustulosis, pyoderma gangrenosum, or severe acne. Psoriatic arthritis, juvenile idiopathic arthritis (JIA), or enthesitis-related arthritis occurs in up to half of patients with CRMO, and inflammatory bowel disease can also be seen in association with the disease.[5,14] Patients with such extraosseous manifestations tend to have greater inflammatory activity.[5]

CRMO can be self-limiting, chronically active, or recurrent. Its course can run over months to multiple years.[15] Significant morbidity can occur in patients who develop lesions in the spinal column or lesions that involve the growing ends of long bones. Untreated spinal lesions can lead to fractures or vertebra plana deformities, which may in turn result in debilitating scoliotic or kyphotic deformities with neurologic manifestations and continued impairment in the growing skeleton.[6] Lesions at the ends of the long bones may lead to physeal bridge formation, which can cause limb-shortening and angular deformities.[3,16] For patients with spinal or growth plate involvement, interventions can help to prevent or mitigate long-term damage.

### Epidemiology

CRMO has previously been thought to be a rare disease, reported in just over 500 patients in the literature.[17] However, its incidence is likely underestimated as a result of underdiagnosis owing to poor awareness of the disease, both in the medical community and in the general public, and to a lack of accepted diagnostic criteria. The exact occurrence of CRMO is unknown, but estimates of its prevalence range from 1:160,000 to 1:2,000,000, with an annual incidence of 1:250,000 to 1:1,000,000.[9,18] Many estimates place the prevalence of CRMO at the same level as that of bacterial osteomyelitis.

There is no clear geographic distribution for CRMO, although the disease is more frequently reported in European populations. However, this may result from underdiagnosis and underreporting in other regions, coupled with an absence of national registry data in some countries.[2,19] Most of the epidemiologic data for CRMO is from "small case studies and regional cohorts," limiting generalizability of the data.[19]

The peak age of onset of CRMO is between 7 and 12 years with an average age of 10 years, although the disease can occur in patients of any age. CRMO is uncommon in children younger than 2 years, and if concerning signs and symptoms are found in younger children, an alternative diagnosis should first be considered.[18] CRMO is more common in girls, demonstrating a 2:1 or as high as 4:1 female to male predominance.[12–14,20–24] Associated autoimmune conditions are seen with varying frequency: cutaneous manifestations occur in 10% to 30%, gastrointestinal disease in 5% to 13%, and arthritis in 5% to 56% of patients.[11–13,25] Male gender, the presence of an associated inflammatory syndrome, multifocal disease, and a long duration of symptoms before diagnosis portend a worse prognosis.[5,13]

### Pathophysiology

The pathophysiology of CRMO is incompletely understood. In normal individuals, exposure to an offending agent yields an immune response that depends on action by both proinflammatory and immune-regulatory cytokines. Immune-regulatory, or antiinflammatory, cytokines are necessary to control immune responses and limit inflammation. In patients with autoinflammatory conditions such as CRMO, dysregulation of the immune response is thought to be caused by an imbalance of cytokine expression with underexpression of regulatory cytokines and overexpression of proinflammatory cytokines.[26,27]

Innate immune cells from untreated patients with more severe manifestations of CRMO, including monocytes and macrophages, have been shown to respond inappropriately to stimulation by inflammatory antigens.[19,26] When exposed to toll-like receptor 4 with lipopolysaccharide (a structure in the outer membrane of gram-negative bacteria), these immune cells failed to produce interleukin-10 (IL-10) and decreased production of its homologue IL-19, both immune-regulatory cytokines. In normal individuals, expression of these cytokines is upregulated in response to such stimuli.

Decreased production of IL-10 and IL-19 in patients with CRMO is thought to result at least in part from diminished activation of 2 mitogen-activated protein kinases (MAPK) called extracellular signal-related kinase (ERK) 1 and ERK2, which in turn leads to decreased recruitment of signaling proteins to IL-10 and IL-19 promoters.[19]

In contrast, expression of IL-20, a proinflammatory cytokine, is increased in patients with CRMO. This increase may result from a combination of diminished inhibition by IL-10 and decreased methylation of an IL-20 promoter. DNA methylation decreases gene expression; hence, reduced methylation of the IL-20 gene may allow for increased IL-20 expression. Expression of the proinflammatory cytokines tumor necrosis factor alpha (TNF-$\alpha$) and IL-6 is also increased in patients with CRMO. Both of these cytokines depend on activation of MAPK pathways, but these pathways are distinct from those of IL-10 and IL-19, and their activation seems to be unaffected.[19,26]

Observations in patients with CRMO and animal models seem to support the notion that the imbalance of these pro- and antiinflammatory cytokines leads to bone inflammation. In addition, some data suggest that this cytokine imbalance, and in particular the overexpression of TNF-$\alpha$, increases interactions between the receptor activator of nuclear factor-$\kappa$B surface receptor and its ligand on osteoclast progenitor cells, leading to increased osteoclast differentiation and activation.[18,19] Increased osteoclastogenesis, in turn, can lead to further inflammatory bone loss and the physical presentation of focal bone pain.[18,28]

Although CRMO is a disease of inflammation, there are inconsistent results when examining the levels of common inflammatory markers such as erythrocyte sedimentation rate (ESR), C-reactive protein (CRP), and antinuclear antibody in patients with active disease. When inflammatory marker levels are abnormal, those most commonly elevated are ESR and CRP; however, their elevation (or a lack thereof) does not correlate with disease severity.[2,16,18]

As a result of its involvement of the growing skeleton, CRMO can lead to chronic and debilitating skeletal deformities. Lesions that involve the metaphyses may disrupt normal chondrocyte apoptosis and endochondral ossification and allow physeal chondrocytes to violate the metaphysis, leading to development of physeal "tongues."[4] Lesions involving the physes can allow vasculature to grow between the metaphysis and the epiphysis; osteoprogenitor cells along these transphyseal vessels deposit bone, resulting in development of physeal bridges.[29] These types of abnormal bone deposition in skeletally immature patients can lead to angular and limb-shortening deformities.

### Diagnosis

Because CRMO typically presents with bone pain, imaging of the affected site is often performed to evaluate for trauma, infection, or a bone lesion. Radiographs are the first-line imaging modality but are insensitive. Radiographic findings vary widely depending on the duration of the flare, including normal findings in early disease (**Fig. 1**). Once the disease is radiographically apparent, its features may mimic neoplastic or aggressive infectious processes, beginning with lytic lesions and periosteal reaction and progressing to adjacent sclerosis (**Figs. 2** and **3**).

MRI is the gold standard for diagnosis of CRMO. MRI is more sensitive and more specific for identification of CRMO lesions than either the clinical examination or other imaging modalities. Targeted MRI can be used to identify lesions when radiographs are negative or to further characterize lesions seen by radiography (see **Figs. 1–3**).

The appearance of CRMO on MRI can be similar to other bone lesions, including infectious osteomyelitis and bone tumors, in that CRMO causes bone marrow edema

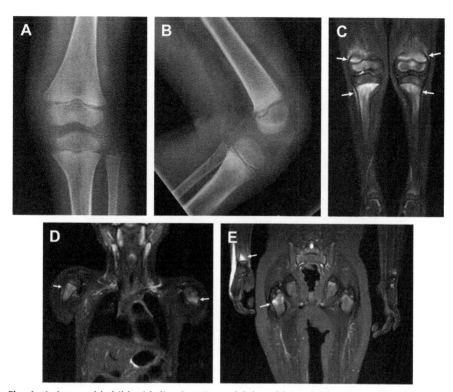

**Fig. 1.** A 4-year-old child with limping. Frontal (*A*) and lateral (*B*) radiographs of the left knee appear normal. Follow-up whole-body survey MRI for unremitting symptoms reveals bone marrow edema in the bilateral distal femoral and bilateral proximal tibial metaphyses (*C*), as well as additional sites of marrow edema in the bilateral proximal humeral metaphyses (*D*), the right distal radial metaphysis and right proximal femur (*E*), and the left distal radial metaphysis (not shown). The (*white arrows*) indicate bone marrow edema in the bilateral distal femoral and bilateral proximal tibial metaphyses in (*C*), bone marrow edema in the bilateral proximal humeral metaphyses in (*D*), and bone marrow edema in the right distal radial metaphysis and right proximal femur in (*E*).

and periosteal inflammation. However, in contradistinction to infectious osteomyelitis, the degree of surrounding soft tissue inflammation is typically less, and soft tissue abscesses are vanishingly rare. In the spine, bacterial osteomyelitis tends to involve the intervertebral disc, whereas CRMO does not. Unlike with malignant bone tumors, soft tissue masses are not seen with CRMO. Bone metastases of other malignancies typically have sharp borders rather than amorphous marrow edema, and leukemia and lymphoma in the bone cause marrow replacement instead of edema. Langerhans cell histiocytosis (LCH) commonly involves the skull, whereas CRMO does not, and LCH is more commonly seen in the diaphyses of long bones than in the periphyseal locations.[4]

When CRMO is suspected on targeted MRI or other imaging, the best next step is to perform a whole-body MRI (WB-MRI) to evaluate for additional lesions (see **Figs. 1–3**). WB-MRI is used in both screening for lesions and monitoring their progression.[4] Studies using WB-MRI at diagnosis have found approximately half of children presenting with unifocal CRMO will have additional asymptomatic lesions on WB-MRI.[30] Lesions are often, but not invariably, symmetric, and characteristic

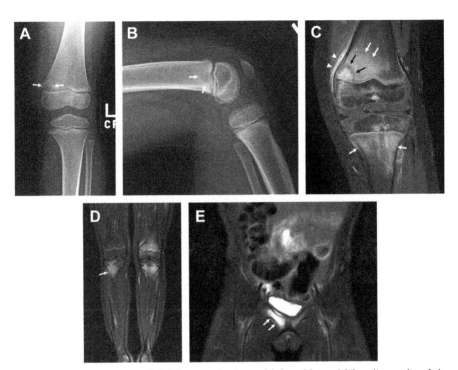

**Fig. 2.** A 4-year-old child with left knee pain. Frontal (*A*) and lateral (*B*) radiographs of the left knee reveal a focal lytic region with subtle sclerotic margins in the medial aspect of the left distal femoral metaphysis (*white arrows*). Targeted MRI of the left knee (*C*) demonstrates bone marrow edema in the metaphyses and epiphyses of the left distal femur and left proximal tibia (*white arrows*), periosteal edema along the left distal femur (*arrowheads*), and a focal hyperintense lesion within the medial metaphysis of the distal femur (*black arrows*) corresponding with the lucent lesion seen on radiographs. Subsequent whole-body survey MRI reveals additional sites of bone marrow edema (*white arrows*) in the right proximal tibia (*D*) and right superior pubic ramus (*E*). The (*white arrows*) in (*A* and *B*) indicate the focal lytic lesion with subtle sclerotic margins in the medial aspect of the left distal femoral metaphysis. The (*white arrows*) in (*D*) indicate an additional site of bone marrow edema in the right proximal tibia. The (*white arrows*) in (i) indicate an additional site of bone marrow edema in the right superior pubic ramus.

disease sites include metaphyses, epiphyses, and metaphyseal and epiphyseal equivalents.[4,14]

Lesional biopsy is performed when imaging is inconclusive, especially when imaging findings overlap with infectious or neoplastic processes. As with imaging, the appearance of CRMO lesions at biopsy differs depending on their duration, and clinicians disagree about the utility of biopsy in diagnosis.[6,14] The predominant histologic features of CRMO are chronic inflammation, bone marrow edema, and/or fibrosis.[16,31] Marrow infiltrates demonstrate predominantly lymphocytes and plasma cells and lack neutrophils, and microbiological sampling yields negative cultures. These findings, along with a lack of response to antibiotics, point away from infectious osteomyelitis.[15,28] In contrast to histologic evaluation of neoplasms, biopsies of CRMO lesions will show evidence of new bone formation and bone remodeling with an absence of blasts or other malignant cells.[16]

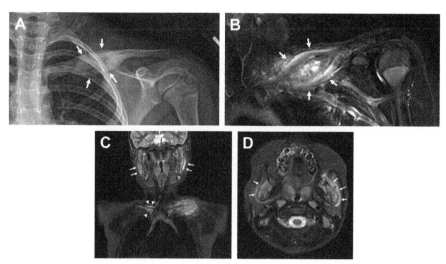

**Fig. 3.** A 7-year-old child with pain along the left clavicle. Frontal radiograph of the left clavicle (*A*) reveals fusiform expansion of the left mid-clavicle with associated patchy sclerosis and overlying periosteal reaction (*white arrows*). Targeted MRI of the left shoulder (*B*) demonstrates expansion and cortical thickening of the left medial to mid-clavicle with heterogeneous marrow edema and surrounding periosteal and soft tissue edema (*white arrows*). Subsequent whole-body survey MRI (*C* and *D*) again demonstrates marrow edema within the left clavicle and reveals additional sites of marrow edema in the right medial clavicle (*arrowheads*), in both mandibles (*white arrows*), and within the bilateral femurs, tibias, fibulas, and feet (not shown).

Universal diagnostic criteria for CRMO do not exist. However, 2 sets of criteria are widely used internationally, the Jansson criteria (**Table 1**) and the Bristol criteria (**Table 2**).[1,8] Both sets of standards use a combination of clinical and imaging findings; the Jansson criteria also include extraosseous manifestations. Use of a criterion-

| Table 1 | |
| :--- | :--- |
| **Jansson clinical scoring system** | |
| **Clinical Risk Factor** | **Score** |
| Normal complete blood count | 13 |
| Normal body temperature | 9 |
| C-reactive protein (CRP) equal to 1 mg/dL or higher | 6 |
| **Radiological Risk Factor** | **Score** |
| Symmetric lesions | 10 |
| Lesions with marginal sclerosis | 10 |
| Vertebral, clavicular, or sternal lesions | 8 |
| Two or more radiologically proven lesions | 7 |
| **Results** | **Score Tally** |
| Total possible score | 63 |
| Probable nonbacterial osteitis (NBO) | 39 or greater |
| Uncertain diagnosis | 29–38 |
| Probably not NBO | 0–28 |

*Data from* Jansson AF, Muller TH, Gliera L, et al. Clinical score for nonbacterial osteitis in children and adults. Arthritis Rheum. Apr 2009; 60(4)1152-9.https://doi.org/10.1002/art.24402.

| Table 2 |  |
| Bristol diagnostic criteria for chronic recurrent multifocal osteomyelitis | |
| **Requires Both** **AND** | **Requires One** |
| --- | --- |
| *1. Typical Clinical Findings* | *Criterion 1* |
| Bone pain | Findings in more than one bone |
| with or without | (or clavicle alone) |
| Localized swelling without significant | plus |
| features of infection/inflammation | C-reactive protein (CRP) < 30 g/L |
| *2. Typical Radiological findings* | *Criterion 2* |
| Radiograph: combination of lytic areas, | Findings are unifocal (other than clavicle) |
| sclerosis, and/or new bone formation | or |
| or | CRP > 30 g/L |
| MRI: bone marrow edema, lytic areas, | plus |
| and/or periosteal reaction | Bone biopsy showing inflammatory |
|  | changes (plasma cells, osteoclasts, |
|  | fibrosis, sclerosis) with no bacterial |
|  | growth (not on antibiotics) |

*Data from* Roderick MR, Shah R, Rogers V, et al. Chronic recurrent multifocal osteomyelitis (CRMO) - advancing the diagnosis. Pediatr Rheumatol Online J. Aug 2016;14(1):47. https://doi.org/10.1186/s12969-016-0109-1.

based clinical scoring system is intended to accelerate diagnosis and reduce the utilization of invasive diagnostic tools such as biopsies.[9]

### Treatment

As with diagnosis of CRMO, there is no clear consensus for treatment of the disorder. Although there are commonly used classes of medications, treatment is largely by trial and error and is tailored to individual patients based on their presentation.

Nonsteroidal antiinflammatory drugs (NSAIDs) are the first-line medications for initial therapy, typically offering at least temporary remission and sometimes yielding permanent remission. The NSAIDs shown most effective in treatment of CRMO are naproxen, diclofenac, indomethacin, and meloxicam.[3] Some patients respond well, with resolution of both symptoms and bone lesions, and develop no further lesions. Many patients will relapse, although the length of time to development of new lesions is varied.[31]

Steroids are often used in the setting of disease relapse but are also sometimes included with initial therapy. Steroids provide symptomatic relief by reducing inflammation, but they do not prevent relapse. For this reason, steroids are usually given in concert with other classes of medications.

When additional sites of disease develop, NSAIDs are often less effective, necessitating introduction of second-line therapies. Second-line therapies include the disease-modifying antirheumatic drug (DMARD) class of biologics and immunosuppressants. Immunosuppressants such as methotrexate and sulfasalazine were used before the advent of biologic agents and have shown efficacy in some patients, meriting continued use.

Biologics, including TNF-$\alpha$ inhibitors such as infliximab and etanercept and complement-mediated cytotoxic drugs such as rituximab, have been widely adopted as second-line medications for CRMO relapses and flares unresponsive to NSAIDs. The biologic class of drugs has been the most effective in long-term reduction of relapses, as these medications directly inhibit the proinflammatory cytokines involved in CRMO.[28] Reports on use of biologics are currently limited to case studies or small group studies, but biologic agents seem to be the most promising treatment of refractory disease. However, the usefulness of biologics is limited for those who suffer from side effects of immunosuppression and superimposed infections.[28]

Recent trials have shown the antigout agent colchicine to be another promising second-line medication as a supplement or alternative to DMARDs because of its low cost and easy administration.[32] Colchicine has been used effectively in treating other autoinflammatory conditions such as familial Mediterranean fever and PFAPA (periodic fever, aphthous stomatitis, pharyngitis, adenitis) syndrome.[32] Specific to diseases such as CRMO, colchicine has been shown to reduce inflammation by regulating receptors on myeloid cells and inhibiting the production of TNF-$\alpha$ and other proinflammatory cytokines.[32]

Bisphosphonates such as zoledronic acid and pamidronate can be given to patients with CRMO at risk for skeletal damage in spinal disease or to those at risk for physeal bridging. Bisphosphonates reduce bone remodeling by inhibiting osteoclasts and suppressing proinflammatory cytokines.[28,31,33] Inhibition of osteoclasts in particular can slow or halt the progression of damage to the vertebral bodies and physes. Although both agents are used in the treatment of CRMO, zoledronic acid has been shown to be a more potent suppressant of bone resorption and inflammation as compared with pamidronate in the setting of osteogenesis imperfecta.[3]

For patients who present initially with isolated bone disease but later develop skin, joint, or gastrointestinal symptoms, DMARDs are effective in controlling the complex extraosseous manifestations of CRMO.

### Sequelae/Natural History

Swift diagnosis of CRMO is important, as delays in treatment increase the risk of long-term sequelae. Children who experience chronic, uncontrolled inflammation without successful treatment can go on to develop arthritis.[31] Those with vertebral lesions are at risk for developing compression fractures and scoliosis and/or kyphosis.[6,7] Lesions along the physes can cause abnormal bone deposition and fibrosis, which can lead to physeal arrest and limb length discrepancies or angular deformities.[3,16]

Once the diagnosis of CRMO has been made, children are followed by pediatric rheumatology and pediatric radiology. The frequency and duration of follow-up imaging vary; no defined interval or length of follow-up has been established. Surveillance WB-MRI is generally performed every 6 to 12 months to assess treatment response and evaluate for new lesions.[2] For those lesions at high risk for resulting skeletal deformities, targeted MRI and radiographs are used to monitor for complications of physeal bridging or vertebral compression fractures.[7,34] Again, no consensus method for tracking disease progression currently exists. Arnoldi and colleagues proposed a scoring system to determine disease severity using both clinical and imaging findings, the radiologic index for nonbacterial osteitis (RINBO) score.[30] In this index, patients are evaluated for clinically active lesions as determined by a rheumatologist and radiologically active lesions detected by WB-MRI, with increasing points assigned for lesion size, extramedullary (periosteal) involvement, and active spinal involvement, intended to correlate with disease activity and severity.[30] Zhao and colleagues recommended using a scoring system incorporating quantitative and qualitative assessment, in which disease activity is defined by a combination of imaging findings and a survey of clinical symptoms and disability obtained from patients, parents, and providers.[3]

Timely diagnosis and early detection of high-risk lesions allow proper treatment to be initiated and escalated with bisphosphonates and biologics as needed, significantly improving outcomes. Unfortunately, despite initial treatment response and apparent disease remission, as many as 60% of cases have been documented to relapse after 5 years.[31] In addition to new bone lesions, extraosseous symptoms, most commonly arthritis and pain amplification syndrome, are documented to have developed up to 5 years after initial bone pain.[7,31] Although there is no clear pattern of involvement, awareness of the potential associated autoinflammatory diseases can be helpful in monitoring children for their development.

Increased physical activity and exercise have been shown to improve symptoms in children with other inflammatory conditions such as JIA, as well as to help lessen bone mineral density loss associated with chronic inflammation. Children with CRMO report lower levels of physical activity in comparison to age-matched controls, thought to result from a combination of symptoms and psychosocial stressors.[20] Long-term, children can go on to develop chronic pain and arthritis, which, along with regular specialist visits, may lead to persistent school absence. These patients risk falling behind in school and being absent from important social experiences.[16,23] Involvement of child psychology may be warranted to mitigate the socioemotional impacts of CRMO.

## FUTURE DIRECTIONS

As researchers attempt to better classify the disease, the heterogeneity of presentation and the possibility of distinct variants of the disorder become more apparent. Some investigators suggest that 3 subsets exist: unifocal bone lesions (CNO), multifocal/recurrent bone lesions (CRMO), and bone lesions plus extraosseous manifestations.[5,13] Others postulate that the disease is binary, presenting as bone lesion only or as "complex" with extraosseous manifestations, and that both lesion location and response to treatments differ across these distinct groups.[5] Still others point to the difficulty in defining clear subsets of CRMO because of the length of time between flares or between isolated bone lesions, as well as the emergence of comorbidities involving other organ systems.

Current research explores classifying CRMO as one phenotype along a wider spectrum of autoinflammatory conditions that share genetic alterations, cytokine dysregulation, and response to pharmaceutical therapies, including SAPHO (synovitis, acne, pustulosis, hyperostosis, osteitis) syndrome, inflammatory bowel disease, palmoplantar pustulosis, familial Mediterranean fever, and PFAPA.[2,5,6,32] These autoinflammatory disorders also share some of the extraosseous manifestations of CRMO, further supporting CNO/CRMO as one disease along a spectrum of autoinflammatory disorders.

Aside from clarity in choosing a name for the disease, arguably the greatest need is for a case definition for CRMO—a universally accepted definition and criteria for measuring and tracking the disease. The paucity of large, multinational cohorts and prospective studies exacerbates the difficulty in achieving a standard classification system. As the medical community begins to recognize the disease and works to standardize its definition and diagnosis, the ultimate goal must be to shorten the time to diagnosis for children affected by this disorder and thereby reduce the long-term complications of the disease.

## SUMMARY

CNO/CRMO is an underrecognized autoinflammatory disorder of the skeletal system resulting from immune dysregulation. Its vague symptoms often result in a delay in diagnosis for days to years, and because of the lack of accepted diagnostic criteria or specific biomarkers, CRMO remains a diagnosis of exclusion. Untreated CRMO has the potential to cause chronic, debilitating skeletal deformities with neurologic manifestations, arthritis, and chronic pain. Diagnosis requires MRI of the symptomatic area as well as WB-MRI for identification of clinically silent lesions. Treatment is primarily through antiinflammatory medications, with NSAIDs comprising first-line therapy and DMARDs used for disease relapse. Bisphosphonates are used when necessary to prevent spinal deformities and growth abnormalities. Early diagnosis and treatment are paramount to lessen disease severity, and involvement of child psychology can be helpful to provide psychosocial support to children with this chronic disease.

## CLINICS CARE POINTS

---

- Initial laboratory test results and radiographs can be normal or inconclusive in the setting of CRMO. MRI is the gold standard for diagnosis, with WB-MRI necessary to detect clinically silent lesions.

- Clinical and radiographic findings of CRMO may mimic neoplastic or aggressive infectious processes.

- NSAIDs are first-line therapy for CRMO. If the disease is incompletely treated or relapses, second-line therapies include disease-modifying antirheumatic drugs with or without bisphosphonates. Steroids can be used at any stage to mitigate inflammation.

- Up to half of patients with CRMO develop other autoinflammatory disorders, including arthritides such as psoriatic arthritis, juvenile idiopathic arthritis, or enthesitis-related arthritis; cutaneous manifestations such as psoriasis, palmoplantar pustulosis, pyoderma gangrenosum, or severe acne; or gastrointestinal manifestations such as inflammatory bowel disease.

---

## DISCLOSURE

The authors have no commercial or financial conflicts of interest to disclose.

## REFERENCES

1. Roderick MR, Shah R, Rogers V, et al. Chronic recurrent multifocal osteomyelitis (CRMO) - advancing the diagnosis. Pediatr Rheumatol Online J 2016;14(1):47.
2. Zhao Y, Ferguson PJ. Chronic nonbacterial osteomyelitis and chronic recurrent multifocal osteomyelitis in children. Pediatr Clin North Am 2018;65(4):783–800.
3. Zhao Y, Chauvin NA, Jaramillo D, et al. Aggressive therapy reduces disease activity without skeletal damage progression in chronic nonbacterial osteomyelitis. J Rheumatol 2015;42(7):1245–51.
4. Aydıngöz Ü, Yıldız AE. MRI in the diagnosis and treatment response assessment of chronic nonbacterial osteomyelitis in children and adolescents. Curr Rheumatol Rep 2022;24(2):27–39.
5. Cebecauerová D, Malcová H, Koukolská V, et al. Two phenotypes of chronic recurrent multifocal osteomyelitis with different patterns of bone involvement. Pediatr Rheumatol Online J 2022;20(1):108.
6. Pastore S, Ferrara G, Monasta L, et al. Chronic nonbacterial osteomyelitis may be associated with renal disease and bisphosphonates are a good option for the majority of patients. Acta Paediatr 2016;105(7):e328–33.
7. Voit AM, Arnoldi AP, Douis H, et al. Whole-body magnetic resonance imaging in chronic recurrent multifocal osteomyelitis: clinical longterm assessment may underestimate activity. J Rheumatol 2015;42(8):1455–62.
8. Jansson AF, Müller TH, Gliera L, et al. Clinical score for nonbacterial osteitis in children and adults. Arthritis Rheum 2009;60(4):1152–9.

9. Taddio A, Zennaro F, Pastore S, et al. An update on the pathogenesis and treatment of chronic recurrent multifocal osteomyelitis in children. Paediatr Drugs 2017;19(3):165–72.

10. Papakonstantinou O, Prountzos S, Karavasilis E, et al. Whole-body magnetic resonance imaging findings and patterns of chronic nonbacterial osteomyelitis in a series of Greek pediatric patients. Acta Radiol Open 2022;11(6). 20584601221106701.

11. Beck C, Morbach H, Beer M, et al. Chronic nonbacterial osteomyelitis in childhood: prospective follow-up during the first year of anti-inflammatory treatment. Arthritis Res Ther 2010;12(2):R74.

12. Borzutzky A, Stern S, Reiff A, et al. Pediatric chronic nonbacterial osteomyelitis. Pediatrics 2012;130(5):e1190–7.

13. Wipff J, Costantino F, Lemelle I, et al. A large national cohort of French patients with chronic recurrent multifocal osteitis. Arthritis Rheumatol 2015;67(4):1128–37.

14. Shah A, Rosenkranz M, Thapa M. Review of spinal involvement in chronic recurrent multifocal osteomyelitis (CRMO): What radiologists need to know about CRMO and its imitators. Clin Imaging 2022;86:1.

15. Bencharef O, Salama T, Aghoutane E, et al. Chronic recurrent multifocal osteomyelitis mimicking a malignant bone tumor: a case report. Pan Afr Med J 2022; 42:150.

16. O'Leary D, Wilson AG, MacDermott EJ, et al. Variability in phenotype and response to treatment in chronic nonbacterial osteomyelitis; the Irish experience of a national cohort. Pediatr Rheumatol Online J 2021;19(1):45.

17. Roderick MR, Sen ES, Ramanan AV. Chronic recurrent multifocal osteomyelitis in children and adults: current understanding and areas for development. Rheumatology 2018;57(1):41–8.

18. Hofmann SR, Kapplusch F, Girschick HJ, et al. Chronic recurrent multifocal osteomyelitis (CRMO): presentation, pathogenesis, and treatment. Curr Osteoporos Rep 2017;15(6):542–54.

19. Hofmann SR, Schnabel A, Rösen-Wolff A, et al. Chronic nonbacterial osteomyelitis: pathophysiological concepts and current treatment strategies. J Rheumatol 2016;43(11):1956–64.

20. Koryllou A, Mejbri M, Theodoropoulou K, et al. Chronic nonbacterial osteomyelitis in children. Children 2021;8(7). https://doi.org/10.3390/children8070551.

21. Jansson AF, Grote V, Group ES. Nonbacterial osteitis in children: data of a German incidence surveillance study. Acta Paediatr 2011;100(8):1150–7.

22. Kaiser D, Bolt I, Hofer M, et al. Chronic nonbacterial osteomyelitis in children: a retrospective multicenter study. Pediatr Rheumatol Online J 2015;13:25.

23. Silier CCG, Greschik J, Gesell S, et al. Chronic non-bacterial osteitis from the patient perspective: a health services research through data collected from patient conferences. BMJ Open 2017;7(12):e017599.

24. Iyer RS, Thapa MM, Chew FS. Chronic recurrent multifocal osteomyelitis: review. AJR Am J Roentgenol 2011;196(6 Suppl):S87–91.

25. Jansson A, Renner ED, Ramser J, et al. Classification of non-bacterial osteitis: retrospective study of clinical, immunological and genetic aspects in 89 patients. Rheumatology 2007;46(1):154–60.

26. Hedrich CM, Morbach H, Reiser C, et al. New insights into adult and paediatric chronic non-bacterial osteomyelitis CNO. Curr Rheumatol Rep 2020;22(9):52.

27. Cox AJ, Zhao Y, Ferguson PJ. Chronic recurrent multifocal osteomyelitis and related diseases–update on pathogenesis. Curr Rheumatol Rep 2017;19(4):18.

28. Eleftheriou D, Gerschman T, Sebire N, et al. Biologic therapy in refractory chronic non-bacterial osteomyelitis of childhood. Rheumatology 2010;49(8):1505–12.
29. Meyers AB. Physeal bridges: causes, diagnosis, characterization and post-treatment imaging. Pediatr Radiol. Nov 2019;49(12):1595–609.
30. Arnoldi AP, Schlett CL, Douis H, et al. Whole-body MRI in patients with non-bacterial osteitis: radiological findings and correlation with clinical data. Eur Radiol. Jun 2017;27(6):2391–9.
31. Schnabel A, Range U, Hahn G, et al. Treatment response and longterm outcomes in children with chronic nonbacterial osteomyelitis. J Rheumatol 2017;44(7): 1058–65.
32. Quintana-Ortega C, Prieto-Moreno Pfeifer A, Palomino Lozano L, et al. Colchicine as rescue treatment in two pediatric patients with chronic recurrent multifocal osteomyelitis (CRMO). Mod Rheumatol Case Rep 2023;7(1):215–8.
33. Simm PJ, Allen RC, Zacharin MR. Bisphosphonate treatment in chronic recurrent multifocal osteomyelitis. J Pediatr 2008;152(4):571–5.
34. Sato TS, Watal P, Ferguson PJ. Imaging mimics of chronic recurrent multifocal osteomyelitis: avoiding pitfalls in a diagnosis of exclusion. Pediatr Radiol 2020; 50(1):124–36.

# Moving?

## Make sure your subscription moves with you!

To notify us of your new address, find your **Clinics Account Number** (located on your mailing label above your name), and contact customer service at:

**Email: journalscustomerservice-usa@elsevier.com**

**800-654-2452** (subscribers in the U.S. & Canada)
**314-447-8871** (subscribers outside of the U.S. & Canada)

**Fax number: 314-447-8029**

**Elsevier Health Sciences Division**
**Subscription Customer Service**
**3251 Riverport Lane**
**Maryland Heights, MO 63043**

*To ensure uninterrupted delivery of your subscription, please notify us at least 4 weeks in advance of move.

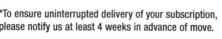

ELSEVIER